STATISTICS for NURSING RESEARCH

A Workbook for Evidence-Based Practice

STATISTICS for NURSING RESEARCH

A Workbook for Evidence-Based Practice

Susan K. Grove, PhD, RN, ANP-BC, GNP-BC
Professor Emerita
College of Nursing and Health Innovation
The University of Texas at Arlington
Arlington, Texas;
Adult and Gerontological NP Consultant
Arlington, Texas

Daisha J. Cipher, PhD
Professor
College of Nursing and Health Innovation
The University of Texas at Arlington
Arlington, Texas

ELSEVIER

Elsevier
3251 Riverport Lane
St. Louis, Missouri 63043

STATISTICS FOR NURSING RESEARCH:
A WORKBOOK FOR EVIDENCE-BASED PRACTICE
FOURTH EDITION

ISBN: 978-0-323-93050-5

Notice

Practitioners and researchers must always rely on their own experience and knowledge in evaluating and using any information, methods, compounds, or experiments described herein. Because of rapid advances in the medical sciences, in particular, independent verification of diagnoses and drug dosages should be made. To the fullest extent of the law, no responsibility is assumed by Elsevier, authors, editors, or contributors for any injury and/or damage to persons or property as a matter of products liability, negligence, or otherwise, or from any use or operation of any methods, products, instructions, or ideas contained in the material herein.

Previous editions copyrighted 2020, 2017, and 2007.

Executive Content Strategist: Lee Henderson
Senior Content Development Specialist: Laura Goodrich
Senior Project Manager: Joanna Souch
Senior Book Designer: Amy Buxton

Printed in India.

Last digit is the print number: 9 8 7 6 5 4 3 2 1

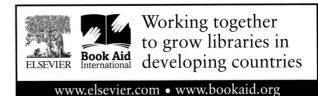

Susan K. Grove
In memory of my husband and sister:

Jay Suggs and Sheryl Grove: You both were the center of my world.

and

To our future:

Jack, Boone, and Cole Appleton

Daisha J. Cipher
To my husband and daughter:

Jason Moore and Gracie Alice Moore, for their love and support

and

To my parents:

John and Joyce Cipher, for their constant encouragement

Preface

With the emphasis in health care today on evidence-based practice, it is more important than ever for nurses to understand essential information about measurement, sampling, and statistical analysis techniques. Having this background enables students and practicing nurses to critically appraise the results of published studies and conduct data analyses to make evidence-based changes in practice.

The fourth edition of this workbook has been significantly revised to meet the needs of students and practicing nurses for basic and advanced statistical knowledge for practice. The revised workbook continues to focus on promoting understanding of statistical methods included in nursing studies and conducting selected statistical analyses for nursing data. This workbook was developed to meet the growing need for statistical knowledge by students in doctor of nursing practice (DNP) programs, master's in nursing programs (e.g., master's in nursing administration, master's in nursing education), and RN-to-BSN and higher-level BSN programs. This workbook provides additional statistical content and practical application of that content to supplement what is provided in *Burns & Grove's The Practice of Nursing Research*, and *Understanding Nursing Research*. The content of this workbook is sufficient to enable graduate and undergraduate nursing students and practicing nurses to do the following:

- Critically appraise the sampling methods and measurement methods in nursing studies.
- Critically appraise the results sections of research articles.
- Understand power analysis and apply it in determining sample size and power of a study to determine relationships among variables and differences between groups.
- Select the most appropriate statistical procedures for analysis of data.
- Calculate selected statistical procedures using statistical software and manually.
- Interpret statistical software output of the results of selected statistical procedures (e.g., mean, standard deviation, Pearson *r*, regression analysis, *t*-test, analysis of variance [ANOVA], chi-square, sensitivity, specificity, and odds ratio).
- Determine statistical significance and clinical importance of analysis results.

The exercises in this fourth edition of *Statistics for Nursing Research* are organized into two parts to help differentiate basic content from more advanced content: Part 1 ("Understanding Statistical Methods") and Part 2 ("Conducting and Interpreting Statistical Analyses"). The exercises in Part 1 were developed to promote understanding of measurement and sampling methods and of how to critically appraise the results sections of current published studies.

Each exercise in Part 1 includes the following sections:

- Statistical Technique in Review
- Research Article
- Introduction
- Relevant Study Results
- Study Questions
- Answers to Study Questions
- Questions for Additional Study

The Statistical Technique in Review at the beginning of each exercise provides a brief summary of the featured technique. The Research Article section then provides a current bibliographic reference to a pertinent published study from the nursing research literature. An Introduction follows to provide the reader with a base from which to interpret the study. A section called Relevant Study Results, based on the cited article, provides a relevant example taken directly from a current, published nursing study. The Study Questions section guides the reader in examining the statistical technique in the research article. The Answers to Study Questions section provides immediate feedback to ensure content mastery or to identify areas needing further study. Finally, Questions for Additional Study can be submitted to the instructor as assigned for additional feedback. Answer Guidelines for Questions for Additional Study are provided for faculty on the Evolve website.

Each exercise in Part 2 features the following content:

- Statistical Formula and Assumptions
- Research Designs Appropriate for the Statistical Application
- Hand Calculations [for selected statistics]
- SPSS Computations [with screen shots]
- Interpretation of SPSS Output
- Final Interpretation in American Psychological Association Format
- Study Questions
- Answers to Study Questions
- Data for Additional Computational Practice
- Questions for Additional Study

The Statistical Formula and Assumptions section at the beginning of each exercise provides the formula and mathematical properties of the statistic. The Research Designs Appropriate for the Statistical Application section lists the potential research designs that might require the calculation of the given statistic. The Hand Calculations section provides the reader with a dataset along with a step-by-step guide to computing the components of the statistic, using the example data. The SPSS Computations section provides instructions on how to compute the statistics using SPSS statistical software and includes screenshots of SPSS at each step. The Interpretation of SPSS Output identifies each portion of statistical output and provides detailed explanations. The Final Interpretation in American Psychological Association Format section provides the reader with an example of how to write the results of the analysis. The Study Questions section guides the reader in examining the statistical technique in the exercise. The Answers to Study Questions section provides immediate feedback to ensure content mastery or to identify areas needing further study. The Data for Additional Computational Practice section provides a new dataset for the reader to practice computing the statistic. Questions for Additional Study query the reader on the data provided for additional computational practice. Answer Guidelines for Questions for Additional Study are provided for faculty on the Evolve website.

We believe that the hands-on approach in this workbook provides students with essential application of statistical content and an ability to assess their understanding of that content. We hope that this revised, expanded statistical workbook provides students and practicing nurses with relevant statistical knowledge for understanding the results of studies and conducting relevant data analyses. We believe that an increased understanding of statistical content provides a stronger background for implementing evidence-based nursing practice.

EVOLVE LEARNING RESOURCES

Resources for both students and instructors are provided on an Evolve website at http://evolve.elsevier.com/Grove/statistics/. For students and instructors, Questions for Additional Study, datasets in SPSS formats, and a Research Article Library with selected research articles are available on the Evolve website. Here, students can submit answers to the Questions for Additional Study for their faculty. For instructors, Answer Guidelines for Questions for Additional Study are provided to help ensure that students have mastered the content.

DISCLAIMER

Data examples used for hand computations present either actual published data (where the individual data values have been made publicly available) or simulated data. In the case of the simulated data examples, the observations were slightly altered to protect the identities of the research participants, so that it would be impossible to identify any participant. However, the statistical results of the analyses of simulated data are wholly consistent with the actual published results. For example, a significant difference yielded by the simulated data mimics the significant differences actually reported in the published studies. No significant effects were manufactured in this textbook.

Acknowledgments

Special thanks are extended to our reviewers, whose statistical knowledge was invaluable in ensuring the quality and accuracy of the information in this workbook. We also appreciate the time and effort that they spent verifying that this book is as current, accurate, and relevant as possible for nursing students and practicing nurses. We also want to thank the students who have provided us comments that have improved the clarity and quality of this text. Any errors that remain are, of course, our own.

Finally, we would like to thank the people at Elsevier who worked tirelessly to produce this book: Lee Henderson, Executive Content Strategist; Laura Goodrich, Senior Content Development Specialist; Amy Buxton, Senior Book Designer; and Joanna Souch, Senior Project Manager.

Susan K. Grove
Daisha J. Cipher

Contents

PART 1

Understanding Statistical Methods

Identifying Levels of Measurement: Nominal, Ordinal, Interval, and Ratio

STATISTICAL TECHNIQUE IN REVIEW

The levels of measurement were identified in 1946 by Stevens, who organized the rules for assigning numbers to objects so that a hierarchy of measurement was established. The **levels of measurement**, from lowest to highest, are nominal, ordinal, interval, and ratio. Fig. 1.1 summarizes the rules for the four levels of measurement that are described in the following sections.

Nominal and Ordinal Levels of Measurement

Variables measured at the **nominal level of measurement** are at the lowest level and must conform to the following two rules: (1) the data categories must be exclusive (each datum will fit into only one category) and (2) the data categories must be exhaustive (each datum will fit into at least one category). Nominal level data might also be called **categorical data,** which means the values are names for categories but not real numbers (Table 1.1; Grove & Gray, 2023). For example, the variable medical diagnosis of heart failure (HF) is measured at the nominal level and includes two categories, *yes* has HF or *no* HF. HF is an example of a dichotomous or binary variable that has only two possible values (see Table 1.1). Variables measured at the nominal level that are frequently described in studies include gender, race/ethnicity, marital status, and medical diagnoses. For some nominal variables, such as medical diagnoses, some study participants might check more than one category because they have more than one medical diagnosis (Gray & Grove, 2021; Kim et al., 2022).

Ordinal level of measurement includes categories that can be rank ordered; like nominal-level measurement, the categories are exhaustive and mutually exclusive (see Fig. 1.1). In ranking categories of a variable, each category must be recognized as higher or lower or better or worse than another category. However, with ordinal level of measurement, you do not know exactly how much higher or lower one participant's value on a variable is in relation to another participant's value. Thus variables measured at the ordinal level are discrete, meaning they do not have a continuum of values with equal distance between them like variables measured at the interval and ratio levels (Grove & Gray, 2023). For example, you could have study participants identify their levels of acute pain as no pain, mild pain, moderate pain, or severe pain. Pain is measured at the ordinal level in this example because the categories can be ranked from a low of no pain to a high of severe pain; however, even though the participants' levels of pain can be ranked, you do not know the differences between the levels of pain. The difference between no pain and mild pain might be less than that between moderate and severe pain. Thus ordinal-level data have unknown, unequal intervals between the categories, such as between the levels of pain (Waltz et al., 2017).

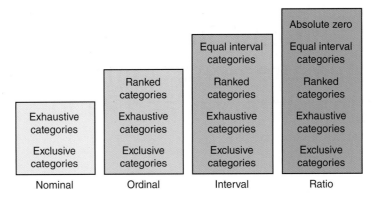

FIG. 1.1 ■ SUMMARY OF THE RULES FOR THE LEVELS OF MEASUREMENT.

TABLE 1.1	MEASUREMENT CONCEPTS	
Concept	**Other Name**	**Description**
Dichotomous	Binary	The variable has only two possible values.
Nominal*	Categorical	Values are names or categories, not real numbers.
Continuous	Ratio	Values use the real number scale, including the values between numerals.
Discrete		Numeric values used are not continuous.

*From the Latin *nomina,* which means name.

Nonparametric Analysis Techniques

Nonparametric or distribution-free analysis techniques are conducted to analyze nominal and ordinal levels of data to describe variables, examine relationships among variables, and determine differences between groups in distribution-free or non-normally distributed samples. The measure of central tendency, which is conducted to describe variables measured at the nominal level, is the mode or the most frequently occurring value in the dataset. The median or middle value in a dataset is calculated to describe variables measured at the ordinal level (see Exercise 8). Descriptive statistical analyses, such as frequencies and percentages, are often calculated to describe demographic variables measured at the nominal and ordinal levels in a study (see Exercise 6). Range is calculated to determine the dispersion or spread of values of a variable measured at the ordinal level (see Exercise 9).

Chi-square analysis is calculated to examine differences in variables measured at the nominal level (see Exercise 19). The Spearman Rank-Order Correlation Coefficient is calculated to examine relationships among variables measured at the ordinal level (see Exercise 20). The Mann-Whitney U and Wilcoxon Signed-Rank tests can be conducted to determine differences among groups when study data are measured at the ordinal level (see Exercises 21 and 22). Nonparametric analyses are also conducted when interval- and ratio-level data are not normally distributed. The process for determining normality of a distribution is presented in Exercise 27. More information about conducting nonparametric analyses is presented in selected exercises of Part 2 of this text. Other nursing textbooks, such as Gray and Grove (2021), Kim et al. (2022), Pett (2016), and Terrell (2021) provide details about conducting and interpreting nonparametric analyses.

Interval and Ratio Levels of Measurement

With **interval level of measurement**, the distances between intervals of the scale are numerically equal. However, there is no absolute zero, which means the score of zero does not indicate the property being measured is absent. Temperature is an example of a variable that is measured at the interval level, because the intervals between the different temperatures on either Fahrenheit or centigrade temperature scales are numerically equal. In addition, zero temperature is not the absence of temperature: it indicates very cold or freezing temperature.

Study participants' scores obtained from multi-item scales are usually considered interval-level measurement. Likert scales are an example of multi-item scales commonly used to collect data about abstract concepts such as anxiety, perception of pain, quality of life, and depression. Each item on the scale has a response set for participants to mark, which might include 1—strongly disagree to 4—strongly agree. The number and type of response options vary based on the scale. The values obtained from each item in the scale are summed to obtain a single score for each study participant. Although the values of each item are technically ordinal-level data, the summed score is often analyzed as interval-level data (Gray & Grove, 2021; Waltz et al., 2017). The Center for Epidemiological Studies Depression Scale is an example of a 20-item, 4-point Likert scale that is used to measure depression in nursing studies (Radloff, 1977), and the data from this scale are considered interval level for analysis.

Ratio level of measurement is the highest form of measurement; it adheres to the same rules as interval-level measurement, with numerically equal intervals on the scale (see Fig. 1.1; Grove & Gray, 2023). In addition, ratio-level measurement has an absolute zero point, where at zero the property is absent, such as zero weight meaning absence of weight. In nursing, many physiologic variables are measured at the ratio level, such as blood pressure, pulse, respiration, body mass index (BMI), and laboratory values (Stone & Frazier, 2017). Variables measured at the interval and ratio levels are also referred to as **continuous variables** (see Table 1.1). The data, if normally distributed, obtained from measuring continuous variables are analyzed with parametric statistics (Grove & Gray, 2023; Kim et al., 2022; Terrell, 2021).

Parametric Analysis Techniques

Parametric statistics are powerful analysis techniques conducted on interval and ratio levels of data to describe variables, examine relationships among variables, and determine differences among groups (Kim et al., 2022; Knapp, 2017). The assumptions of parametric statistics are introduced here and discussed in more detail for the parametric analysis techniques conducted in Part 2 of this text. If study data do not meet the assumptions outlined as follows, then researchers conduct nonparametric analyses to address the study questions and hypotheses (Gray & Grove, 2021; Pett, 2016).

Assumptions for parametric analyses:

1. The distribution of scores in a sample is expected to be normal or approximately normal.
2. The variables are continuous, measured at the interval or ratio level.
3. The data can be treated as though obtained from a random sample.
4. All observations within each sample are independent (Gray & Grove, 2021; Kim et al., 2022; Terrell, 2021).

Parametric analysis techniques are the same for variables measured at either the interval or the ratio level of measurement. For example, means and standard deviations can be calculated to describe study variables measured at the interval or the ratio level (see Exercises 8 and 9). Pearson correlation coefficient (Pearson r; see Exercise 13) is computed to determine relationships between variables, and the t-test (see Exercises 16 and 17) or analysis of variance (ANOVA; see Exercise 18) are calculated to determine significant differences among groups. **Significant results** are those in keeping with the outcomes predicted by the researcher, where the *null hypothesis is rejected*. Significant results are usually identified by * or p values less than or equal to alpha (α), which is often set at 0.05 in nursing research (Grove & Gray, 2023; Heavey, 2019). The symbol ≤ 0.05 means less than or equal to 0.05, so any p values ≤ 0.05 are considered significant. Because the analysis techniques are similar for variables measured at the interval and ratio levels, these levels of measurement are sometimes referred to as interval/ratio level. In addition, these variables are identified as continuous in this text (see Table 1.1).

RESEARCH ARTICLE

Source

Ha, F. J., Toukhsati, S. R., Cameron, J. D., Yates, R., & Hare, D. L. (2018). Association between the 6-minute walk test and exercise confidence in patients with heart failure: A prospective observational study. *Heart & Lung, 47*(1), 54–60. https://doi.org/10.1016/j.hrtlng.2017.09.006

Introduction

Ha and colleagues (2018, p. 54) conducted a descriptive correlational study to examine "the association between a single 6-min walk test (6MWT) and exercise confidence in HF [heart failure] patients." The sample included HF patients from an outpatient clinic, who completed the Cardiac Depression Scale (CDS) and an Exercise Confidence Scale before and after the 6MWT. The CDS was a 26-item Likert scale developed to measure depressive symptoms in cardiac patients. The scale included response sets that ranged from "1 = Not at all tearful" to "7 = Very easily tearful," with higher numbers indicating increased severity of symptoms. The Exercise Confidence Scale is a self-reported measure of confidence of cardiac patients to perform a range of physical activities on a scale of 0 to 100 (where 0 = "Quite uncertain," 50 = "Moderately certain," and 100 = "Completely certain"). The Exercise Confidence Scale is a multi-item rating scale, and the values obtained from this scale are analyzed as interval-level data (Gray & Grove, 2021; Waltz et al., 2017).

"The 6MWT was associated with a significant improvement in exercise confidence in HF patients. Exercise confidence is associated with age, gender, duration of HF, New York Heart Association (NYHA) class, and severity of depressive symptoms" (Ha et al., 2018, p. 59). The researchers recommended further controlled studies to determine whether the 6MWT and exercise confidence translate into improved exercise adherence and physical functioning in HF patients.

Relevant Study Results

"There were 106 participants, most of whom were male (82%) with a mean age of 64 ± 12 years (Table 1.2). Almost three-quarters (72%) had a history of reduced EF [ejection fraction] (<40%) and one-quarter (25%) had preserved EF (≥40%). . . . Approximately one-third of patients (36/106; 34%) were depressed (CDS ≥ 95) and the prevalence of depression increased with greater NYHA class (NYHA class I, 11%; NYHA class II, 44%; NYHA class III, 64%). . . . There were no significant differences detected in any clinical characteristics between patients with HFrEF [heart failure with reduced ejection fraction] or HFpEF [heart failure with preserved ejection fraction].

One hundred two patients (96%) had complete data for Baseline Exercise Confidence. Participant mean scores indicated higher Baseline Exercise Confidence for Walking (70 ± 25), Climbing (75 ± 30), and Lifting Objects of Graded Weight (71 ± 29) than for Running (35 ± 30). Total Exercise Confidence exceeded the midpoint of the Exercise Confidence Scale, indicating greater than 'moderate certainty' to complete exercise activities overall (62 ± 24). Total Exercise Confidence and all subscales were inversely associated with age, NYHA class, CDS score, and 6MWD. . . . Additionally, duration of HF was inversely associated with Climbing and Lifting Confidence, while BMI [body mass index] was inversely associated with Walking Confidence. Male participants had significantly higher scores compared with females for the Total Exercise Confidence" (Ha et al., 2018, pp. 56–57).

TABLE 1.2 PATIENT DEMOGRAPHIC AND CLINICAL CHARACTERISTICS	
Patient Demographic and Clinical Characteristics	**Total (%) _N_ = 106**
Age, mean years ±	64 ± 12
Sex, female	19 (18)
Etiology, ischemic	36 (34)
Type of HF	
HFrEF	76 (72)
HFpEF	27 (25)
Not documented	3 (3)
Duration of HF, years ± SD	3.8 ± 3.6
NYHA Class	
I	35 (33)
II	58 (55)
III	11 (10)
Not specified	2 (2)
BMI, kg/m^2	31 ± 7
Comorbidities	
Hypertension	71 (67)
Diabetes mellitus	40 (38)
CAD	37 (35)
Previous stroke	8 (8)
COPD	9 (9)
CKD (stage 3–5)	37 (35)
Current Therapy	
ACE-I/ARB	90 (85)
Beta (β) blocker	100 (94)
Aldosterone antagonist	55 (52)
Antidepressant	15 (14)
Device Therapy	
ICD	16 (15)
Pacemaker	16 (15)
CDS score, mean ± SD	86 ± 27
Depressed (CDS ≥ 95)	36 (34)
6MWD	
Feet ± SD	1325 ± 384
Meters ± SD	404 ± 117

6MWD, 6-min walk test distance; ACE-I, angiotensin-converting enzyme inhibitor; ARB, angiotensin-II receptor blocker; BMI, body mass index; CAD, coronary artery disease; CDS, Cardiac Depression Scale; CKD, chronic kidney disease; COPD, chronic obstructive pulmonary disease; eGFR, estimated glomerular filtration rate; HF, heart failure; HFpEF, heart failure with preserved ejection fraction; HFrEF, heart failure with reduced ejection fraction; ICD, implantable cardioverter defibrillator; NYHA, New York Heart Association; SD, standard deviation.

From Ha, F. J., Toukhsati, S. R., Cameron, J. D., Yates, R., & Hare, D. L. (2018). Association between the 6-minute walk test and exercise confidence in patients with heart failure: A prospective observational study. _Heart & Lung, 47_(1), 57.

STUDY QUESTIONS

All of the study questions in this section refer to Ha et al. (2018) article except question 6.

1. Identify the level of measurement for the sex or gender demographic variable. Also identify the level of measurement for the BMI physiologic variable in this study.

2. Identify the level of measurement for the type of HF variable in this study. Provide a rationale for your answer.

3. Examine the results for the type of HF variable in Table 1.2. Were any data missing for this demographic variable? Provide a rationale for your answer.

4. What is the mode for the comorbidities demographic variable? What is the meaning of these results?

5. Identify the level of measurement for the demographic variable age. Provide a rationale for your answer.

6. In a hypothetical study, researchers used the following item to measure registered nurses' (RNs) income:

   a. Less than $70,000

   b. $70,000 to 89,999

   c. $90,000 to 109,999

   d. $110,000 to 130,000

   e. $130,000 or greater

   What level of measurement is this income variable? Does the income variable follow the rules outlined in Fig. 1.1? Provide a rationale for your answer.

7. What are the frequency and percent for the male sex or gender variable? Discuss the representativeness of this sample for males and females.

8. Are parametric or nonparametric statistical techniques conducted to analyze nominal-level data in Table 1.2? Provide a rationale for your answer.

9. How was exercise confidence measured in this study? What was the level of measurement for the exercise confidence variable in this study? Provide a rationale for your answer.

10. Jafri and colleagues (2022) examined the cardiovascular outcomes of patients who participated in a home-based clinical rehabilitation program. The highest risk factor or comorbidity was hypertension (HTN), with 141 (90%) of the participants experiencing HTN. How does this result compare with the Ha et al. (2018) study results for HT?

Answers to Study Questions

1. The sex or gender demographic variable was measured at the nominal level and included two categories, male and female, that cannot be rank ordered (see Fig. 1.1). BMI was measured at the ratio level because it is a continuous physiologic variable with an absolute zero (see Fig. 1.1; Grove & Gray, 2023; Stone & Frazier, 2017).

2. The type of HF demographic variable was measured at the nominal level. The HF categories included in this study (HFrEF, HFpEF, and not documented) were exclusive (each cardiac patient fit into only one category) and exhaustive (all cardiac patients fit into one category). The types of HF cannot be ranked, because one category is not clearly higher or lower than another category, resulting in a nominal level of measurement rather than an ordinal one (see Fig. 1.1; Waltz et al., 2017).

3. No data were missing for the types of HF variable. The frequencies and percentages for the types of HF categories were as follows: HFrEF was $n = 76$ (72%), HFpEF was $n = 27$ (25%), and not documented was $n = 3$ (3%). The two common types of HF (HFrEF and HFpEF) included most of the study participants ($n = 103$, 97%) and the other HF patients ($n = 3$, 3%) fit into the open category of not documented. No data were missing for this demographic variable, because the frequencies in the categories added to the sample size $N = 106$, 100% (Grove & Gray, 2023).

4. The mode for the comorbidities variable for this sample of cardiac patients was hypertension, $n = 71$ (67%). These results indicate that many of the patients with HF have hypertension and should be closely monitored and managed for this comorbidity.

5. The level of measurement for the participants' age was ratio, because age has an underlying continuum of years in this study. Each year includes the same equal intervals of 12 months or 365 days. Age has an absolute zero, because zero indicates the absence of age for a person. Age might also be called a continuous variable because it has a continuum of values (see Table 1.1; Gray & Grove, 2021).

6. In this hypothetical study, the income variable is measured at the ordinal level. The income categories are exhaustive, ranging from less than $70,000 to greater than $130,000. The two open-ended categories ensure that all salary levels are covered. The categories are not exclusive, because categories (d) and (e) both include a $130,000 salary, so study participants making $130,000 might mark either (d) or (e) or both categories, resulting in erroneous data. Category (e) could be changed to > $130,000, making the categories exclusive. The categories can be rank ordered from the lowest salary to the highest salary without a continuum of values, which is consistent with ordinal data (Grove & Gray, 2023; Waltz et al., 2017).

7. The sample was composed of 82% males (see the study narrative) and the frequency of males in the study was $n = 87$ (106 [sample size] – 19 [number of females]). The sample was predominately males, making the results representative of the male gender. The study included only 19 females (18% of the sample), which limits the representativeness of the study results for females with HF.

8. Nonparametric statistics—frequencies and percentages—were conducted to analyze the nominal-level data in Table 1.2. Nominal data are sorted into categories that are mutually exclusive and exhaustive, and only nonparametric analysis techniques can be conducted on this level of data (Kim et al., 2022; Pett, 2016). Parametric analyses are conducted on variables measured at the interval or ratio level (Grove & Gray, 2023; Terrell, 2021).

9. Exercise confidence of the patients with HF was measured with the Exercise Confidence Scale that included four subscales focused on Walking, Climbing, Lifting Objects of Graded Weight, and Running (see the study narrative). This was a rating scale with values ranging from 0 to 100. The patients' scores for the Total Exercise Confidence Scale and the subscales were considered interval-level data and analyzed with parametric statistics, such as means and *SDs* (see the study narrative; Waltz et al., 2017).

10. The highest risk factor or comorbid condition was hypertension (HTN) in both studies. Ha et al. (2018) reported 67% of the study participants had HTN compared with 90% in the Jafri et al. (2022) study. HTN is a common risk factor for patients with cardiovascular diseases (CVDs); therefore HTN needs to be monitored and managed appropriately in patients with CVDs.

Questions for Additional Study

Name: _____ Class: _____

Date: _____

Follow your instructor's directions to submit your answers to the following questions for additional study. Your instructor may ask you to write your answers below and submit them as a hard copy for evaluation. Alternatively, your instructor may ask you to submit your answers online.

1. In Table 1.2 of the Ha et al. (2018) study, identify the level of measurement for the current therapy variable. Provide a rationale for your answer and discuss if the categories of current therapy were exclusive and exhaustive.

2. Identify the mode for the current therapy variable. What is the meaning of these results?

3. What is the level of measurement for the demographic variable duration of HF? Provide a rationale for your answer.

4. What statistics were conducted to describe the body mass index (BMI) of the cardiac patients in this sample? Discuss whether these analysis techniques were appropriate or inappropriate.

5. How many cardiac patients participated in the Ha et al. (2018) study? Determine the frequency and percentage of those patients who did not have a pacemaker. Round your answer to the nearest whole percent (%).

6. What is the level of measurement for the NYHA class variable? Provide a rationale for your answer.

7. What level of measurement is the Cardiac Depression Scale (CDS) score? Provide a rationale for your answer.

8. Is the prevalence of depression linked to the NYHA class? Discuss the clinical importance of this result.

9. What frequency and percentage of cardiac patients in the Ha et al. (2018) study were not being treated with an antidepressant? Show your calculations and round your answer to the nearest whole percent (%).

10. Jafri and colleagues (2022) conducted a study to examine the cardiovascular outcomes of patients who were referred to a home-based cardiac rehabilitation program. Depression was measured with the Patient Health Questionnaire (PHQ-9) with the pre-rehabilitation score being 6 and the post-score was 5 ($p < 0.01$). What implications do these results have for clinical practice?

Understanding the Sampling Section of a Research Report: Population, Sampling Criteria, Sample Size, Refusal Rate, and Attrition Rate

STATISTICAL TECHNIQUE IN REVIEW

Sampling or eligibility criteria include a list of requirements or characteristics essential for membership in the target population. Sampling criteria include both inclusion and exclusion criteria. **Inclusion sampling criteria** are the requirements identified by the researcher that must be present for an element or participant to be included in a sample. **Sampling exclusion criteria** are the requirements identified by the researcher that eliminate or exclude participants from being in a sample. Researchers may identify from very broad sampling criteria to very specific criteria. Broad sampling criteria can promote a large, diverse, or heterogeneous population, although specific sampling criteria promote a smaller, more homogeneous population (Grove & Gray, 2023).

A **population** is the particular group of elements or individuals who are being studied, such as central catheters, adults with diabetes, or overweight children. The sampling criteria determine the **target population**, and the sample is selected from the **accessible population** or the available potential study participants within the target population. The **sample** is the focus of a particular study. Fig. 2.1 demonstrates the relationships among the concepts of population, target population, accessible population, sample, and study elements (Gray & Grove, 2021). The **study elements** are the participants, objects, or events that might be included in the sample for a study. When the study is completed, researchers determine the extent to which the findings can be generalized or transferred from the sample to the accessible population. If the findings from a study are significant and consistent with the findings from previous studies, the findings might be generalized to the target population (Kazdin, 2022).

The **sample size** is the number of individuals or elements that participate in a study. An adequate sample size is essential for identifying significant relationships among variables or differences between groups. **Power** is the probability that a given statistic can detect relationships or differences that exist in the population studied (Gray & Grove, 2021; Kim et al., 2022). Put another way, statistical power refers to the probability of rejecting the null hypothesis when it is actually false. "Statistical power is indexed on a scale of 0.00 to 1.00, with zero indicating there is no chance of rejecting a false null hypothesis and 1.00 indicating the false null hypothesis will be rejected 100% of the time it is studied" (Taylor & Spurlock, 2018, p. 263). Large samples increase the power of the statistics conducted so that researchers might accurately accept or reject the null hypotheses for their study. **Power analysis** is a statistical technique conducted to determine the sample size needed to detect significant relationships and differences between groups in a study. A power analysis includes the following four elements: (1) alpha or level of significance set by the researcher, usually at 0.05; (2) standard power for a

Population

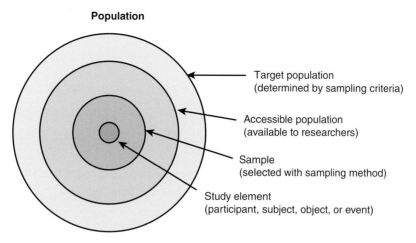

Target population
(determined by sampling criteria)

Accessible population
(available to researchers)

Sample
(selected with sampling method)

Study element
(participant, subject, object, or event)

FIG. 2.1 ▦ LINKING POPULATION, SAMPLE, AND ELEMENT IN A STUDY.

study is usually 0.80 or 80%; (3) effect size (strength of relationships among variables or extent of group differences); and (4) sample size (Aberson, 2019; Cohen, 1988). A study effect size should be based on the results of similar studies or determined by conducting a pilot study (Gray & Grove, 2021). The process for conducting and interpreting power analyses is presented in Exercises 24 and 25 of this text.

Researchers need to identify a large enough accessible population to ensure an adequate sample is obtained after accounting for refusal and attrition rates. **Refusal rate** is the percentage of potential participants who decline to be in a study. The refusal rate is calculated using the following formula:

Refusal rate = (Number refusing to participate ÷ Number of individuals approached) × 100%

Example: Refusal rate = (5 decline to participate ÷ 50 approached) × 100% = 0.1 × 100% = 10%

Attrition rate is the percentage of participants who drop out of a study after the sample size has been determined based on the sampling criteria. Attrition can occur actively, when participants choose to drop out of a study for a variety of reasons, or passively, when participants are lost to follow-up. The attrition rate is calculated by dividing the number of participants who dropped out of the study by the total number of individuals in the study sample. Because study attrition happens for a variety of reasons, researchers must anticipate this rate and increase the number of participants recruited into a study to ensure an adequate sample size (Grove & Gray, 2021).

Attrition rate = (Number dropping out of a study ÷ Total sample size) × 100%

Example: Attrition rate = (4 dropped out of study ÷ 80 sample size) × 100% = 0.05 × 100% = 5%

The refusal and attrition rates decrease the sample's representativeness of the target population. Therefore refusal and attrition rates greater than 10% to 15% are of concern, and researchers should report the reasons people provided for declining to take part in or for dropping out of a study. Researchers need to take these rates into consideration when determining the findings for their study. Sample attrition also reduces the final sample size and decreases the power of the statistical analyses conducted to detect significant relationships among variables and differences between groups (Aberson, 2019). Attrition from intervention and control groups in a study should be low and the group sizes approximately equal to maintain statistical power (Gray & Grove, 2021; Kim et al., 2022).

RESEARCH ARTICLE

Source

Ayar, D., & Sabancioğullari, S. (2022). The effect of a solution-oriented therapy on the depression levels and the perceived social support of depressive patients. *Archives of Psychiatric Nursing, 36,* 62–69. https://doi.org/10.1016/j.apnu.2021.11.004

Introduction

Ayar and Sabancioğullari (2022) conducted a randomized controlled trial (RCT) with a repeated measures design. The experimental group received the Solution-Oriented Therapy Programme (SOTP) intervention and the control group received routine nursing care. The depression levels of the participants were measured with the Beck Depression Inventory (BDI) and perceived social support was measured with the Perceived Social Support Inventory (PSSI). The participants' depression and social support were measured three times: before the intervention, after the intervention, and 3 months later. These researchers found that the participants in the experimental or intervention group demonstrated significant improvement in their BDI and PSSI scores compared with the control group. The sampling process from this RCT is presented as an example in the following study excerpt and is diagrammed in Fig. 2.2.

Relevant Study Results
"Research Population and Sample

The present research was executed in the inpatient units of a public hospital, which is located in the city center. Within the scope of the study, the quantity of samples was determined as 57 with G*POWER, 0.7 effect size, 0.80 power, and a 0.05 error margin. The depressive patients were allocated to the study as experimental ($n = 28$) or control ($n = 29$) groups by utilizing simple random sampling.

Inclusion Criteria

Depressive patients who were undergoing inpatient treatment, who were diagnosed with depressive disorder, who had recurrent depressive disorder at least 6 months ago, who were between the ages of 18 and 60, who were taking inpatient treatment in the psychiatry clinics, who had a Beck Depression Inventory (BDI) score between 30 and 45, and who knew how to read and write were included in the study.

Exclusion Criteria

Depressive patients who had comorbid psychiatric disorders, who had psychotic symptoms, who had chronic organic illnesses, who had alcohol and/or substance abuse or addiction, and who took part in any support group or psychotherapy were excluded from the present research" (Ayar & Sabancioğullari, 2022, p. 63).

"Research Procedure

...The SOTP is a consultative approach developed to help depressive patients concentrate on their resources and strengths. The researcher has received theoretical/practical training and supervision about solution-oriented therapy with a certification, so she designed the SOTP for the current study. .... The depressive patients in the control group were provided with routine clinical care. .... The patients in the experimental group were asked not to share information about the interventions applied in the program, the recommendations given, and homework with other patients. In addition, the patients in the experimental and control groups were

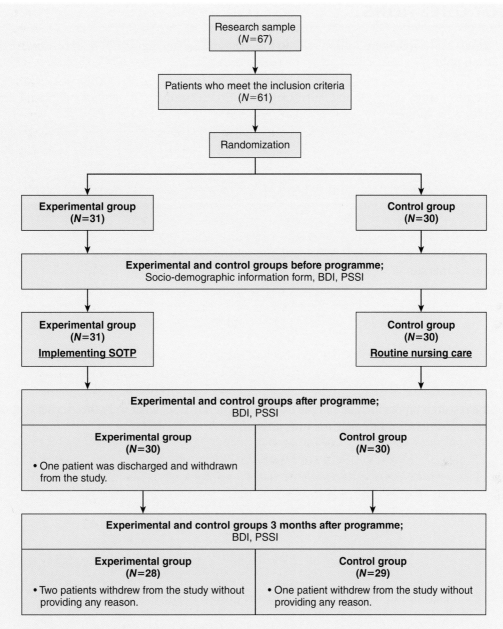

FIG. 2.2 ■ **RESEARCH PROCEDURE.** *BDI,* Beck Depression Inventory; *PSSI,* Perceived Social Support Inventory; *SOTP,* Solution-Oriented Therapy Programme. Ayar, D., & Sabancioğullari, S. (2022). The effect of a solution-oriented therapy on the depression levels and the perceived social support of depressive patients. *Archives of Psychiatric Nursing, 36,* 64. https://doi.org/10.1016/j.apnu.2021.11.004

called at different times for measurements and interviews, and interviews were held in different places (Fig. 2.2).

Ethics

Each stage of the study was executed in line with the ethical principles. Before the application of treatment, permission/approval was obtained from the University Non-Interventional Clinical Research Ethics Committee. . . . Moreover, verbal and written informed consent forms were collected from the participants of the study. The depressive patients were unaware of which research group they were allocated" (Ayar & Sabancioğullari, 2022, pp. 63–65).

STUDY QUESTIONS

The questions in the following section refer to the Ayar and Sabancioğullari (2022) research article except for question 6.

1. What type of study did Ayar and Sabancioğullari (2022) conduct? What dependent and independent variables were studied?

2. What population was studied? What was the setting for this study? Were these appropriate for the purpose of this study?

3. Did the research report include sample exclusion criteria? If so, what were these criteria and were they appropriate? Provide a rationale for your answer.

4. Describe the groups in this study. How were the groups formed?

5. How many participants were in each group of the study? What was the attrition number and rate for the experimental group? Was attrition a weakness in this study? Provide a rationale for your answer.

6. Calculate a refusal rate for a hypothetical study where researchers approached 250 potential participants and 235 consented to be in the study. Show your calculations and round your answer to the nearest tenth of a percent.

7. Was Fig. 2.2 helpful in identifying the sample size of the RCT and in determining the group sizes for the pretest, posttest, and follow-up assessment at 3 months? Discuss the importance of these diagrams in understanding the sampling process in quasi-experimental and experimental studies.

8. Define the term *power* as used in research. What is the usual power level for conducting a power analysis? What level of significance is often used for conducting a power analysis?

9. Did Ayar and Sabancioğullari (2022) obtain official approval to conduct their study? Did the study participants provide consent to be included in this study?

10. Identify three design strategies used to reduce the potential for bias and error in this study and increase the credibility of the findings.

Answers to Study Questions

1. This study was an RCT with a repeated measures design. The independent variable or intervention was the SOTP. The dependent or outcome variables were depression level and perceived social support.

2. The population studied included patients with depression and the setting was inpatient units of an urban, public hospital. The population and setting were appropriate to address the study purpose that was focused on the effect of SOTP intervention on the depression levels and perceived social support of hospitalized patients with depression.

3. Yes, the sample exclusion criteria were clearly identified with a header as "Depressive patients who had comorbid psychiatric disorders, who had psychotic symptoms, who had chronic organic illnesses, who had alcohol and/or substance abuse or addiction, and who took part in any support group or psychotherapy" (Ayar & Sabancioğulları, 2022, p. 63). These are relevant exclusion criteria that reduce the effects of extraneous variables to increase the validity of the design and the accuracy of the study findings. RCT is conducted with a strong design and relevant sampling criteria to determine the effectiveness of the intervention being tested (Gray & Grove, 2021; Kazdin, 2022).

4. This study included an experimental group that received the SOTP intervention and a control group that received routine care (see Fig. 2.2). Participants were randomly assigned to the experimental and control groups, resulting in independent groups (Grove & Gray, 2023).

5. Initially the experimental group included 31 participants and the control group included 30 participants. Three months after the SOTP was implemented, the experimental group included 28 participants. The attrition number is 3 and the attrition rate = $(3 \div 31) \times 100\% = 0.097 \times 100\% = 9.7\%$. The attrition rate for the experimental group is not a weakness because it is small (less than 10%) and will probably have limited effects on the study results (Aberson, 2019; Kazdin, 2022).

6. Refusal rate = (number of participants declining to participate in a study ÷ by the number of potential participants approached) $\times$ 100%. The number declining to participate = $250 - 235 = 15$. Refusal rate = (15 refused to participate ÷ 250 potential participants approached) $\times$ 100% = $0.06 \times 100\% = 6\%$ (Grove & Gray, 2023).

7. Graphics, such as Fig. 2.2, provide quality reporting of the sampling process in RCTs and other quasi-experimental and experimental studies. This type of figure can be used to identify the number of potential participants, indicate those meeting sample criteria, refusal numbers and rates, numbers in each group, attrition numbers and rates, and final size of study groups. A sampling algorithm, such as Fig. 2.2, is considered the standard for reporting RCTs by the Preferred Reporting Items for Systematic reviews and Meta-Analysis (PRISMA) 2020 Statement (Page et al., 2021).

8. Power is the probability that a given statistic can detect differences or relationships that exist in the population studied. Put another way, statistical power refers to the probability of rejecting the null hypothesis when it is false (Taylor & Spurlock, 2018). With adequately powered statistical analyses, researchers can more accurately accept or reject the null hypotheses in their study. The minimum acceptable power is usually set at 0.80 or 80% for power analysis and the level of significance or alpha (α) is typically set at 0.05 (Aberson, 2019; Gray & Grove, 2021).

9. Yes, the researchers executed the study according to ethical principles and obtained the approval to conduct the study from the University Non-Interventional Clinical Research Ethics Committee. Verbal and written informed consent forms were obtained from each of the study participants.

10. You might have listed any of the following design strategies. RCT is considered a gold standard for examining differences between intervention and control groups in studies. The sampling criteria were very specific, which increased the similarities of the study participants and reduced the potential for error in determining group differences. A power analysis was conducted to determine an adequate sample size for this study. The participants were randomly assigned to the intervention and control groups, decreasing the potential for bias. The patients in the experimental group were asked to not share information with those in the control group and the outcome variables were measured at different times. The BDI and PSSI are considered quality methods for measuring the study outcomes (Gray & Grove, 2021; Kazdin, 2022; Kim et al., 2022).

Questions for Additional Study

Name: _____ Class: _____

Date: _____

Follow your instructor's directions for submitting answers to the following questions. Your instructor may ask you to write your answers below and submit them as a hard copy for evaluation. Alternatively, your instructor may ask you to submit your answers online.

1. What were the sample inclusion criteria identified by Ayar and Sabancıoğullari (2022) in their study? Discuss the appropriateness of these criteria.

2. Sample inclusion and exclusion criteria are developed to determine what type of population? What is the accessible population? Document your answer.

3. Compare the attrition numbers and rates for the experimental and control groups at the 3-month follow-up in this study. Was the attrition rate for the experimental and control groups in this study a strength or weakness? Provide rationale and documentation for your answer.

4. Calculate the attrition rate for a hypothetical study that included a sample of 166 patients treated for heart failure (HF) in a cardiac center. A total of 15 study participants could not be contacted after hospital discharge; 10 participants became too ill to continue in the study; and 4 died. Round your answer to the nearest tenth of a percent.

5. Is the attrition rate calculated in Question 4 a study strength or weakness? Provide a rationale for your answer.

6. The intervention and control groups had unequal numbers. Is this a study strength or weakness? Provide a rationale for your answer.

7. Discuss the results of the power analysis conducted for this study. Was the reporting of the power analysis information complete? Provide a rationale for your answer.

8. What was the sample size for the Ayar and Sabancioğullari (2022) study? Was the sample size adequate to obtain credible results? Provide a rationale for your answers.

9. What were the strengths of the SOPT intervention implemented in this study?

10. Are the findings from this study ready for use in practice? Provide a rationale for your answer.

Identifying Probability and Nonprobability Sampling Methods in Studies

STATISTICAL TECHNIQUE IN REVIEW

A **sampling method** is the process of selecting people, events, behaviors, or other elements that are representative of the population being studied (Grove & Gray, 2023). The sampling methods implemented in research are usually categorized as either probability (random) or nonprobability (nonrandom). Tables 3.1 and 3.2 identify the common probability and nonprobability sampling methods applied in quantitative, qualitative, mixed methods, and outcomes studies in nursing (Gray & Grove, 2021; Heavey, 2019; Kazdin, 2022). **Quantitative research** is an objective research methodology used to describe variables, examine relationships or associations among variables, and determine cause-and-effect interactions between independent and dependent variables (Creswell & Creswell, 2023; Grove & Gray, 2023; Shadish et al., 2002). **Qualitative studies** are scholarly, rigorous approaches used to describe life experiences, cultures, and social processes from the perspective of the persons involved (Creswell & Báez, 2021; Creswell & Poth, 2018). **Mixed methods studies** include methodologies from both quantitative and qualitative research to better understand the area of study (Creswell & Clark, 2018). **Outcomes research** is a rigorous scientific method used to investigate the end results of health care. The sampling method used in a study is based on the type of research, the study problem and purpose, study design, population studied, and the expertise and experiences of the researchers.

Probability Sampling Methods

Probability sampling, also known as random sampling, requires that every member or element of the study population has an equal and independent opportunity to be chosen for inclusion in a study. Probability sampling involves identifying the **sampling frame** or each

TABLE 3.1   PROBABILITY SAMPLING METHODS, COMMON APPLICATIONS, AND SAMPLE REPRESENTATIVENESS IN NURSING RESEARCH

Sampling Method	Common Application(s)	Sample Representativeness
Simple random sampling	Quantitative and outcomes research	Provides strong representativeness of the target population that increases with sample size.
Stratified random sampling	Quantitative and outcomes research	Provides strong representativeness of the target population that increases with control of stratified variable(s).
Cluster sampling	Quantitative and outcomes research	Is less representative of the target population than simple random sampling and stratified random sampling, but representativeness increases with sample size.
Systematic sampling	Quantitative and outcomes research	Is less representative of the target population than simple random sampling and stratified random sampling, but representativeness increases with sample size.

person or element in a study's target population and then randomly selecting a sample from that population (see Fig. 2.1 in Exercise 2). Thus probability sampling allows every person of the study population to be represented without researcher bias and minimizes sampling error. The purpose of sampling in quantitative research is to obtain study participants who are as representative of the target population as possible. The sample's representativeness of the study population is increased by probability sampling. A large sample with a low refusal rate and minimal attrition has strong representativeness of the sample (Aberson, 2019; Cohen, 1988). Four probability sampling designs commonly used to select random samples in quantitative and outcomes studies include simple random sampling, stratified random sampling, cluster sampling, and systematic sampling (Gray & Grove, 2021; Kazdin, 2022; Kim et al., 2022). Table 3.1 identifies these probability sampling methods, their common applications in studies, and the sample's representativeness of the study population.

Simple random sampling is achieved by random selection of members from the sampling frame. The random selection can be accomplished in many different ways, the most common being a computer program to randomly select the sample from the sampling frame. Another example would be to assign each potential participant a number and then randomly select numbers from a random numbers table to fulfill the required number needed for the sample. Random sampling helps to ensure the sample is representative of the study population and that the study has adequate power to detect a difference or identify relationships if they are present (see Exercise 24). This sampling method is strongly representative of the target population, and the representativeness increases with sample size (Aberson, 2019).

Random sampling is not to be confused with **random assignment of study participants to groups**, which is a design strategy to promote more equivalent groups (i.e., intervention and control groups) at the beginning of a study and to reduce the potential for error (Gray & Grove, 2021; Kazdin, 2022; Shadish et al., 2002). Researchers should clearly indicate the sampling method and the process for group assignment in their research report.

Stratified random sampling is used when the researcher knows some of the variables within a population that will affect the representativeness of the sample. Some examples of these variables include age, gender, race/ethnicity, medical diagnosis, and severity of illness. The study participants are selected randomly based on their classification into the selected stratum of a variable. The strata identified ensure that all levels of the variable(s) are represented in the sample. For example, age could be the variable, and, after stratification, the sample might include equal numbers of participants in the established strata of age ranges: 18 to 39, 40 to 59, 60 to 79, and 80 years of age or older. Stratified random sampling is a strong sampling method that is representative of the target population, and the representativeness increases with control of the stratified variable(s) (Gray & Grove, 2021; Kazin, 2022).

Researchers use **cluster sampling** (also referred to as complex sampling) in two different situations: (1) when the time and travel necessary to use simple random sampling would be prohibitive; and (2) when the specific elements of a population are unknown, therefore making it impossible to develop a sampling frame. In either of these cases, a list of institutions or organizations associated with the elements of interest can often be obtained. To conduct cluster sampling, a list of all the states, cities, institutions, or organizations associated with the elements of the population is developed. The states, cities, institutions, or organizations are then randomly selected from the list to form the sample. However, the data collected from study participants from the same institution are likely to be correlated and thus not completely independent (Gray & Grove, 2021). Therefore cluster sampling produces a sample that is not as representative of the study population as with simple random sampling and stratified random sampling (see Table 3.1; Kazdin, 2022).

Systematic sampling requires an ordered list of the members of a population. Individuals are selected through a process that accepts every *k*th member on the list using a randomly selected starting point. k is calculated based on the size of population and the sample size desired. For example, if the population has 1000 potential participants and a sample size of 100 is desired, then $k = 1000 \div 100 = 10$, which means that every 10th person or unit on a list is invited to participate in the study. The initial starting point must be random for the sample to be considered a probability sample. Also, steps must be taken to ensure that the original list was not ordered in any way that could affect the study results. Probability sampling methods are more commonly used in quantitative and outcomes studies to increase the representativeness of a study sample.

Nonprobability Sampling Methods

Nonprobability sampling is a nonrandom sampling technique that does not extend equal opportunity for selection to all members of the study population. You should never assume a probability sampling method was used in a study; rather, the researchers must identify the sampling method as probability or nonprobability for their study. In addition, researchers should describe the process for accomplishing the sampling method in a study. In clinical research, nonprobability sampling methods are used much more frequently than probability sampling methods because of the limited availability of potential subjects (Holmes, 2018). The common nonprobability sampling methods applied in nursing research include convenience, quota, purposive, network, and theoretical sampling (see Table 3.2). Convenience sampling is

TABLE 3.2 NONPROBABILITY SAMPLING METHODS, COMMONLY APPLICATIONS, AND SAMPLE REPRESENTATIVENESS IN NURSING RESEARCH

Sampling Method	Common Application(s)	Representativeness, Insight, Understanding
Convenience sampling	Quantitative, qualitative, mixed methods, and outcomes research	There is questionable representativeness of the target population, which improves with increasing sample size for quantitative and outcomes research. This method is used in qualitative and mixed methods research to identify participants who are likely to have experience with the research topic.
Quota sampling	Quantitative, mixed methods, and outcomes research; rarely qualitative research	Use of stratification for selected variables in quantitative and outcomes research makes the sample more representative than convenience sampling. In mixed methods research, participants of different ages, ethnic groups, or severity of illness may be selected to increase the depth and richness of the study findings.
Purposeful or purposive sampling	Qualitative and mixed methods research; rarely quantitative research	Focus is on insight, description, and understanding of a phenomenon, situation, process, or cultural element with specially selected participants who can provide quality data to address the study purpose.
Network or snowball sampling	Qualitative and mixed methods research; rarely quantitative research	Focus is on insight, description, and understanding of a phenomenon, situation, process, or cultural element in a difficult-to-access population. Intent is to identify additional participants who contribute to the study focus.
Theoretical sampling	Qualitative research	Focus is on obtaining quality participants with different perspectives, of an adequate number for developing a relevant framework, model, or theory in a selected area of study.

the most frequently used sampling method in quantitative, qualitative, mixed methods, and outcomes nursing studies (Creswell & Clark, 2018; Creswell & Creswell, 2023; Creswell & Poth, 2018; Kazdin, 2022).

Researchers obtain a **convenience sample** by enrolling study participants who meet sample criteria, are accessible, and are willing to participate in a study (Grove & Gray, 2023; Kazdin, 2022). Individuals are enrolled in a study until the target sample size is obtained. Convenience sampling does not allow for the opportunity to control for sampling errors or biases. To counter the inability to control for biases, researchers must carefully examine the population being studied and adjust the sampling criteria to appropriately address the identified biases. For example, researchers might include only individuals with a new diagnosis of type 2 diabetes in their study of the effects of diet education on hemoglobin A1c values. This sampling criterion of newly diagnosed diabetic patient decreases the potential for errors or biases created by previous diabetic education and other management strategies that patients might have experienced in the past to control their type 2 diabetes.

Researchers use **quota sampling** to ensure adequate representation of types of individuals who are likely to be underrepresented, such as women, minorities, the elderly, or the poor. A convenience sampling method is used in conjunction with quota sampling to help ensure the inclusion of the identified participant type. Quota sampling can be used to mimic the known characteristics of the population or to ensure adequate numbers of participants in each stratum. This sampling strategy is like stratified random sampling and is more frequently applied in quantitative than in qualitative studies. Quota sampling is recognized as more representative of the target population than convenience sampling because of the decreased opportunity for sampling error or bias (see Table 3.2; Grove & Gray, 2023; Kim et al., 2022).

Purposive, network, and theoretical sampling methods are more commonly used in qualitative and mixed methods research rather than in quantitative and outcomes studies. **Purposive sampling** occurs when the researcher consciously selects participants, elements, events, or incidents to include in a study. Those selected by the researchers are information-rich cases or those from whom a lot of information can be obtained (see Table 3.2; Creswell & Báez, 2021; Creswell & Poth, 2018). Researchers usually try to include typical and atypical cases in the sample. This type of sampling has been criticized because the researcher's judgments in the selection of cases cannot be evaluated. However, this sampling method can be a good way to explore new areas of study.

Network or snowball sampling makes use of social networks and the fact that friends often have common characteristics. The researcher identifies a few study participants who meet the sampling criteria and then asks them to assist in recruiting others with similar characteristics. Network sampling is useful for gathering samples that are difficult to obtain, have not been previously identified for study, or can help the researcher explore a particular area of interest or focus. Sampling errors or biases are inherent in networking samples because the study participants are not independent of one another (Gray & Grove, 2021).

Theoretical sampling is used in the research process to advance the development of a theory and is more commonly used in grounded theory studies. Data are gathered from individuals or groups who can provide relevant information for theory generation. For example, a researcher might interview family members and patients to develop a theory of surviving a near-death experience. The researcher continues to seek study participants and collects data until saturation of the theoretical concepts and relationships has occurred. **Saturation of data** occurs when collecting data from new study participants does not add new knowledge regarding the study purpose. Participant diversity in the sample is promoted to ensure that the developed theory is applicable to a range of behaviors and settings (Charmaz, 2014; Creswell & Poth, 2018).

STUDY QUESTIONS

Directions: Answer the following questions with a clear, appropriate response. For each question that includes an excerpt about sampling from a research article, provide the following information: (1) decide whether the sampling method presented is either a *probability* or *nonprobability sampling method*; (2) identify the *specific sampling method* used—that is, simple random, stratified random, cluster, or systematic sampling for probability samples (see Table 3.1) or convenience, quota, purposive, network, or theoretical sampling for nonprobability samples (see Table 3.2); and (3) provide a *rationale for the sampling method* you selected. Some of the examples might include *more than one sampling method* to obtain the study sample.

1. Study excerpt: Bronas et al. (2022) conducted a randomized controlled trial (RCT) to examine the effect of an exercise training program on cognitive function for individuals with chronic kidney disease (CKD). "The study population is community-dwelling men and women with CKD, between 60 and 80 years of age, with preclinical cognitive impairment. . . . A sample size of 12 per group is recommended for pilot studies estimating the mean and variability of continuous outcomes. . . . It is anticipated that 17 participants will be randomized to a 6-month home-based exercise program and 17 participants randomized to the usual care control group" (Bronas et al., 2022. p. 76).
   Source: Bronas, L. G., Hanna, M., Lash, J. P., Ajilore, O., Zhou, X. J., & Lamar, M. (2022). Exercise training and cognitive function in kidney disease: Protocol for a pilot randomized controlled trial. *Nursing Research, 71*(1), 75–82. https://doi.org/10.1097/NNR.0000000000000554

2. How were the groups formed in the Bronas et al. (2022) study? Was group assignment a study strength or weakness? Provide a rationale for your answer.

3. Study content: Chatreewatanakul et al. (2022) conducted a qualitative study to explore the lived experience of symptom recognition and management among exacerbation chronic obstructive pulmonary disease (COPD) patients. The participants were 20 COPD patients recruited from a hospital outpatient medical clinic who were living with COPD and had the potential to provide in-depth, rich data.

   Source: Chatreewatanakul, B., Othaganont, P., & Hickman, R. (2022). Early symptom recognition and symptom management among exacerbation COPD patients: A qualitative study. *Applied Nursing Research, 63,* 151522. https://doi.org/10.1016/j.apnr.2021.151522

4. Study excerpt: Han et al. (2018) conducted a pilot study to examine the effects of a tailored lifestyle intervention on body composition, obesity-related biomarkers, and lifestyle modification for women at high risk for breast cancer. "Seventy-three women were approached for the study. Of those, 30 were determined to be eligible, and 16 consenting participants completed the baseline study visit. These participants were then randomized through a computer-generated table with stratification based on menopausal status, with eight assigned to each group" (Han et al., 2018, p. 981).

   Source: Han, C. J., Korde, L. A., Reding, S., Allott, K., Van Doren, M., Schwarz, Y., Vaughan, C. & Reding, K. W. (2018). Investigation of a lifestyle intervention in women at high risk of breast cancer. *Western Journal of Nursing Research, 40*(7), 976–996. https://doi.org/10.1177/0193945917697227

5. Was the sample for the Han et al. (2018) study representative of the population of women at high risk for breast cancer? Provide a rationale for your answer.

6. Currin-McCulloch et al. (2022) conducted a qualitative study to explore the unique physical and psychosocial losses and grief response of young adults (YA) living with advanced cancer. The population included YA treated for a stage III or IV cancer between the ages of 18 and 39 years. "Initial participant recruitment included outreach to YA cancer treatment centers and support organizations that were willing to share the study requirements and recruitment procedures. ... After purposive sampling and data analysis of the first 5 participants' interviews, the primary investigator (PI) incorporated Glaser's theoretical sampling methods to guide the recruitment of new comparison groups that would fulfill exploration of the necessary physical, social, or psychological factors needed to elaborate and test the budding conceptual framework" (Currin-McCulloch et al., 2022, p. E356).

   Source: Currin-McCulloch, J., Kaushik, S., & Jones, B. (2022). When will I feel normal? *Cancer Nursing*, *45*(2), E355–E363. https://doi.org/10.1097/NCC.0000000000000977

7. Study excerpt: Hurley et al. (2018) examined the relationship between 804 registered nurses' personal health practices and their perceptions of themselves as role models for health promotion. "The population from which the study sample was drawn included all registered nurses in Tennessee ($n = 61,829$) listed in the Tennessee Board of Nursing 2015 database. After approval from East Tennessee State University's Institutional Review Board, a simple random sample was drawn from the database. Inclusion criteria were active registered nurse licensed in the state of Tennessee, and a valid email in the database."

   Source: Hurley, S., Edwards, J., Cupp, J., & Phillips, M. (2018). Nurses' perceptions of self as a role model of health. *Western Journal of Nursing Research*, *40*(8), 1131–1147. https://doi.org/10.1177/0193945917701396

8. Rekisso et al. (2022) conducted a quantitative study to describe nurses' attitudes toward the nursing profession from five randomly selected public hospitals. "The sample size was determined $n = 357$ with considering 10% of nonresponse rate. Study participants were recruited using a systematic random sampling method and drawn every 6th interval of the study population of sampling frame" (Rekisso et al., 2022).

   Source: Rekisso, A. D., Mengistu, Z., & Wurjine, T. H. (2022). Nurses' attitudes towards the nursing profession and associated factors in selected public hospitals, Addis Ababa, Ethiopia, 2021: A cross-sectional study. *BMC Nursing*, *21*(1), 1–9. https://doi.org/10.1186/s12912-022-00808-2

9. Study excerpt: "A cross-sectional study was conducted with a sample of qualified nurses recruited from two hospitals. . . . The sample was representative of qualified nurses within the target population. . . . A two-stage sampling approach was taken. The first stage involved the selection of different work areas within two teaching hospitals. . . . The second stage involved the random selection of a sample of nurses from each of these work areas. . . . Nurses were randomly selected from the nursing off-duty (work roster) using a random generator application. . . . In total 300 nurses were invited to participate in the study. . . . A response rate of 70% was obtained ($n = 210$); however, only $n = 203$ of the returned questionnaires were completed properly and thus included in these analyses" (McCarthy et al., 2018, pp. 117–118).

   Source: McCarthy, V. J., Wills, T., & Crowley, S. (2018). Nurses, age, job demands and physical activity at work and at leisure: A cross-sectional study. *Applied Nursing Research, 40*, 116–121. https://doi.org/10.1016/j.apnr.2018.01.010

10. Study excerpt: "We analyzed data from two statewide cross-sectional surveys of California registered nurses conducted in 2013 and 2016. The survey samples were randomly selected from the California Board of Registered Nursing's (BRN) up-to-date lists at the time. The sampling was stratified by region (Northern counties, Sacramento region, Central 5-county San Francisco Bay Area, remainder of the San Francisco Bay Area, Central Valley and Sierra, Central Coast, Los Angeles, Inland Empire, and Border counties). . . . The sampling within each stratum was proportional to the population size of the registered nurses in the region" (Lee et al., 2021, Methods section).

    Source: Lee, S. J., Kang, K. J., & Lee, J. H. (2021). Safe patient handling legislation and changes in programs, practices, perceptions, and experience of musculoskeletal disorders by hospital characteristics: A repeated cross-sectional survey study. *International Journal of Nursing Studies, 113*, 103791. https://doi.org/10.1016/j.ijnurstu.2020.103791

Answers To Study Questions

1. Nonprobability; convenience sampling method. Bronas et al. (2022) did not identify the sampling method in their study, but it was consistent with convenience sampling (see Table 3.2; Grove & Gray, 2023). The study participants with CKD were recruited from the community and asked to participate in the study. With convenience sampling, participants are recruited because they meet sample criteria and are available, accessible, and willing to participate, as in a study. Often when the sampling method is not identified, convenience sampling was used in a study. The random assignment of participants to groups is part of the design and should not be confused with simple random sampling (Grove & Gray, 2023).

2. The groups were formed by random assignment of participants to either the intervention or control group. Random assignment to groups is a study strength that promotes equivalence of the groups and reduces the potential for bias and errors that might affect the study results. Random assignment of participants to groups is an effective strategy used in quasi-experimental and experimental studies to determine the effectiveness of an intervention (Gray & Grove, 2021; Kazdin, 2022).

3. Nonprobability; purposive or purposeful sampling method. Chatreewatanakul et al. (2022) conducted a qualitative study; often purposive sampling is used to identify participants with in-depth, rich knowledge of the research topic (see Table 3.2; Creswell & Poth, 2018).

4. Nonprobability; quota sampling method. A total of 30 women who met sample criteria were asked to participate but only 16 consented. The women were randomized into groups with stratification by menopause status. The initial sample is one of convenience that was strengthened by stratification by menopause status, resulting in quota sampling (Grove & Gray, 2023; Kazdin, 2022).

5. Answers may vary, but the best response is that the sample has limited representativeness of the population of women at high risk for breast cancer. Nonprobability sampling decreases representativeness of the population; however, quota sampling is the strongest of nonprobability sampling methods for promoting representativeness (see Table 3.2; Gray & Grove, 2021). The sample size for the pilot study was small at 16 because 14 (46.7%) of the women approached for the study refused to participate. The small sample size and high refusal rate reduce the representativeness of the sample (Aberson, 2019).

6. Nonprobability; purposive and theoretical sampling. Currin-McCulloch et al. (2022) clearly identified that their qualitative study included purposive and theoretical sampling to develop a framework for YA with advanced cancer (Creswell & Poth, 2018). This sampling combination is often used with grounded theory studies. The initial participants were identified using a purposive sample to select individuals with rich, in-depth information related to the study topic. Theoretical sampling was used to identify participants who might provide details to expand the conceptual framework being developed.

7. Probability; simple random sampling method. The sampling frame and method were identified by Hurley et al. (2018). The sampling frame was all RNs in the Tennessee Board of Nursing 2015 database who were randomly selected for study participation. The researchers should have identified how the sample was randomly selected, but it was probably done by a computer program.

8. Probability; systematic sampling method. Rekisso et al. (2022) clearly identified that systematic sampling was used to obtain their sample from five randomly selected public hospitals. The sampling interval was every sixth nurse from the population sampling frame. However, the researchers needed to provide more detail about the development of the sampling frame and if the initial starting point was random for this systematic sampling process (Gray & Grove, 2021; Kazdin, 2022).

9. Probability; cluster sampling method. McCarthy et al. (2018) identified their sampling approach as having two stages. The first stage involved the selection of nursing units, which is done with cluster sample to identify the settings for the study participants. The second stage involved randomly selecting nurses from these units. This multistage process of sampling is consistent with cluster sampling when the sampling frame of potential participants is not available. The researchers also identified how the nurses were randomly selected from the hospital units (Gray & Grove, 2021; Kim et al., 2022).

10. Probability; stratified random sampling. Lee et al. (2021) conducted a survey of RNs who were randomly selected from the sampling frame of the California BRN. However, the process for random selection of the RNs was not described but was probably achieved by computer program. The study included proportional stratified random sampling because the number of RNs included in each stratum is proportional to the RN population of each region (Gray & Grove, 2021; Kazdin, 2022).

Follow your instructor's directions to submit your answers to the following questions for additional study. Your instructor may ask you to write your answers below and submit them as a hard copy for evaluation. Alternatively, your instructor may ask you to submit your answers online.

Directions: Answer the following questions with a clear, appropriate response. For each question that includes an excerpt about sampling from a research article, provide the following information: (1) decide whether the sampling method presented is either a *probability* or *nonprobability sampling method*; (2) identify the *specific sampling method* used—that is, simple random, stratified random, cluster, or systematic sampling for probability samples (see Table 3.1) or convenience, quota, purposive, network, or theoretical sampling for nonprobability samples (see Table 3.2); and (3) provide a *rationale for the sampling method* you selected. Some of the examples might include *more than one sampling method* to obtain the study sample.

1. Study excerpt: Mensinger et al. (2022) described the psychological responses of nurses working in hospitals during the COVID-19 pandemic in the United States (U.S.). "Participants were recruited using a snowballing strategy including outreach to alumni of the authors' university, news media, professional and trade organizations, social media, and outreach to facilities that treated COVID-19 patients. Registered nurses working throughout the U.S. and the U.S. territories (Puerto Rico, Guam, and the U.S. Virgin Islands) were eligible for the study. The primary sample described in this paper includes 467 hospital-based registered nurses (RNs) enrolled between May 5, 2020, and June 15, 2020" (Mensinger et al., 2022, Methods section).

    Source: Mensinger, J. L., Brom, H., Havens, D. S., Costello, A., D'Annunzio, C., Durning, J. D., Bradley, P. K., Copel, L., Maldonado, L., Smeltzer, S., Yost, J., & Kaufmann, P. (2022). Psychological responses of hospital-based nurses working during the COVID-19 pandemic in the United States: A cross-sectional study. *Applied Nursing Research, 63,* 151517. https://doi.org/10.1016/j.apnr.2021.151517

2. Study excerpt: Loew et al. (2018) conducted a mixed-methods study of college women to define responsible sexual behaviors. Phase I of the study was quantitative and Phase II was qualitative. "Participants in this study were all women who had, or might have, sex with men; that is, women not in exclusively same-sex partnerships. All participants were 18 to 35 years old, English-speaking, and attended a large, public, Midwestern university. More than 2000 women completed Phase 1 of the study, a survey; of these approximately 900 volunteered to participate in the Phase II interviews. Women were selected from this pool to be interviewed using a purposive maximum variation sampling strategy. . . . Based on survey data, women were sampled based on variation in their knowledge and use of emergency contraception and on some aspects of sexual history. . . . Theoretical sampling was used to select potential participants based on the data as they were collected, including women who had experienced a pregnancy termination or 'false alarm' pregnancy. . . . This process yielded a sample of 35 women who represented a wide range of experiences. When saturation was reached, recruitment and data collection ended" (Loew et al., 2018, p. 1151).

   Source: Loew, N., Mackin, M. L., & Ayres, L. (2018). Collegiate women's definitions of responsible sexual behavior. *Western Journal of Nursing Research, 40*(8), 1148–1162. https://doi.org/10.1177/0193945917706508

3. Study excerpt: Xiao et al. (2022) conducted a correlational study to determine if school bullying was associated with suicidal risk in children and adolescents. "In the two study sites, a two-stage simple random clustering sampling method with probability proportionate to sample size (PPS) design was used to select study subjects: in stage one, altogether 19 primary, secondary, and senior high schools were randomly chosen from all schools within the two cities; in stage two, based on the required sample size, 2–4 classes in each grade of the chosen school were further randomly selected, all students within the chosen class were initially included" (Xiao et al., 2022, p. 393).

   Source: Xiao, Y., Ran, H., Fang, D., Che, Y., Donald, A. R., Wang, S., Peng, J., Chen, L., & Lu, J. (2022). School bullying associated suicidal risk in children and adolescents from Yunnan, China: The mediation of social support. *Journal of Affective Disorders, 300,* 392–399. https://doi.org/10.1016/j.jad.2022.01.032

4. Study excerpt: Mansfield et al. (2018) conducted a correlational study to examine the association between parental knowledge of human papillomavirus (HPV) and their intentions to have their daughters vaccinated. "This study used HINTS [Health Information National Trends Survey] 2006-2007 because it was the only dataset that assessed the outcome variable, intention to vaccinate for HPV. . . . HINTS's probability-based sample design used a random-digit dialing to conduct telephone surveys and a nationwide address list to administer surveys via mail. A subsampling screening tool, Westat's Telephone Research Center (TRC), was used to identify working residential numbers. A total of 3,767 telephone interviews were then completed, and 325 were partially completed ($n = 4,092$); 3,473 mail surveys were completed and 109 were partially completed ($n = 3,582$). The final total sample was 7,674 participants" (Mansfield et al., 2018, p. 481).

   Source: Mansfield, L. N., Onsomu, E. O., Merwin, E., Hall, N. M., & Harper-Harrison, A. (2018). Association between parental HPV knowledge and intentions to have their daughters vaccinated. *Western Journal of Nursing Research*, 40(4), 481–501. https://doi.org/10.1177/0193945916682953

5. Was the sample identified in the Mansfield et al. (2018) study representative of parents' intentions to have their daughters vaccinated? Provide a rationale for your answer.

6. Study excerpt: Dickson et al. (2021) conducted a mixed methods study to describe the self-care practices in older working populations with cardiovascular disease (CVD). "A convenience sample of 108 older adults with CVD were enrolled from clinical and community settings in a large urban region in Northeast United States. . . . Individuals were excluded if they had: 1) history of a prior neurological event (e.g., stroke, head injury, encephalopathy); or 2) self-employment status. A sample size of 108 was calculated to achieve adequate ($\geq 80\%$) power for the quantitative aims of this study. For the qualitative data collection, a purposive sample ($n = 40$) from the total sample were recruited . . . to ensure that cases for the qualitative analysis emerged that provided the maximum heterogeneity on specific attributes (e.g., age, race, CVD diagnosis and occupation)" (Dickson et al., 2021, p. 448).

   Source: Dickson, V. V., Jun, J., & Melkus, G. D. (2021). A mixed methods study describing the self-care practices in an older working population with cardiovascular disease (CVD): Balancing work, life, and health. *Heart & Lung, 50*(3), 447–454. https://doi.org/10.1016/j.hrtlng.2021.02.001 0147-9563

7. Study excerpt: "This study was a part of a multi-site prospective observational study of COPD [chronic obstructive pulmonary disease] patients to explore the relationship between depression, inflammation, and functional status. . . . Participants were recruited from various sources including outpatient clinics from three medical centers, pulmonary rehabilitation programs, a research database maintained by the investigators, queries of medical records and pulmonary function tests, Better Breathers Club, community pulmonary practices, advertisements, study website, and other referrals." A total of 282 patients with COPD were included in the study (Lee et al., 2018, p. 150).

   Source: Lee, J., Nguyen, H. Q., Jarrett, M. E., Mitchell, P. H., Pike, K. C., & Fan, V. S. (2018). Effect of symptoms on physical performance in COPD. *Heart & Lung, 47*(2), 149–156. https://doi.org/10.1016/j.hrtlng.2017.12.007

8. Study excerpt: "The population in this study were the people who will undergo the 1st dose of COVID-19 vaccination totaling 503 respondents. The sample in this study was part of the population that met the inclusion and exclusion criteria. Inclusion criteria are willing to be respondents, aged 18-45 years, not being chronically ill, and having a family. Exclusion criteria are currently undergoing treatment for mental disorders. The sampling technique used is accidental sampling" (Fadlilah et al., 2022, p. 39).

   Source: Fadlilah, S., Setiawan, D. I., Murdhiono, W. R., Wiyani, C., Mindarsih, E., Lustiyati, E. D., & Susanto, R. (2022). The anxiety facing the 1st dose of COVID-19 vaccination and related factors. *International Medical Journal, 29*(1), 38–42.

9. Was the sample in the Fadlilah et al. (2022) study representative of the target population? Provide a rationale for your answer.

10. Study excerpt: Macartney and colleagues (2018) studied the concussion symptoms in 136 adolescents: 74 females and 62 males. "A retrospective chart review was completed between 11/21/2014 to 11/20/2015. A purposive sample of all patients who visited the CHEO [Children's Hospital of Eastern Ontario] concussion clinic during the study period [was] included. Patients were excluded if symptoms records were not documented . . . CHEO's concussion clinic opened in the fall of 2014. The clinic provides care to patients less than nineteen years old who remain symptomatic at least four weeks post injury" (Macartney et al., 2018, p. 59).

   Source: Macartney, G., Simoncic, V., Goulet, K., & Aglipay, M. (2018). Concussion symptoms prevalence, severity, and trajectory: Implications for nursing practice. *Journal of Pediatric Nursing*, *40*(1), 58–62. https://doi.org/10.1016/j.pedn.2018.03.006

Understanding Reliability of Measurement Methods

STATISTICAL TECHNIQUE IN REVIEW

The **reliability** of a measurement method or instrument denotes the consistency of the measures obtained of an attribute, concept, or situation in a study or clinical practice. Broadly, reliability is concerned with the dependability, consistency, stability, precision, and reproducibility of a measurement method (Bartlett & Frost, 2008; Gray & Grove, 2021; Kazdin, 2022). An instrument that demonstrates strong reliability in the measurement of a variable or concept has less random error (Bialocerkowski et al., 2010). For example, the Center for Epidemiologic Studies Depression Scale (CES-D) was developed through research to diagnose depression in mental health patients (Radloff, 1977). Over time, different versions of the CES-D have been developed; and these versions have proven to be quality measures of depression in clinical practice and in research for children, adolescents, adults, and the elderly (Armenta et al., 2014; Cosco et al., 2017; Jiang et al., 2019; Siddaway et al., 2017). If a scale like the CES-D consistently measures a concept, then it is considered reliable. However, when a scale produces inconsistent scores with repeat testing of study participants or has low reliability values, it is considered unreliable, resulting in increased measurement error (Bandalos, 2018; Waltz et al., 2017).

Reliability testing examines the amount of random error in an instrument that is used in a study. Because all measurement methods contain some error, reliability exists in degrees and usually is expressed as a correlation coefficient. *Estimates of reliability are specific to the sample being tested*. High reliability values reported for an established instrument do not guarantee that reliability will be satisfactory in another sample or with a different population. Researchers need to perform reliability testing on each instrument used in a study to ensure that it is reliable for that study sample (Bialocerkowski et al., 2010; Kazdin, 2022). The three most common types of reliability testing reported in healthcare studies are stability reliability, equivalence reliability, and internal consistency or homogeneity. Table 4.1 summarizes these types of reliability testing (Grove & Gray, 2023).

Stability Reliability

Stability reliability is concerned with the consistency of repeated measures of the same variable or attribute with the same scale or measurement method over time. Stability is commonly referred to as **test-retest reliability** because of the repeated measurement of a variable over time. Reliability testing examines the amount of random error in a measurement technique, and a quality measurement method should have acceptable reliability for a study sample (Gray & Grove, 2021). For example, if a scale is being used to measure stress in a study, the study participants given this scale should mark the items similarly if they are given the same stress scale at a later time (e.g., 1–2 days later). If the participants complete the scale in a similar way

TABLE 4.1	DETERMINING THE RELIABILITY AND READABILITY OF MEASUREMENT METHODS
Quality Indicator	**Description**

Reliability	**Stability reliability:** Focused on the reproducibility of scores with repeated measures of the same concept or attribute with an instrument or scale over time. Stability is usually examined with test-retest reliability.
	Equivalence reliability: Includes interrater reliability and alternate forms reliability.
	    Interrater or interobserver reliability: Comparison of raters in determining their equivalence in rating variables or events in a study. Interobserver reliability is focused on the agreement between two or more observers in a study.
	    Alternate forms reliability: Correlation between different forms of the same instrument to determine their equivalence in measuring a concept.
	Internal consistency: Degree of homogeneity or consistency of items within a multi-item scale. Each item on a scale is correlated with all other items to determine the consistency of an instrument in measuring a concept. Cronbach's alpha coefficient is the frequently conducted statistic reported for internal consistency of a multi-item scale.

Precision	**Precision of physiologic measure:** Degree of consistency or reproducibility of the measurements made with physiologic instruments or equipment on the same variables under specified conditions. The smaller the change sensed in the instrument, the greater the precision in the measurement equipment.
Readability	**Readability level:** Conducted to determine the participants' ability to read and comprehend the items on an instrument. Researchers should report the level of education needed to read the instrument. Readability level must be appropriate to promote reliability and validity of an instrument.

from one time to the next, this indicates adequate test-retest reliability, which is designated by an intraclass correlation coefficient (ICC). The ICC values vary based on the test-retest reliability of the scale, the changes in the participants over time, and the changes in the administration of the scale. However, the higher the correlation coefficient obtained in a study, the stronger the test-retest reliability for the measurement method (Kim et al., 2022). Koo and Li (2016, p. 161) recommend evaluating the ICC "level of reliability using the following general guideline: Values less than 0.50 are indicative of poor reliability, values between 0.50 and 0.75 indicate moderate reliability, values between 0.75 and 0.90 indicate good reliability, and values greater than 0.90 indicate excellent reliability."

Equivalence Reliability

Equivalence reliability includes interrater reliability and alternate forms reliability (see Table 4.1). **Interrater reliability** is the comparison of two raters or judges to determine their equivalence in rating variables or events in a study. **Interobserver reliability** is focused on the agreement between two or more observers in a study (Bandalos, 2018). There is no absolute value less than which interrater reliability is unacceptable because the behaviors or situations being judged or observed vary in complexity and abstractness (Bialocerkowski et al., 2010; Gray & Grove, 2021). However, any Pearson r value less than 0.70 should generate concern about the reliability of the data, data gatherer, or both. The interrater reliability value should be reported in the research report and ideally should be 0.80 (80%) to 0.90 (90%) or higher, which means the raters are approximately equivalent during the study (Gray & Grove, 2021; Kazdin, 2022).

The kappa statistic or (kappa coefficient) is the most commonly used statistic to determine interobserver agreement in a study (Viera & Garrett, 2005). A kappa of 1 indicates perfect observer agreement that is never achieved because of measurement error, and a kappa of 0 indicates agreement equivalent to chance. Viera and Garrett (2005) recommended the following values be used when interpreting kappa: 0.01 to 0.20, slight agreement; 0.21 to 0.40, fair agreement; 0.41 to 0.60, moderate agreement; 0.61 to 0.80, substantial agreement; and 0.81 to 0.99, almost perfect agreement.

Comparison of two versions of a test or scale is referred to as **alternate-forms reliability** or **parallel-forms reliability** (see Table 4.1; Waltz et al., 2017). Alternative forms of tests are developed for normative knowledge testing such as the Scholastic Aptitude Test (SAT), which is used as a college entrance requirement. There are many forms of this test, with a variety of items included on each. These alternate forms of the SAT were developed to measure students' knowledge consistently and protect the integrity of the test. Multiple forms of the Graduate Record Exam (GRE) have been developed and used for entrance to graduate school. For most scales, the development of two comparable versions of a scale is difficult and not often done (Bannigan & Watson, 2009; Waltz et al., 2017).

Internal Consistency

Internal consistency, also known as homogeneity reliability testing, is used primarily with multi-item scales, where each item on a scale is correlated with all other items on the scale to determine consistency of measurement (see Table 4.1). The principle is that each item should be consistently measuring a concept, such as depression, and so should be correlated with the other items on the scale. The Cronbach's alpha coefficient is the most commonly used measure of internal reliability for scales with multiple items. Cronbach's alpha coefficients range from 0.00 to 1.00, where 1.00 indicates perfect reliability and a coefficient of 0.00 indicates no reliability or chance (Bandalos, 2018; Waltz et al., 2017).

A Cronbach's alpha coefficient ≥ 0.80 indicates a strong reliability for a scale that has been used in a variety of studies. The stronger correlation coefficients, which are closer to 1.00, indicate less random error and a more reliable scale. For example, the CES-D has strong internal consistency reliability, with Cronbach's alphas ranging from 0.84 to 0.90 in field studies (Armenta et al., 2014; Cosco et al., 2017; Jiang et al., 2019). For relatively new scales, a reliability of 0.70 is considered acceptable because the scale is being refined and used with a variety of samples. Reliability coefficients of <0.60 indicate limited instrument reliability or consistency in the measurement of a variable or concept with higher potential for error (Waltz et al., 2017).

Cronbach's alpha coefficient can be used to calculate the error for a scale with a specific population. The alpha coefficient is squared and subtracted from 1.00 to determine the potential for error in the scores from a scale. The formula and example are presented as follows:

1.00 − (Cronbach's alpha)^2 = measurement error   **100% × error = Percentage of error**

1.00 − (0.80)^2 = 1.00 − 0.64 = 0.36   **100% × 0.36 = 36%**

Many scales have subscales that comprise the concept measured, and the reliability of the subscales should also be included in a research report. The subscales of instruments usually have lower reliability coefficients (0.60–0.70) than the total scale. The number of items in the total scale provides a more stable measurement of a concept in a study than the subscales, with fewer items (Gray & Grove, 2021; Waltz et al., 2017). If the data are dichotomous (yes or no responses) the Kuder-Richardson formula 20 (K-R 20) is used to estimate internal consistency (Waltz et al., 2017). A research report should include the results from stability, equivalence, and homogeneity reliability testing done on a measurement method from previous research and for the present study (Gray & Grove, 2021; Waltz et al., 2017).

Precision

Precision is the degree of consistency or reproducibility of measurements made with physiologic equipment or devices. There should be close agreement in the replicated physiologic measures of the same variable or element under specified conditions (Ryan-Wenger, 2017; Stone & Frazier, 2017). The precision of most physiologic equipment is determined by the manufacturer and is a part of the quality-control testing done by the agency using the device. To promote precision in physiologic measures or devices, researchers develop protocols to ensure consistent collection of physiologic data, transfer of specimens, and analysis of physiologic data or specimens. The physiologic equipment used to collect and analyze physiologic data should be recalibrated and maintained as indicated by the manufacturer.

Test-retest reliability is appropriate for physiologic variables that have minimal fluctuations, such as lipid levels, bone mineral density, or weight of adults (Ryan-Wenger, 2017). Test-retest reliability can be inappropriate if the variables' values frequently fluctuate with various activities, such as with pulse, respirations, and blood pressure (BP). However, test-retest is a good measure of precision if the measurements are taken in rapid succession. For example, the national BP guidelines encourage taking three BP readings 1 to 2 minutes apart and then averaging them to obtain the most precise and accurate measure of BP (Todkar et al., 2021). Higher levels of precision (0.90–0.99) are important for physiologic measures that are used to monitor critical physiologic functions, such as arterial pressure and oxygen saturation (Stone & Frazier, 2017).

Readability

Readability level is an essential element of the reliability and validity of an instrument. Assessing the grade level for reading an instrument is simple and takes seconds with the use of a readability formula, of which there are more than 30. These formulas count language elements in the document and use this information to estimate the degree of difficulty a reader may have in comprehending the text. The formulas provide an overview of the readability of a document based on estimated grade level, ease of reading, and grammar in the document. Readability formulas are now a standard part of word-processing software. When researchers determine the readability level of their measurement methods are appropriate for a study population, this strengthens the reliability and validity of the instruments in the study. Often a scale needs to be at the sixth-grade level for certain adults to be able to comprehend and complete it (Waltz et al., 2017). Study participants must be able to read and understand the items on a scale in order to complete the items consistently and accurately.

The concepts of reliability and validity (see Exercise 5) should be evaluated together to determine the quality of a measurement method. An instrument that has low reliability cannot be valid because it is inconsistent in its measurement of the study variable or concept. However, an instrument can be reliable but not necessarily valid. For example, a Likert scale that was developed to measure pain has a Cronbach's alpha of 0.84, but it is actually more focused on measuring stress and anxiety than pain, resulting in low validity for the scale. The measurement of study variables with reliable and valid measurement methods is essential for obtaining quality study results and findings. The questions in this exercise will help you critically appraise the reliability of scales and the precision of physiologic measures in published studies (Grove & Gray, 2023; Waltz et al., 2017). Some of the sources in this exercise are older because frequently used quality instruments are developed over years.

RESEARCH ARTICLE

Source

Williams, S. G., Turner-Henson, A., Langhinrichsen-Rohling, J., & Azuero, A. (2017). Depressive symptoms in 9th graders: Stress and physiological contributors. *Applied Nursing Research*, 34(1), 24–28. https://doi.org/10.1016/j.apnr.2017.01.001

Introduction

Williams et al. (2017) conducted a predictive correlational study to determine whether stressful life events, perceived stress, and bullying were predictive of depressive symptoms in ninth graders. In addition, cortisol values and diurnal rhythm were examined in these adolescents.

"A non-probability, convenience sampling method was used; the resulting sample consisted of 143 9th graders recruited from two public suburban southeastern U.S. high schools" (Williams et al., 2017, p. 25). Nurses may encounter adolescents with depressive symptoms in many settings, but school is an optimal site to screen for these symptoms. The measurement methods for depressive symptoms, bullying, and cortisol values are presented in the following study excerpt.

Relevant Study Results

"Depressive symptoms were measured with the Center for Epidemiologic Studies Depression Survey (CESD-10). . . . The CESD-10 was chosen due to the applicability for adolescent populations and the length of the measure (10 questions). In a study of $n = 156$ adolescents, reliability of CESD-10 was found to be $\alpha = 0.85$ (Bradley et al., 2010). Reliability for the current study was $\alpha = 0.86$. . . .

Bullying was measured using the Personal Experiences Checklist (PECK), a 32-item Likert scale instrument that was previously used in adolescents ages 8 to 15 years (Hunt et al., 2012). This self-report instrument is scored from 0 to 4: 0 (never), 1 (rarely), 2 (sometimes), 3 (most days), and 4 (every day). Bullying behaviors included the following number of items, internal consistency, and test-retest coefficients: verbal/relational bullying (11 items, $\alpha = 0.90$, $r = 0.75$); physical bullying (9 items, $\alpha = 0.91$, $r = 0.61$); cyberbullying (8 items, $\alpha = 0.90$, $r = 0.86$); and cultural bullying (4 items, $\alpha = 0.78$, $r = 0.77$). High scores indicate more bullying. Reliability for the overall scale was $\alpha = 0.94$ in the current study. . . .

Cortisol diurnal rhythm (cortisol change from morning to afternoon) was assessed by collecting salivary specimens during an elective course in the morning school hours (8 am– 11 am) and again in the afternoon school hours (12 pm–3 pm). When collecting saliva, 9th graders were asked to refrain from eating or drinking anything except water for approximately 1 h before sample collection. Upon arrival to the testing room, the participants were instructed to rinse their mouth thoroughly with water 5 to 10 min before the sample was collected to minimize potential pH variability and bacterial contamination. Specimens were collected using a passive drool approach to collect saliva in a cryo vial using a saliva collection aid for a period of 3 min while under the principal investigator's supervision" (Williams et al., 2017, p. 25).

STUDY QUESTIONS

1. What types of reliability testing are commonly presented in nursing research reports to demonstrate the consistency or the stability of instruments in measuring study variables? Why is reliability testing important? Document your answer.

2. What statistical techniques are commonly used to determine internal consistency or homogeneity reliability for scales with ordinal-, interval-, or ratio-level data and for scales with nominal-level data? Provide a rationale for your answer.

3. If the Cronbach's alpha coefficient was 0.52 for a multi-item pain perception scale to measure pain in adolescents, is this value a study strength or weakness? Provide a rationale for your answer. Include the percentage of random error for this scale and round your answer to the nearest whole percent.

4. What type of reliability testing is appropriate to conduct on the CESD-10 scale to determine homogeneity? Provide a rationale for your answer.

5. What reliability value was reported for the CESD-10 scale in this study and was this reliability value satisfactory? Provide a rationale for your answer.

6. Calculate the percentage of random error for the CESD-10 scale in the Williams et al. (2017) study. Show your calculations and round to the nearest whole percent.

7. What type of scale is the PECK? Was this scale appropriate to gather data on bullying from adolescents? Provide a rationale for your answer.

8. What is stability reliability and what was the stability reliability value reported for the verbal/relational bullying subscale of the PECK reported in the Williams et al. (2017) study? Was this reliability value a strength or weakness? Provide a rationale for your answer.

9. Why is the readability level or value of a measurement method important to include in a research report? Discuss the relevance of Williams et al. (2017), including a readability level for the PECK scale used in their study.

10. "When collecting saliva, 9th graders were asked to refrain from eating or drinking anything except water for approximately 1 h before sample collection" (Williams et al., 2017, p. 25). Discuss the importance of this statement in this study.

Answers to Study Questions

1. The three most common types of reliability testing reported in nursing studies are (1) stability reliability, (2) equivalence reliability, and (3) internal consistency or homogeneity (see Table 4.1; Gray & Grove, 2021). Reliability testing determines the consistency of an instrument in measuring a variable and the potential for measurement or random error. An instrument with strong reliability and limited potential for error provides consistent data about a concept or variable. If an instrument has limited reliability in a study, reviewers need to question the results and findings related to the instrument (Bandalos, 2018; Waltz et al., 2017).

2. Cronbach's alpha coefficient is calculated to determine the homogeneity or internal consistency of multi-item scales with ordinal, interval, or ratio levels of data in a study. A Cronbach's alpha value should be determined for every multi-item scale and its subscales used in a study, because the scales' reliability should be examined for a particular study sample (Bandalos, 2018; Kazdin, 2022). The Kuder-Richardson formula 20 (K-R 20) is calculated to determine the internal consistency of instruments with data measured at the nominal level. Researchers also need to discuss the reliability of the scales used in their study based on previous research (Gray & Grove, 2021; Waltz et al., 2017).

3. If Cronbach's alpha coefficient is 0.52, then the scale has a 0.52 internal consistency reliability and a 0.7296 (72.96% or 73%) measurement error. The measurement error calculation follows: $1.00 - (0.52)^2 = 1.00 - 0.2704 = 0.7296$. The measurement error rate is determined by multiplying the measurement error by 100%; thus $100\% \times 0.7296 = 72.96\%$ rounded to 73% error. The measurement error rate was to be rounded to the nearest whole percent. This scale has a high potential for measurement error, which means that researchers should question the results obtained from the adolescents in this study using this pain perception scale. In addition, the reliability of this scale should be reported as a limitation in the study (Bandalos, 2018; Gray & Grove, 2021). Further research is needed to identify a reliable scale to measure pain perception in adolescents (Waltz et al., 2017).

4. The CESD-10 is a 10-item Likert scale developed to measure depression in adolescents. Multi-item scales are tested for homogeneity or internal consistency using Cronbach's alpha coefficient (see Table 4.1; Bialocerkowski et al., 2010; Waltz et al., 2017). Multi-item scales might be considered ordinal- or interval-level measurements based on the construction of the scale. Thus the Cronbach's alpha coefficient is the appropriate statistic to conduct to determine the internal consistency of the CESD-10 scale (Bandalos, 2018; Gray & Grove, 2021).

5. The CESD-10 had a reliability $\alpha = 0.86$ for the Williams et al. (2017) study. A reliability value greater than 0.80 is strong and indicates the scale had evidence of adequate reliability in this study (Armenta et al., 2014; Bialocerkowski et al., 2010; Waltz et al., 2017).

6. The percentage of random error for the CESD-10 scale in the Williams et al. (2017) study was 26%. The calculations for measurement error are: $1.00 - (0.86)^2 = 1.00 - 0.7396 = 0.2604$. The measurement error rate is calculated by $100\% \times 0.2604 = 26.04\%$, which is rounded to the closest whole percent of 26%.

7. Yes, the PECK is a Likert scale that is appropriate to gather data on bullying from adolescents. Williams et al. (2017, p. 25) reported, "Bullying was measured using the PECK, a 32-item Likert scale instrument that was previously used in adolescents ages 8 to 15 years (Hunt et al., 2012)." The reliability for the PECK in this study was $\alpha = 0.94$. Thus the PECK has a history of being used with adolescents, and the internal consistency reliability was very strong in this study (Gray & Grove, 2021; Kazdin, 2022; Waltz et al., 2017).

8. Stability reliability is concerned with the consistency of repeated measures of the same variable or concept with the same scale or measurement method over time. Stability is commonly referred to as test-retest reliability because of the repeated measurements of a variable over time (see Table 4.1). The test-retest coefficient for verbal/relational bullying was $r = 0.75$. This test-retest reliability value is a strength and indicates the repeated measurement of bullying over time with PECK results in a stable value. The strong test-retest value reduces the potential for measurement error using the PECK in this study (Grove & Gray, 2023; Waltz et al., 2017).

9. Researchers reporting appropriate reading levels or readability scores for their measurement methods in a study enhance the reliability and validity of the instruments. Study participants must be able to read and understand the items on an instrument to complete it consistently and accurately (Bandalos, 2018; Gray & Grove, 2021). The measurement section for the PECK scale would have been strengthened by Williams et al. (2017) reporting the readability level of the PECK scale to ensure the reading level was less than the ninth-grade level. Study participants have varying levels of reading capability, so documenting a sixth- to seventh-grade level of reading would have strengthened the reliability and validity of the PECK used in this study (Gray & Grove, 2021; Waltz et al., 2017).

10. This statement indicates how precision was achieved in the collection of the saliva specimens. Precision is the degree of consistency or reproducibility of measurements obtained with physiologic instruments. Williams et al. (2017) documented the protocol that was followed to ensure consistent collection of salivary specimens that were uncontaminated by food and drinks in this study (Ryan-Wenger, 2017; Waltz et al., 2017).

Questions for Additional Study

Name: _____ Class: _____

Date: _____

Follow your instructor's directions to submit your answers to the following questions for additional study. Your instructor may ask you to write your answers below and submit them as a hard copy for evaluation. Alternatively, your instructor may ask you to submit your answers online.

1. Based on the information provided from the Williams et al. (2017) study, which of the two scales have the higher Cronbach's alpha coefficient for this study? Which of these two scales has the greater random error? Provide rationales for your answers.

2. What types of reliability testing were provided for the cyberbullying subscale of the PECK? Were the reliability values a study strength or weakness? Provide a rationale for your answer.

3. Calculate the percentage of random error for the cyberbullying subscale of the PECK. Show your calculations and round your answer to the nearest whole percent.

4. Would you consider the CESD-10 a reliable measure of depression in this population of ninth-grade adolescents? Provide a rationale for your answer and document with relevant sources.

5. What are the Cronbach's alphas for the four subscales for the PECK used to measure bullying in the Williams et al. (2017) study? Did these subscales have adequate reliability in this study? Provide a rationale for your answer.

6. Which subscale of the PECK had the lowest Cronbach's alpha? What is the random error for this subscale? Show your calculations and round to the nearest whole percent.

7. Williams et al. (2017, p. 25) reported the PECK "was previously used in adolescents ages 8 to 15." Based on readability, do you think the PECK is acceptable for the population in this study? Provide a rationale for your answer.

8. Could you assume that the PECK would be a reliable scale to measure bullying in college students? Provide a rationale for your answer.

9. Did Williams et al. (2017) provide a clear discussion of the reliability of the CESD-10 and PECK scales in their study? Provide a rationale for your answer.

10. Was the collection of saliva for cortisol values precise? Provide a rationale for your answer.

Understanding Validity of Measurement Methods

STATISTICAL TECHNIQUE IN REVIEW

Types of Validity Examined for Measurement Methods

A measurement method has **validity** if it accurately reflects the concept it was developed to measure. In examining validity, we focus on the appropriateness, meaningfulness, and usefulness of the measurement method in capturing the aspects of a selected concept. Validity, like reliability, is not an all-or-nothing phenomenon; it is measured on a continuum. No instrument is completely valid, so researchers determine the degree of validity of an instrument rather than whether validity exists or not (DeVon et al., 2007; Waltz et al., 2017).

Many types of validity exist, but this text focuses on the types most commonly reported in nursing studies, which include content validity, construct validity, and criterion-related validity (Bannigan & Watson, 2009; Grove & Gray, 2023). Table 5.1 provides a brief overview of content, construct, and criterion-related validity that are discussed in more depth in the following pages.

Content Validity

Content validity examines the extent to which a measurement method includes all the major elements relevant to the concept being measured. The evidence for content validity of an instrument or scale includes the following: (1) how well the items of the scale reflect the description of the concept in the literature, which is usually called **face validity**; (2) the content experts' evaluation of the relevance of items on the scale that might be reported as an index; and (3) the study participants' responses to scale items (Bandalos, 2018; Gray & Grove, 2021; Kazdin, 2022; Waltz et al., 2017).

Construct Validity

Construct validity focuses on determining whether the instrument measures the theoretical construct that it purports to measure, which involves examining the fit between the conceptual and operational definitions of a variable (see Chapter 8 in Grove & Gray, 2023). Construct validity is developed using several methods such as (1) convergent validity, (2) divergent validity, (3) validity from factor analysis, (4) validity from contrasting groups, and (5) successive verification validity (see Table 5.1; Gray & Grove, 2021; Waltz et al., 2017). **Convergent validity** is examined by comparing two scales or instruments that measure the same concept or construct, such as comparing a new instrument with an existing instrument. The two instruments are administered to a sample at the same time, and the results are evaluated with correlational analyses. If the measures or scales have moderate positive correlational values (0.40–0.50) or strong (0.60 or greater) correlational values, the validity of each instrument is

TABLE 5.1	EXAMINING THE VALIDITY OF MEASUREMENT METHODS
Quality Indicator	**Description**
Validity	**Content validity:** Examines the extent to which a measurement method includes all the major elements relevant to the construct being measured.
	Face validity: Type of content validity that verifies an instrument looks like it is valid or gives the appearance of measuring the construct for which it was developed.
	Construct validity: Focuses on determining whether an instrument measures the theoretical construct that it purports to measure, which involves examining the fit between the conceptual and operational definitions of a variable.
	Convergent validity: Type of construct validity where two scales measuring the same concept are administered to a group at the same time and the study participants' scores on the scales should be positively correlated. For example, individuals completing two scales to measure depression should have positively correlated scores.
	Divergent validity: Type of construct validity where two scales that measure opposite concepts, such as hope and hopelessness, administered to participants at the same time should result in negatively correlated scores on the scales.
	Validity from factor analysis: Type of construct validity that determines whether an instrument includes the elements of the concept being measured by conducting exploratory and/or confirmatory factor analysis. Factor analysis is conducted to determine whether the items in an instrument are related and cluster together to form factors that reflect the elements or subconcepts of the concept being measured.
	Validity from contrasting (known) groups: Type of construct validity where an instrument or scale is given to two groups that are expected to have opposite or contrasting scores, where one group scores high on the scale and the other scores low.
	Successive verification validity: Validity is achieved when an instrument is used in studies with a variety of study participants in various settings.
	Criterion-related validity: Validity that is strengthened when a study participant's score on an instrument can be used to infer his or her performance on another variable or criterion.
	Predictive validity: The extent to which an individual's score on a scale or instrument can be used to predict future performance or behavior on a criterion.
	Concurrent validity: Focuses on the extent to which an individual's score on an instrument or scale can be used to estimate his or her present or concurrent performance on another variable or criterion.
Accuracy	**Accuracy of physiologic measures:** Addresses the extent to which the physiologic instrument or equipment measures what it is supposed to measure in a study; comparable to validity for multi-item scales.

strengthened (see Chapter 16 in Gray & Grove, 2021; Waltz et al., 2017). For example, the Center for Epidemiological Studies Depression Scale (CES-D) has shown positive correlations ranging from 0.40 to 0.80 with the Hamilton Rating Scale for Depression (Sharp & Lipsky, 2002). Jiang et al. (2019) correlated the responses of 2068 university student responses on a 14-item CES-D with those on the Beck Depression Inventory-II (BDI-II) and found a convergent validity value of 0.744. Thus the CES-D has documented convergent validity with the Hamilton Rating Scale for Depression and the BDI-II.

Divergent validity is examined when participants complete two scales, at the same time, that measure opposite concepts. For example, the scores from two different scales, one measuring hope and the other measuring hopelessness, could be correlated to identify divergent validity. If the scores from the two measurement strategies have a moderate to strong negative correlation (such as −0.40 to −0.80), the divergent validity of both scales is strengthened (Waltz et al., 2017). Convergent validity of scales is examined more frequently than divergent validity (Bandalos, 2018; Gray & Grove, 2021).

Validity from factor analysis is conducted to determine whether an instrument includes the elements of the concept being measured. To employ factor analysis, the instrument must be administered to a large, representative sample of participants at one time. Usually, the data are initially analyzed with **exploratory factor analysis (EFA)** to examine relationships among the various items of the instrument (Bandalos, 2018; Waltz et al., 2017). Scale items that are closely related are clustered into a factor. Determining and naming the factors identified through EFA require detailed work on the part of the researcher in interpreting the EFA results and in comparing them to the relevant literature. Researchers can validate the number of factors in the instrument by conducting **confirmatory factor analysis (CFA)**. The factors confirmed through CFA are the subconcepts or subscales of a scale that can be examined in a study (Gray & Grove, 2021; Kim et al., 2022). Cosco et al. (2017) conducted a CFA of the 20-item CES-D scale and found it to include four subconcepts: (1) depressed affect, (2) somatic/vegetative factors, (3) positive affect, and (4) interpersonal. This four-factor structure is consistent with the original work conducted by Radloff (1977). If the factor analysis results identify the essential elements of the concept to be measured by an instrument, then the validity of the instrument is strengthened (Gray & Grove, 2021; Waltz et al., 2017).

Validity from contrasting groups is tested by identifying groups that are expected or known to have contrasting scores on an instrument and then asking the groups to complete the instrument (see Table 5.1). If the two groups have contrasting scores on the instrument, then the validity of the instrument is strengthened. For example, researchers could compare the scores on the CES-D scale (Radloff, 1977) for a group of patients diagnosed with depression and a group of individuals who do not have a depression diagnosis. If the groups have contrasting scores, then the depression scale is thought to measure the concept of depression, and the validity of the scale is strengthened (Gray & Grove, 2021; Kim et al., 2022). **Successive verification validity** is achieved when an instrument is used in studies with a variety of study participants in various settings (Grove & Gray, 2023). The validity of instruments is determined over time, with some of the strongest instruments developed over 20 to 30 years ago, resulting in older sources for scales used in studies.

Criterion-Related Validity

Criterion-related validity is examined by using a study participant's score on an instrument or scale to infer her or his performance on a criterion. Criterion validity is strengthened when the participants' scores on a scale are successful in determining their behaviors on a variable or criterion. Criterion-related validity includes validity from the prediction of future events and prediction of concurrent events (see Table 5.1). **Validity from the prediction of future events** is achieved when the scores on an instrument can be used to predict future behaviors, attitudes, and events (Bandalos, 2018; Waltz et al., 2017). For example, fall risk assessment scales have been developed to predict the fall potential of elderly patients. The positive relationship of the scale score with the incidence of falls in the elderly strengthens the validity of this scale to determine the risk for falling. Thus elderly with high fall risk assessment scores require additional interventions to prevent their falling.

Validity from prediction of concurrent events can be evaluated by examining the ability to predict the concurrent value of one instrument based on the value obtained on an instrument to measure another concept. For example, researchers might use the results from a self-esteem scale to predict the results on a coping scale. Thus, if study participants with high self-esteem scores had high coping scores, this would add to the validity of the self-esteem scale (Gray & Grove, 2021; Waltz et al., 2017).

In summary, there are a variety of ways to add to the validity of an instrument, and an instrument's validity needs to be discussed in the measurement section of a study. The validity of an instrument should be provided from instrument development (i.e., psychometric) research and from studies using it. In addition, a study might focus on examining an instrument's validity if limited information is available. Stating that a scale is *valid* is insufficient information for the reader to assess the validity of the scale (Grove & Gray, 2023). An instrument must be both valid and reliable to provide a quality measurement of a concept in a study (Bandalos, 2018; Bannigan & Watson, 2009; Gray & Grove, 2021; Waltz et al., 2017).

Accuracy of Physiologic Measures

The accuracy of physiologic and biochemical measures is similar to the validity of scales used in research. **Accuracy** involves determining the closeness of the agreement between the measured value and the true value of the physiologic variable being measured. New measurement devices are compared with existing standardized methods (i.e., gold standard) of measuring a biophysical property or concept (Gray & Grove, 2021; Ryan-Wenger, 2017). For example, measures of oxygen saturation with a pulse oximeter were correlated with arterial blood gas measures of oxygen saturation to determine the accuracy of the pulse oximeter. There should be a strong, positive correlation (≥ 0.95) between pulse oximeter and blood gas measures of oxygen saturation to support the accuracy of the pulse oximeter. Accuracy of physiologic measures depends on the quality of the measurement equipment or device, detail of the data collection plan, and expertise of the data collector (Ryan-Wenger, 2017). Researchers need to report the accuracy of the physiologic and biochemical measures used in their studies (Stone & Frazier, 2017).

RESEARCH ARTICLE

Source

Williams, S. G., Turner-Henson, A., Langhinrichsen-Rohling, J., & Azuero, A. (2017). Depressive symptoms in 9th graders: Stress and physiological contributors. *Applied Nursing Research*, *34*(1), 24–28. https://doi.org/10.1016/j.apnr.2017.01.001

Introduction

Williams and colleagues (2017) conducted a predictive correlational study to determine whether stressful life events, perceived stress, and bullying were predictive of depressive symptoms in 9th graders. In addition, cortisol values and cortisol diurnal rhythm were examined in these adolescents. "A non-probability, convenience sampling method was used; the resulting sample consisted of 143 9th graders recruited from two public suburban southeastern U.S. high schools" (Williams et al., 2017, p. 25). Nurses may encounter adolescents with depressive symptoms in many settings, but school is an optimal site to screen for these symptoms.

The Williams et al's (2017) article was the focus of Exercise 4 and included content relevant to the reliability of the measurement methods in this study. This exercise includes relevant content focused on the validity of the measurement methods for depressive symptoms, stressful life events, and cortisol values that are presented in the following study excerpt.

Relevant Study Results

"Depressive symptoms were measured with The Center for Epidemiologic Studies Depression Survey (CESD-10) that has been used to measure four factors related to depressive symptoms including: positive/negative affect, somatic symptoms, retarded activity, and interpersonal issues. CESD-10 scores range from 0 to 30 with scoring from 0 to 3: 0 (rarely), 1 (some of the time), 2 (occasionally or moderate amount), 3 (all the time) for each item. A score of 10 or greater indicates need for referral (clinically meaningful). The CESD-10 was chosen due to the applicability for adolescent populations and the length of the measure (10 questions). . . . Reliability for the current study was $\alpha = 0.86$.

Stressful life events (SLE) and the impact of these events or Life Change Units (LCU) were measured with The Coddington (1972) Life Events Scale for Adolescents (CLES-A). The CLES-A, designed for adolescents aged 13–19 years, had validity and reliability determined with test-retest reliability ($\alpha = 0.84$) . . . and interclass correlation ($r = 0.63$). . . . Reliability for the current study was $\alpha = 0.76$.

Cortisol diurnal rhythm (cortisol change from morning to afternoon) was assessed by collecting salivary specimens during an elective course in the morning school hours (8 am–11 am) and again in the afternoon school hours (12 pm–3 pm). When collecting saliva, 9th graders were asked to refrain from eating or drinking anything except water for approximately 1 h before sample collection. Upon arrival to the testing room, the participants were instructed to rinse their mouth thoroughly with water 5–10 min before the sample was collected to minimize potential pH variability and bacterial contamination. Specimens were collected using a passive drool approach to collect saliva in a cryo vial using a saliva collection aid for a period of 3 min while under the principal investigator's supervision. Specimens were kept on ice during data collection and then frozen at $-20\,°C$ until shipped to Salimetrics, LLC on dry ice. Duplicate analysis of saliva was completed with an ELISA/EIA assay, calibration range of 0.012–3.00 $\mu g/dL$ and a sensitivity of $<0.003\ \mu g/dL$ to determine the cortisol levels. The expected range of salivary cortisol for adolescents aged 12–18 years is 0.021–0.883 $\mu g/dL$ for morning and 0.0–0.259 $\mu g/dL$ for afternoon, and the correlation between saliva and serum cortisol is $r(47) = 0.91$, $p<0.0001$ (Salimetrics LLC, 2013)" (Williams et al., 2017, p. 25).

STUDY QUESTIONS

1. Define validity for measurement methods. What are the three major categories of measurement validity discussed in this exercise?

2. What type of validity is examined when a scale is initially developed? Provide a rationale for your answer.

3. Identify the types of validity that contribute to the construct validity of an instrument or scale. Which of these types of validity involves comparing the values from two scales? Provide a rationale for your answer.

4. A measurement method that predicts the length of stay for patients hospitalized for heart failure (HF) has which type of validity? Provide a rationale for your answer.

5. Which scale would probably have stronger validity for the measurement of the concept of depression in the Williams et al. (2017) study: (1) the Hamilton Depression Scale developed over 30 years ago for adults; or (2) the CESD scale developed by Radloff in 1977, refined for use with different age groups, and used frequently in studies? Provide a rationale for your answer.

6. What scale was used to measure stressful life events in the Williams et al. (2017) study? What type of validity information was provided for this scale?

7. Was the validity information provided for the CLES-A adequate in this research report? Provide a rationale for your answer.

8. Give an example of how validity from contrasting groups might have been developed for the CLES-A.

9. The CLES-A had a reliability of $\alpha = 0.76$ for this study. Is there a link between reliability and validity for a scale used in a study? Provide a rationale for your answer.

10. Williams et al. (2017, p. 27) reported, "This study's results identify that 9th graders' perception of stress, bullying, and sexual orientation explained 59% of the variance of depressive symptoms." Discuss how the findings from this study might be used in clinical practice. Locate the Williams et al.'s (2017) article in your online library system and compare your ideas with what is included in the study.

Answers to Study Questions

1. The validity of a measurement method is determined by how accurately it measures the abstract concept it was developed to measure. The three categories of measurement validity presented in this text are content validity, construct validity, and criterion-related validity (see Table 5.1; Grove & Gray, 2023; Waltz et al., 2017).

2. Content validity is examined during the initial development of a scale. Researchers identify a concept like resilience that they want to measure for individuals with chronic illnesses. A review of the literature is conducted to define and identify possible subconcepts of this concept. Using this content, researchers develop possible items for a scale to measure resilience. The scale items are reviewed by experts for completeness, conciseness, clarity, and readability and refined as needed. Face validity is a type of content validity (Bandalos, 2018; Gray & Grove, 2021; Waltz et al., 2017).

3. Construct validity includes convergent validity, divergent validity, validity from factor analysis, validity from contrasting groups, and successive verification validity (Gray & Grove, 2021). Convergent validity involves determining the relationship between two instruments that measure the same concept, such as two scales to measure depression. Divergent validity involves comparing the scores from two scales that measure opposite concepts, such as scales measuring resilience and hopelessness. The data for these two types of validity need to be collected from the same sample at approximately the same time (Waltz et al., 2017).

4. Criterion-related validity is examined when an instrument predicts the future event length of stay for hospitalized patients with HF. The predictive criterion validity of the scale is strengthened if it can be used to successfully predict a future event such as length of stay of patients with HF (Bandalos, 2018; Waltz et al., 2017). Identifying patients at risk for prolonged hospital stay will direct nurses in how to best manage their care.

5. The CESD scale probably has stronger validity than the Hamilton Depression Scale because it was developed and refined over 45 years to measure depression (Radloff, 1977). In addition, the CESD scale has been refined for use with different age groups, and the CESD-10 is considered "applicable for adolescent populations" (Williams et al., 2017, p. 25). A depression scale for adults would probably not be as valid as the CESD-10 in measuring depression in adolescents (Waltz et al., 2017). The CESD-10 also has stronger successive verification validity, with its use in a variety of studies with different populations in various settings (Gray & Grove, 2021).

6. The CLES-A was used to measure stressful life events in this study. Content validity was addressed by indicating that the CLES-A measured "Stressful life events (SLE) and the impact of these events or Life Change Units (LCU)" (Williams et al., 2017, p. 25). The CLES-A was designed for adolescents 13 to 19 years of age, which adds to the scale's validity. In addition, the CLES-A has successive verification validity because it was used in previous studies.

7. No, the validity information provided for the CLES-A was not adequate in this study. Only limited, vague information on content and successive verification validity was provided. The researchers indicated the scale had validity, but no specific information was provided, so the validity of the scale cannot be evaluated (Grove & Gray, 2023; Waltz et al., 2017).

8. Answers will vary. You need to identify two groups that you think would have different or contrasting values on the CLES-A (Bandalos, 2018; Waltz et al., 2017). For example, you might contrast the scores of the CLES-A for 9th graders in private school versus those in public school. Students who are home-schooled might be contrasted with those in formal school settings using the CLES-A. These groups might be expected to have different stressful life events.

9. Yes, there is a link between reliability and validity for a scale in a study. A scale must be reliable or consistently measuring a concept in a study if it is to be valid. The CLES-A had an acceptable (0.76) but not strong (≥ 0.80) reliability in this study (see Exercise 4; Grove & Gray, 2023).

10. Williams et al. (2017, p. 27) made the following recommendations for clinical practice: "It is important for nurses to recognize that 9th graders may be vulnerable and to seek them out for inquiry. Nurses should also advocate for screening of depressive symptoms in settings where 9th graders are readily accessible to try and identify and to refer for post screening follow-up and treatment if necessary." The 9th grade students also need to be monitored for bullying and supported in the school setting.

Follow your instructor's directions to submit your answers to the following questions for additional study. Your instructor may ask you to write your answers below and submit them as a hard copy for evaluation. Alternatively, your instructor may ask you to submit your answers online.

1. Discuss the importance of accuracy for a physiologic measure used in a study.

2. Does the CESD-10 scale have evidence of successive verification validity in the Williams et al. (2017) study? Provide a rationale for your answer.

3. Did the CESD-10 in the Williams et al. (2017) study present evidence of validity from factor analysis? Provide a rationale for your answer.

4. Did the CESD-10 have evidence of criterion-related validity in the Williams et al. (2017) study? Provide a rationale for your answer.

5. Provide an example of how convergent validity might have been examined for the CESD-10.

6. Explain the types of validity that were discussed related to the CESD-10 scale in the Williams et al. (2017) study.

7. Was the information on validity provided for the CESD-10 adequate in this study? Provide a rationale for your answer.

8. Williams et al. (2017, p. 25) reported, "Specimens were collected . . . under the principal investigator's supervision. Specimens were kept on ice during data collection and then frozen at $-20°C$ until shipped to Salimetrics, LLC on dry ice." What does this statement indicate about the precision of the saliva specimens collected?

9. How was accuracy determined in the measurement of cortisol levels in the Williams et al. (2017) study? Provide a rationale for your answer.

10. Was the description of the measurement of cortisol diurnal rhythm adequate in this study? Provide a rationale for your answer.

Understanding Frequencies and Percentages

STATISTICAL TECHNIQUE IN REVIEW

Frequency is the number of times a score or value for a variable occurs in a set of data. **Frequency distribution** is a statistical procedure that involves listing all the possible values or scores for a variable in a study. Frequency distributions are used to organize and examine data for data entry errors and coding or computer programming errors (Gray & Grove, 2021). In addition, frequencies and percentages are used to describe demographic or attribute variables and the major variables measured in a study at the nominal or ordinal levels (see Exercise 1; Grove & Gray, 2023; Waltz et al., 2017).

Percentage can be defined as a portion or part of the whole or a named amount in every hundred measures. For example, a sample of 100 study participants might include 40 females and 60 males. In this example, the whole is the sample of 100 participants, and gender is described as including two parts, 40 females and 60 males. A percentage is calculated by dividing the smaller number, which would be a part of the whole, by the larger number, which represents the whole. The result of this calculation is then multiplied by 100%.

Formula for Percentage

Percentage (%) = (part of the whole or sample ÷ the whole or entire sample) × 100%

For example, if 14 nurses out of a total of 62 are working on a given day, you can divide 14 by 62 and multiply by 100% to calculate the percentage of nurses working that day. Calculations: $(14 \div 62) \times 100\% = 0.2258 \times 100\% = 22.58\% = 22.6\%$. The answer also might be expressed as a whole percentage, which would be 23% in this example. You need to read the directions for answering questions to determine the number of decimal places to include in the final answer (Grove & Gray, 2023).

A **cumulative percentage distribution** involves the summing of percentages from the top of a table to the bottom. Therefore the bottom category has a cumulative percentage of 100% (Grove & Gray, 2023). Cumulative percentages can also be used to determine percentile ranks, especially when discussing standardized scores. For example, if 75% of a group scored equal to or lower than a particular examinee's score, then that examinee's rank is at the 75th percentile. When reported as a percentile rank, the percentage is often rounded to the nearest whole number. **Percentile ranks** can be used to analyze ordinal data that can be assigned to categories that can be ranked. Percentile ranks and cumulative percentages might also be used in any frequency distribution where study participants have only one value for a variable. For example, demographic characteristics are usually reported with the frequency (*f*) or number of participants and percentage (%) of participants for each level of a demographic variable. Income level is presented as an example for 200 individuals in a study in Table 6.1.

TABLE 6.1 FREQUENCIES AND PERCENTAGES			
Income Level	Frequency (*f*)	Percentage (%)	Cumulative %
1. <$60,000	20	10%	10%
2. $60,000–$79,999	50	25%	35%
3. $80,000–$99,999	80	40%	75%
4. $100,000–$120,000	40	20%	95%
5. >$120,000	10	5%	100%

In data analysis, percentage distributions can be used to compare findings from different studies that have different sample sizes, and these distributions are usually arranged in tables in order either from greatest to least or least to greatest percentages (Heavy, 2019; Kim et al., 2022).

RESEARCH ARTICLE

Source

Mensinger, J. L., Brom, H., Havens, D. S., Costello, A., D'Annunzio, C., Durning, J. D., Bradley, J. D., Copel, L., Maldonado, L., Smeltzer, S., Yost, J., & Kaufmann, P. (2022). Psychological responses of hospital-based nurses working during the COVID-19 pandemic in the United States: A cross-sectional study. *Applied Nursing Research, 63,* 151517. https://doi.org/10.1016/j.apnr.2021.151517

Introduction

Mensinger and colleagues (2022) conducted a study to describe the well-being of hospital-based registered nurses (RNs) in the United States working during the initial phase of the novel coronavirus of 2019 (COVID-19). The study included a cross-sectional design with a sample of 467 RNs. A cross-sectional design involves simultaneous examination of groups of study participants in various stages in a process, such as nurses' well-being during the COVID-19 pandemic, with the intent of inferring trends over time (Gray & Grove, 2021). Well-being was measured using the following tools: Generalized Anxiety Disorder-7, Patient Health Questionnaire-2 for depressive symptoms, Impact of Events Scale-Revised for traumatic stress, and the Insomnia Severity Index" (Mensinger et al., 2022, Abstract). The demographic variables described in this study are compared with the National Workforce Survey data obtained from the CHAMPS Registry. The prevalence of psychological symptoms in this study are compared with meta-analyses of these symptoms globally (Batra et al., 2020; Li et al., 2021). The Mensinger et al. (2022) study results are presented in the following research excerpt.

Relevant Study Results

"The demographic characteristics of hospital-based RNs are described in Table 6.2. The second column of this table shows comparisons of our sample to the National Workforce Survey data on variables available. The CHAMPS hospital-based RN sample identified mostly as female (92%) and white (91%); 69% were under the age of 45 years. Ninety-three percent served in direct patient care with 26% identifying their primary work as taking place on a COVID-19 designated unit and another 26% identifying their primary site as the intensive care unit (ICU). Compared to the characteristics of the meta-analyses, our sample [was] comprised of a greater proportion of females (70% vs. 92%). However, they were relatively similar in age; data were available to calculate a weighted mean of 34.7 years for the Li study. This

TABLE 6.2	DEMOGRAPHIC CHARACTERISTICS		
Characteristic	**N**	**(%)**	**2020 National Workforce Survey**
Overall	467	(100)	
Gender			
Male	38	(8.1)	(9.4)
Female	429	(91.9)	(90.5)
Gender nonconforming	0	(0)	(0.1)
Race/Ethnicity			
White Non-Hispanic	425	(91.0)	(80.6)
Black/African American	9	(1.9)	(6.7)
Latinx/Hispanic	9	(1.9)	(5.6)
Asian/Pacific Islander	9	(1.9)	(7.6)
Multiracial/Mixed identities	8	(1.7)	(2.1)
Other	6	(1.3)	(2.3)
Native American/Alaskan Native	1	(0.2)	(0.5)
Age (Years)			
18–29	156	(33.4)	(8.4)
30–44	166	(35.5)	(28.6)
45–59	111	(23.8)	(31.7)
60 and over	34	(7.3)	(31.2)
Marital Status			
Unmarried	211	(45.2)	
Married	256	(54.8)	
Education			
Associate's degree/Registered Nurse diploma	36	(7.7)	(28.1)
Bachelor's degree	338	(72.4)	(48.1)
Graduate degree	92	(19.7)	(17.1)
Type of Hospital			
Large/metropolitan	240	(51.4)	
Suburban/regional	175	(37.5)	
Rural/community-based	52	(11.1)	
Supervisory Role			
Yes	55	(11.8)	
No	411	(88.2)	
Direct Patient Care			
Yes	436	(93.4)	(68.6)
No	31	(6.6)	(31.4)
Living Alone			
Yes	59	(12.6)	
No	408	(87.4)	
Primary Work Unit			
COVID–designated	117	(25.8)	
Intensive Care Unit	117	(25.8)	
Emergency Department	55	(12.1)	
Other	165	(36.3)	
Region			
Northeast	351	(75.3)	
South	57	(12.2)	
Midwest	34	(7.3)	
West	24	(5.2)	

compares with a mean (*SD*) of 38.1 (12.4) years for present study's CHAMPS hospital RNs. Additionally, the samples of the meta-analyses were primarily from Asian countries and included other healthcare workers with nurses comprising approximately 45% of their participants.

To answer our first study aim, we present the rates of each symptom category (anxiety, depression, insomnia, and traumatic stress) and the 95% confidence intervals (CIs) for the CHAMPS hospital-based RN sample in the upper portion of Table 6.3. These rates are based on 'moderate' degrees of symptom severity, as discussed in the measures section. . . .

To answer our second study aim, we present the global prevalence rates of the symptoms captured in two recently published meta-analyses (Batra et al., 2020; Li et al., 2021) in the lower portions of Table 6.3. . . . [The] findings showed that compared to global rates reported in Batra et al. (2020) and Li et al. (2021), respectively, our sample of U.S. hospital-based RNs experienced significantly more traumatic stress (54.6% vs. 11.4%; $p < 0.001$) and (54.6% vs. 21.5%; . . . $p < 0.001$). Rates of insomnia were also significantly higher in the CHAMPS hospital-based RN sample compared to the Batra et al. meta-analysis (27.8% vs. 32.4%; . . . $p < 0.033$); the Li et al. review did not report on insomnia. Depressive symptoms were significantly more common in CHAMPS hospital-based RNs (54.6% vs. 31.8%; . . . $p < .001$) compared to the Batra et al. global rates and the rates reported by Li et al. (54.6% vs. 21.7%; . . . $p < .001$). While rates of anxiety symptoms reported in CHAMPS hospital-based RNs (37.3%) did not differ from the 34.4% reported in the Batra et al. review . . ., they were significantly higher than the 22.1% reported in the Li et al. review" (Mensinger et al., 2022, Results section).

TABLE 6.3   PREVALENCE OF PSYCHOLOGICAL SYMPTOMS

CHAMPS Hospital RNs (U.S.)		
Psychological Outcome	**N**	**Prevalence**
Anxiety (GAD–7 ≥ 10)	418	37.3%
Depression (PHQ–2 ≥ 2)	416	54.6%
Insomnia (ISI ≥ 15)	438	32.4%
Traumatic stress (IES-R ≥ 26)	421	54.6%
Batra et al. (Global)		
Anxiety	51,596	34.4%
Depression	53,164	31.8%
Insomnia	18,546	27.8%
Traumatic stress	3,676	11.4%
Li et al. (Global)		
Anxiety	97,333	22.1%
Depression	97,333	21.7%
Insomnia	NA	NA
Traumatic stress	97,333	21.5%

RNs, registered nurses; GAD-7, Generalized Anxiety Disorder-7; PHQ-2, Patient Health Questionnaire-2 for depressive symptoms; ISI, Insomnia Severity Index; IES-R, Impact of Events Scale-Revised for traumatic stress.

STUDY QUESTIONS

1. What are the frequency and percentage of females in the Mensinger et al. (2022) sample?

2. Compare the percentages of females in the Mensinger et al. (2022) study with the National Workforce Survey results. Are these percentages significantly different? Provide a rationale for your answer.

3. What is the largest educational category for the Mensinger et al. (2022) study? How does this compare with the National Workforce Survey? What do these results indicate?

4. Are the majority of nurses in the Mensinger et al. (2022) study in supervisory roles? Provide a rationale for your answer.

5. In the Mensinger et al. (2022) study, what are the frequency and percentage of nurses working in the COVID-designated areas and the ICUs? Provide your calculations and round your answer to the appropriate whole percentage.

6. What are the cumulative frequency and percentage for the demographic variable Type of Hospital? Show your calculations.

7. In the Mensinger et al. (2022) study, the variable depression had missing data for 51 nurses. What percentage of the nurses had missing data for depression? Provide your calculations and round your answer to the appropriate whole percent.

8. Are the results for anxiety similar for the nurses in the three research reports presented in Table 6.3? Provide a rationale for your answer.

9. Identify the frequencies and percentages for the insomnia symptom in the Mensinger et al. (2022) study and the meta-analyses by Batra et al. (2020) and Li et al. (2021). Was there a significant difference in the insomnia symptoms in the Mensinger et al. (2022) study versus the Batra et al. (2020) meta-analysis? Provide a rationale for your answer.

10. Are the psychological symptoms reported what you might expect nurses to experience in the COVID-19 pandemic? Provide internet sites and other sources that can support your answer.

Answers to Study Questions

1. Mensinger et al. (2022) reported their study included 429 female nurses, which was 91.9% of the sample ($N = 467$) (see Table 6.2).

2. The 2020 National Workforce Survey was 90.5% female, which was very similar to the Mensinger et al. (2022) study that was 91.9% female. Based on the similar percentages, the two groups of nurses are probably not significantly different. However, no results are provided in the Mensinger et al. (2022) study to indicate if these groups are significantly different for any of the demographic variables.

3. The largest educational category for the Mensinger et al. (2022) study is bachelor's degree ($n = 338$, 72.4%). The National Workforce Survey group included 48.1% bachelor-prepared nurses and 28.1% nurses with an associate's degree or diploma. The Mensinger et al. (2022) sample only included 7.7% associate- or diploma-prepared RNs. Thus the educational level of the nurses in this study is higher than the National Workforce Survey group.

4. No, the majority of the RNs are not in supervisory roles, as indicated by $n = 55$, 11.8%. The majority of the RNs were providing direct patient care ($n = 436$, 93.4%), as presented in Table 6.2.

5. The frequency and percentage of RNs working in both the COVID-designated units and the ICUs need to be calculated using the results in Table 6.2.

$$117 \text{ RNs in COVID units} + 117 \text{ RNs in ICUs} = 234 \text{ RNs}$$

$$234 \text{ RNs} \div 467 \text{ sample size} (100\%) = 0.501 \times 100\% = 50.1\% \text{ or } 50\%$$

6. Cumulative frequency or number of nurses working in hospitals in the Mensinger et al. (2022) study = 240 + 175 + 52 = 467 or the size of the sample. This demographic variable has no missing data. Cumulative percentage = 51.4% + 37.5% + 11.1% = 100%.

7. The percentage of RNs with missing depression data was calculated as follows: $51 \div 467 (100\%) = 0.109 \times 100\% = 10.9\%$ or 11%.

8. Yes, the percentage of RNs with anxiety in the Mensinger et al. (2022) study was 37.3%, which was similar to the 34.4% anxiety reported by Batra et al. (2020). Li et al. (2021) had a smaller incidence (22.1%) of anxiety reported (see Table 6.3).

9. Mensinger et al. (2022) reported insomnia was experienced by 438 RNs or 32.4% of the sample. In their meta-analysis, Batra et al. (2020) reported 18,546 (27.8%) RNs experienced insomnia. Li et al. (2021) did not include the psychological symptom of insomnia, so NA is reported in Table 6.3. Yes, Mensinger et al. (2022) reported "Rates of insomnia were also significantly higher in the CHAMPS hospital-based RNs (27.8% vs. 32.4%; $p < 0.033$)." Alpha in this study was set at 0.05; the p value is less than alpha, so the results are significantly different for insomnia in these two studies (Grove & Gray, 2023; Kim et al., 2022).

10. Yes, the psychological symptoms of anxiety, depression, insomnia, and traumatic stress are common symptoms you would expect RNs to report during the COVID-19 pandemic. The meta-analysis by Batra et al. (2020) identified these same psychological symptoms as being common for RNs during the pandemic. Li et al. (2021) also identified the symptoms of anxiety, depression, and traumatic stress. The meta-analyses had extremely large samples, providing support for the psychological symptoms of anxiety, depression, and stress commonly experienced by nurses during the pandemic. An online article identified stress, insomnia, and distress as common psychological symptoms for RNs during the pandemic, https://www.ncbi.nlm.nih.gov/pmc/articles/PMC8701954/. You might find other websites that discuss this topic.

Questions for Additional Study

Follow your instructor's directions to submit your answers to the following questions for additional study. Your instructor may ask you to write your answers below and submit them as a hard copy for evaluation. Alternatively, your instructor may ask you to submit your answers online.

1. What are the frequency and percentage of nurses providing direct patient care in the Mensinger et al. (2022) sample?

2. Compare the percentages of nurses providing direct patient care in the Mensinger et al. (2022) study with the National Workforce Survey results. How different are these percentages and what do these results indicate?

3. What is the predominant race(s) for the RNs in both the Mensinger et al. (2022) study and the National Workforce Survey? What do these results indicate?

4. Identify the type of hospital where the largest number and percentage of nurses worked. Is this result what you might expect? Provide a rationale for your answer.

5. What frequency and percentage of nurses are under 45 years of age? Provide your calculations.

6. Identify the frequencies and percentages for the nurses from the different regions in the United States.

7. How representative is the Mensinger et al. (2022) sample of the U.S. regions? Should the study findings be generalized to all U.S. regions? Provide a rationale for your answer.

8. In the Mensinger et al. (2022) study, the variable of anxiety had missing data for 49 nurses. What percentage of the nurses had missing data for anxiety? Provide your calculations and round your answer to one decimal place.

9. Identify the percentages of RNs who experienced traumatic stress in the Mensinger et al. (2022) study, meta-analysis by Batra et al. (2020), and meta-analysis by Li et al. (2021). Are these results for traumatic stress significantly different for the U.S. hospital-based RNs versus the traumatic stress reported in the meta-analyses by Batra et al. and Li et al.? Provide a rationale for your answer.

10. What were the two most prevalent psychological symptoms reported in the meta-analyses? Are these psychological symptoms reflective of RNs globally during the COVID-19 pandemic? Provide a rationale for your answer.

Interpreting Line Graphs

STATISTICAL TECHNIQUE IN REVIEW

Tables and figures are commonly used to present findings from studies or to provide a way for researchers to become familiar with research data. Using figures, researchers are able to illustrate the results from descriptive and correlational data analyses, assist in identifying patterns in data, identify changes over time, and interpret exploratory findings (American Psychological Association, 2020). A **line graph** is a figure that is developed by joining a series of plotted points with a line to illustrate how a variable changes over time or how one variable changes in relation to another (Kim et al., 2022; Terrell, 2021). A line graph figure includes a horizontal scale, or x-axis, and a vertical scale, or y-axis. The x-axis is often used to document time, and the y-axis is used to document the mean scores or values for a variable (Gray & Grove, 2021; Plichta & Kelvin, 2013). For example, researchers might include a line graph to illustrate a relationship between anxiety and pain values for a sample of postsurgical patients. Line graphs might also be used to identify changes in experimental and comparison groups values for a selected variable.

Fig. 7.1 presents a line graph that documents time in weeks on the x-axis and mean weight loss in pounds on the y-axis for an experimental group consuming a low-carbohydrate diet and a control group consuming a standard diet. This line graph illustrates the trend of a steady increase in the mean weight lost by the experimental or intervention group and minimal mean weight change by the control group. It is important to note that sometimes, the slope of a line (or the amount by which a line deviates from the horizontal axis) in a line graph does not represent significant effects. Alternatively, sometimes lines do not indicate large changes, but may represent significant effects in large samples (Gray & Grove, 2021; Kim et al, 2022).

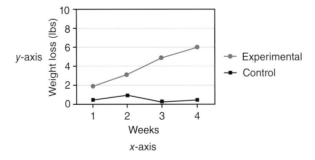

FIG. 7.1 ■ LINE GRAPH COMPARING EXPERIMENTAL AND CONTROL GROUPS FOR WEIGHT LOSS OVER FOUR WEEKS.

RESEARCH ARTICLE

Source

Donnelly, M. R., Grigorian, A., Swentek, L., Arora, J., Kuza, C. M., Inaba, K., Kim, D., Lekawa, M., & Nahmias, J. (2022). Firearm violence against children in the United States: Trends in the wake of the COVID-19 pandemic. *Journal of Trauma & Acute Care Surgery, 92*(1), 65–68. https://doi.org/10.1097/TA.0000000000003347

Introduction

Donnelly and colleagues (2022) conducted a study to examine the firearm violence against children before and during the COVID-19 pandemic and to determine the types of firearm violence that occurred against children in the United States (U.S.). The historical firearm data were obtained from the Gun Violence Archive, which includes the details of the current trends and types of child-involved shootings. This is an independent organization for evidence-based firearm research and includes information from over 7500 sources. Only firearm incidents with children younger than 18 were included, excluding suicides from firearms. The primary outcome focused on the number of child-involved shooting incidents and the secondary outcomes focused on the number of fatal and nonfatal firearm incidents over time. Donnelly et al. (2022, p. 66) hypothesized an increase in "total, fatal, and nonfatal child-involved shootings during the COVID-19 pandemic." Direct quotes from this study are included in the following section.

Relevant Study Results

"**METHODS**

. . . U.S. Census population reports were used to weigh the rates of firearm violence per 100,000 children. The number of children in the United States during each year was recorded and these numbers were used in calculations for 2016 to 2019. Summary data for 2020 were not yet available. Therefore, 2020 projected pediatric population data were used from a report released by the Federal Interagency Forum on Child and Family Statistics. . . . A linear trendline was fit to 2016 to 2019 data to show projected versus actual 2020 firearm violence.

The Giffords Law Center Annual Gun Law Scorecard grades each state using a point system to evaluate their gun legislation based on specific laws and policies. The points are tabulated, and the states are ranked from 1, which is the state with the strongest gun laws, to 50, which is the state with the weakest gun laws. We compared the top 25 stronger gun law states to the bottom 25 weaker gun law states.

Mann-Whitney U tests were performed to compare median monthly trends and types of child-involved firearm violence incidents between 2018 and 2020, as well as between 2019 and 2020. . . . Statistical significance was set as $p < 0.05$ (Table 7.1)" (Donnelly et al., 2022, p. 66).

"**RESULTS**

There was a total of 1,076 child-involved shootings in 2020, 811 in 2019 and 803 in 2018. The median total child-involved shooting incidents per 100,000 children per month increased from 2018 to 2020 (0.095 vs. 0.124, $p = 0.003$), as well as from 2019 to 2020 (0.097 vs. 0.124, $p = 0.010$). From 2018 to 2020, child killed by adult (0.020 vs. 0.034, $p = 0.024$) incidents increased. Consistent, increasing trends in child killed by adult (0.021 vs. 0.034, $p = 0.049$) were also found between 2019 and 2020. . . . Total child-involved shooting incidents, as well as both fatal and nonfatal child-involved shooting incidents per 100,000 per year (2016–2020), all exceeded the projected number of incidents extrapolated from the 2016 to 2019 data

TABLE 7.1   MANN-WHITNEY *U* TEST OF POSTCOVID-19 (2020) CHILD-INVOLVED INCIDENTS TO HISTORICAL DATA PER MONTH PER 100,000 CHILDREN ACROSS THE UNITED STATES

Median	2020	2018	*p*	2019	*p*
All incidents	0.124	0.095	**0.003**	0.097	**0.010**
Fatal incidents	0.039	0.031	0.068	0.288	0.068
Nonfatal incidents	0.073	0.060	**0.007**	0.066	0.128
Child killed by a child	0.003	0.004	0.630	0.005	0.347
Child injured by child	0.006	0.008	0.242	0.007	0.551
Child killed by self	0.005	0.005	0.590	0.003	0.101
Child injured by self	0.009	0.007	0.089	0.006	**0.045**
Child killed by an adult	0.034	0.020	**0.024**	0.021	**0.049**
Child injured by an adult	0.061	0.049	**0.010**	0.051	0.160

Data in bold emphasis indicate statistical significance.
From: Donnelly, M. R., Grigorian, A., Swentek, L., Arora, J., Kuza, C. M., Inaba, K., Kim, D., Lekawa, M., & Nahmias, J. (2022). Firearm violence against children in the United States: Trends in the wake of the COVID-19 pandemic. *Journal of Trauma & Acute Care Surgery, 92*(1), 66. https://doi.org/10.1097/TA.0000000000003347

(Fig. 7.2). . . . Compared with weaker gun law states, stronger gun law states were associated with decreased monthly total child-involved shooting incidents between 2018 and 2020 (. . . *p* < 0.001)" (Donnelly et al., 2022, p. 66).

"DISCUSSION

. . . This study found an overall increasing rate of child-involved shootings for the year of 2020 during the COVID-19 pandemic. During this time, children were more likely to be fatally injured by an adult with a firearm. In addition, the strength of gun laws was shown to be associated with decreased rates of pediatric firearm violence. Given that access to social support systems and community safety nets has been hindered by the pandemic, implementation of stronger gun laws across all states may help reduce the number of fatal and nonfatal child-involved shooting incidents" (Donnelly et al., 2022, p. 68).

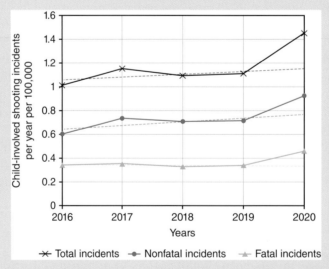

FIG. 7.2 ▪ RATE OF TOTAL, FATAL, AND NONFATAL CHILD-INVOLDED INCIDENTS PER 100,000 CHILDREN PER YEAR (2016–2020). From: Donnelly, M. R., Grigorian, A., Swentek, L., Arora, J., Kuza, C. M., Inaba, K., Kim, D., Lekawa, M., & Nahmias, J. (2022). Firearm violence against children in the United States: Trends in the wake of the COVID-19 pandemic. *Journal of Trauma & Acute Care Surgery, 92*(1), 67. https://doi.org/10.1097/TA.0000000000003347

STUDY QUESTIONS

1. What is the purpose of a line graph? What elements are included in a line graph?

2. Review Fig. 7.2 and identify the focus of the x-axis and the y-axis. What is the time frame for this line graph?

3. What variables are presented on the line graph in Fig. 7.2? Are these variables relevant to the focus of this study? Provide a rationale for your response.

4. Review Fig. 7.2 and identify when the greatest change occurred in total firearm incidents with children. Discuss the value of this line graph.

5. State the null hypothesis for the total firearm incidents with children from 2018 to 2020.

6. Was the null hypothesis in Question 5 accepted or rejected? Provide a rationale for your response.

7. Was there a significant change in the incidence of children killed by adults from 2018 to 2020? Provide a rationale for your answer. What does this result mean?

8. How many children were killed by adults with firearms in 2018 and 2020? Show your calculations.

9. Was there a significant difference in the fatal firearms incidents with children between 2019 and 2020? Provide a rationale for your response. What does this result mean?

10. Was the sample size adequate in this study? Provide a rationale for your response.

Answers to Study Questions

1. A line graph is a figure developed to illustrate the results from descriptive data analyses, to identify patterns in data over time, or to demonstrate how one variable changes in the experimental group versus the control group (see Fig. 7.1; Kim et al., 2022; King & Eckersley, 2019). For example, a line graph might include an x-axis to document time (first 5 days after surgery) in a study and a y-axis to identify the mean scores or values for ambulation of postsurgical patients. The mean scores for variables are plotted and connected with a line to show change over time. More than one variable and more than one group can be included on a line graph.

2. In Fig. 7.2, the x-axis represents time in years and the y-axis represents child-involved shooting incidents per year per 100,000 children. The years covered in this line graph include 2016, 2017, 2018, 2019, and 2020. These are years before and during the COVID-19 pandemic.

3. The variables on the line graph include total firearm incidents, nonfatal incidents, and fatal incidents involving children. Yes, these variables are relevant because they are the focus of the primary and secondary outcomes of the Donnelly et al. (2022) study. The primary outcome focused on the total number of child-involved shooting incidents and the secondary outcomes focused on the number of fatal and nonfatal firearm incidents over time.

4. The greatest change in total firearm incidents with children occurred between 2019 and 2020. The line graph provides a visual representation of the changes taking place in total firearm incidents from 2016 to 2020. Minimal change occurred from 2016 to 2019, with the greatest change in 2019 to 2020.

5. Null hypothesis: *There is no change in the total firearm incidents with children from 2018 to 2020 in the United States.*

6. The null hypothesis was rejected because the total firearm incidents with children from 2018 to 2020 increased significantly ($p = 0.003$). The level of significance for this study was set at alpha (α) $= 0.05$. The p value of 0.003 is less than $\alpha = 0.05$, indicating a significant result. When results are significant, the null hypothesis is rejected (Grove & Gray, 2023; Terrell, 2021).

7. Yes, there was a significant change in the incidence of children killed by adults from 2018 to 2020. Donnelly et al. (2022, p. 66) reported: "From 2018 to 2020, child killed by adult (0.020 vs. 0.034, $p = 0.024$) incidents increased." This is a significant result because the $p = 0.024$ is less than $\alpha = 0.05$ set for this study (Grove & Gray, 2023; Kim et al., 2022). This result indicates that the children killed by adults significantly increased in the wake of the COVID-19 pandemic. This serious social problem requires further investigation and development of interventions to manage it.

8. In 2018, a total of 2000 children were killed by adults with firearms. The calculations are as follows: $0.20 \times 100,000 = 2000$. In 2020 a total of 3400 children were killed by adults. The calculations are $0.034 \times 100,000 = 3400$.

9. There was a nonsignificant change in the fatal firearms incidents with children between 2019 and 2020 as indicated by the results (0.288 vs. 0.039, $p = 0.068$) (see Table 7.1). The $p = 0.068$ is greater than $\alpha = 0.05$, indicating a nonsignificant result. This result supports a nonsignificant change in fatal firearms incidents with children from 2019 to 2020. The line graph of fatal incidents in Fig. 7.2 shows limited change in these incidents from 2019 to 2020 (Kim et al., 2022; Terrell, 2021).

10. Yes, the sample size for this study was adequate (Aberson, 2019; Cohen, 1988). This study involved a secondary data analysis of firearm incidents from the Gun Violence Archive that included data for all 50 U.S. states. The specific number of incidents examined was not identified but the rate of firearm violence was weighted per 100,000 children. In this study, the researchers examined the total sample of firearm incidents in the U.S., providing a representative sample of the U.S. but not of other countries (Aberson, 2019; Gray & Grove, 2021; Plichta & Kelvin, 2013).

Name: _____ Class: _____

Date: _____

Follow your instructor's directions to submit your answers to the following questions for additional study. Your instructor may ask you to write your answers below and submit them as a hard copy for evaluation. Alternatively, your instructor may ask you to submit your answers online.

1. How many total firearm incidents with children occurred in 2018, 2019, and 2020? What do these results demonstrate?

2. Review Fig. 7.2 and discuss the trend of nonfatal firearm incidents per 100,000 children from 2018 to 2020. Was there a significant change in nonfatal firearm incidents for this time frame? Provide a rationale for your response.

3. State the null hypothesis for the nonfatal firearm incidents with children between 2019 and 2020 in the United States.

4. Was there a significant change in the child nonfatal firearm incidents between 2019 and 2020? Provide a rationale for your answer. Was the null hypothesis in Question 3 accepted or rejected?

5. State the null hypothesis for the fatal firearm incidents per 100,000 children from 2018 to 2020 in the United States.

6. Was the null hypothesis in Question 5 accepted or rejected? Provide a rationale for your response. What do these results mean?

7. Was there a significant difference in the firearm incidents of a child injured by self between 2019 and 2020? Provide a rationale for your response. What does this result mean?

8. Donnelly et al. (2022, p. 66) hypothesized an "increase in total, fatal, and nonfatal child-involved shootings during the COVID-19 pandemic." Was this hypothesis accepted or rejected? Provide a rationale for your response.

9. Was there a significant difference between the states with stronger versus weaker gun laws? Provide a rationale for your response. What is the meaning of this result?

10. What implications for practice do you note from the Donnelly et al. (2022) study?

Measures of Central Tendency: Mean, Median, and Mode

STATISTICAL TECHNIQUE IN REVIEW

Mean, median, and mode are the three **measures of central tendency** used to describe study variables. These statistical techniques are calculated to determine the center of a distribution of data, and the central tendency that is calculated is determined by the level of measurement of the data (i.e., nominal, ordinal, interval, or ratio; see Exercise 1). The **mode** is a category or value that occurs with the greatest frequency in a distribution of data. Thus the mode is always a score in a distribution of sample data. The mode is the only acceptable measure of central tendency for analyzing nominal-level data, which are not continuous and cannot be ranked (see Fig. 1.1 in Exercise 1; Grove & Gray, 2023). Most distributions of values in a study are **unimodal**, or have one mode, and frequencies progressively decline as they move away from the mode. A **symmetric curve**, like the one in Fig. 8.1, is unimodal, and the left side of the curve is a mirror image of the right side of the curve. The mode, median, and mean are essentially equal. If a distribution has two scores that occur more frequently than others (two modes), the distribution is called **bimodal**. A distribution with more than two modes is **multimodal** (Gray & Grove, 2021; Kim et al., 2022).

The **median** *(MD)* is a score that lies in the middle of a rank-ordered list of values of a distribution. If a distribution consists of an odd number of scores, the *MD* is the middle score that divides the rest of the distribution into two equal parts, with half of the values falling above the middle score and half of the values falling below this score. In a distribution with an even number of scores, the *MD* is half of the sum of the two middle scores of that distribution. If several scores in a distribution are of the same value, then the *MD* will be the value of the middle score.

The *MD* is the most precise measure of central tendency for ordinal-level data and for non-normally distributed or skewed interval- or ratio-level data. Curves that are not symmetric are

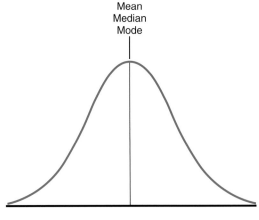

Mean
Median
Mode

FIG. 8.1 ■ SYMMETRICAL CURVE

referred to **asymmetric or skewed**. A curve may be positively skewed, which means that the largest portion of data is below the mean (Fig. 8.2). For example, data on the length of enrollment in hospices are **positively skewed**. Most people die within the first few days or weeks of enrollment, whereas increasingly smaller numbers survive as time increases. A curve can also be negatively skewed, which means that the largest portion of data is above the mean (see Fig. 8.2). For example, data on the occurrence of chronic illness by age in a population are **negatively skewed**, with most chronic illnesses occurring in older age groups. In a **skewed distribution**, the mean, median, and mode are not equal. In a positively skewed distribution, the mean is greater than the median, which is greater than the mode. In a negatively skewed distribution, the mean is less than the median, which is less than the mode (see Fig. 8.2). However, in some skewed distributions of data, the mode and median are equal (Gray & Grove, 2021; Kim et al., 2022).

The following calculation can be conducted to locate the median in a distribution of values.

$$\text{Median }(MD) = (N+1) \div 2$$

N is the number of scores

$$\text{Example: } N = 31 \quad \text{Median} = \frac{31+1}{2} = 32 \div 2 = 16\text{th score}$$

$$\text{Example: } N = 40 \quad \text{Median} = \frac{40+1}{2} = 41 \div 2 = 20.5\text{th score}$$

In the first example, the sample includes an odd number of study participants ($N = 31$), so the median is an actual score in the distribution (16th score). In the second example, the sample includes an equal number of participants ($N = 40$), so the median is halfway between the 20th and the 21st scores in the sampling distribution (Grove & Gray, 2023; Terrell, 2021). Thus the median is sometimes a score in a distribution of sample data and sometimes not.

The **mean** ($\overline{X}$) is the arithmetic average of all scores of a sample, that is, the sum of its individual scores divided by the total number of scores. The mean is the most accurate measure of central tendency for normally distributed data measured at the interval and ratio levels and is only appropriate for these levels of data (Gray & Grove, 2021). The mean is sometimes but often not a score in a distribution of sample data. In a normal distribution as presented in Fig. 8.1, the mean, median, and mode are essentially equal (see Exercise 27 for determining the normality of a distribution). The mean is sensitive to extreme values, such as outliers. An **outlier** is a value in a dataset that is unusually low or unusually high in context of the rest of the sample data. Outliers can result in skewed distributions of data and skewness interferes with the validity of many statistical analyses. Therefore statistical procedures have been developed to measure the skewness of the distribution of the sample being studied (see Exercise 27). If a study has outliers, the mean is most affected by these, so the median might be the measure of central tendency included in a research report (Grove & Gray, 2023).

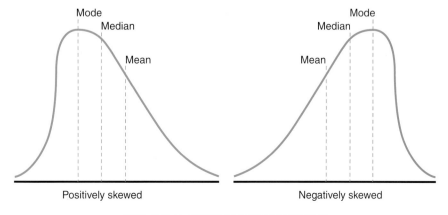

FIG. 8.2 ■ **SKEWED DISTRIBUTIONS**

The formula for the mean is:

$$\text{Mean} = \bar{X} = \frac{\sum X}{N}$$

$\sum X$ is the sum of the raw scores in a study
N is the sample size or number of scores in the study

RESEARCH ARTICLE

Source

Oshvandi, K., Movaheditabar, E., Naghshtabrizi, B., Mohammadi, Y., & Shamsizadeh, M. (2021). The effect of video-based educational program on satisfaction and comfort in patients undergoing transradial coronary angiography: A single-blinded, randomized controlled trial. *Journal of Vascular Nursing, 39*(2), 27–32. https://doi.org/10.1016/j.jvn.2021.01.001

Introduction

Oshvandi and colleagues (2021) conducted a randomized controlled trial (RCT) to determine the effect of a video-based educational program on satisfaction and comfort in patients undergoing a transradial coronary angiography (TCA). A total of 89 patients were recruited and randomly assigned to either the intervention or control group. All the TCA procedures were performed by one cardiologist, and patients who needed an analgesic to reduce pain were excluded from the study to reduce the potential for error (Gray & Grove, 2021). Satisfaction was measured with the Patient Satisfaction Questionnaire (PSQ; a four-point Likert scale), and comfort was measured with a visual analog scale (VAS). VAS is a 100-mm line that patients mark to indicate their experiences, such as comfort level, that results in ratio-level data. Oshvandi et al. (2021, p. 27) reported that "after the intervention, the mean scores of satisfaction and comfort in the intervention group were higher than in the control group ($p < 0.001$). Video-based educational strategies should be integrated into the nursing interventions to improve patients' health status."

Relevant Study Results

"In this study, the video-based educational program was conducted at 24 hours before the TCA, and the content of the educational package was presented to the patients by a video projector. The content of the educational package included the following: introduction of the catheterization laboratory atmosphere, being familiar with the equipment in the catheterization laboratory and the healthcare professionals working there, understanding and being familiar with the angiography procedure (how it is implemented, contrast injection, vascular access, etc.) and the care before, during, and after angiography. The training lasted about 40 minutes. At the end of the education, patients received a pamphlet of educational content, and the researcher also answered their questions" (Oshvandi et al., 2021, p. 28).

"Results

Demographic and clinical characteristics of the participants

In this study, a total of 89 patients were selected and then divided into two groups: intervention ($n = 44$) and control ($n = 45$). Mean and standard deviation of age in the intervention and the control group were 56.34 ± 10.23 and 60.18 ± 9.08, respectively. In terms of age, the *t*-test showed no significant difference between the two groups. In terms of gender, most participants in the intervention (59.1%) and the control group (76.2%) were male. More than 85% of patients in both groups were married. Most patients in the intervention (75%) and the control group (64.4%) were not smokers. The two groups were homogenous in terms of demographic characteristics. Further information is included in Table 8.1.

TABLE 8.1 DEMOGRAPHIC INFORMATION OF THE POPULATION IN THE INTERVENTION AND CONTROL GROUPS

Groups Characteristics	Intervention n (%)	Control n (%)	p-value
Age			
35–55	20 (22.5)	12 (13.5)	
56–70	24 (27)	33 (37.1)	
Mean (SD)	56.34 (10.23)	60.18 (9.08)	.36* t = .90
Gender			.76†
Male	26 (59.1)	62 (76.2)	Df = 1
Female	18 (40.9)	37 (23.8)	
Marital Status			.51‡
Married	38 (86.4)	38 (84.4)	Df = 2
Lone	6 (11.4)	7 (15.6)	
Job			.48†
Homemaker	14 (31.8)	14 (31.1)	Df = 6
Free jobs	12 (27.3)	12 (26.7)	
Employee	4 (9.1)	2 (4.4)	
Retired	8 (18.2)	15 (33.3)	
Construction worker	6 (13.6)	2 (4.4)	
Educational Level			.53†
Illiterate	20 (45.5)	13 (28.9)	Df = 5
Elementary	12 (27.3)	14 (31.1)	
Prediploma	2 (4.5)	5 (11.1)	
Diploma	5 (11.4)	8 (17.8)	
BSc	5 (11.4)	5 (11.1)	
Smoking			.17†
Yes	11 (25)	16 (35.6)	Df = 5
No	33 (75)	29 (64.4)	
Insurance			.309†
Yes	43 (97.7)	45 (100)	Df = 1
No	1 (2.3)	0 (0)	
Systole (mm Hg)			t = −.15
Mean	119.61	118.93	.15*
SD	17.12	24.7	
Diastole (mm Hg)			t = −.90
Mean	72.3	73.78	.36*
SD	10.73	13.01	
Body Mass Index (kg/m²)			.15†
Mean	26.5	26.63	t = −.13
SD	4.15	4.7	
HTN in Family			.55†
Yes	23 (52.3)	21 (46.7)	Df = 2
No	21 (47.7)	24 (53.3)	

BSc = Bachelor of Science; Df = degrees of freedom; HTN = hypertension; SD = standard deviation; t = t-test.
* Independent sample t test.
†Chi-square.
‡ Fisher's exact test.
Oshvandi, K., Movaheditabar, E., Naghshtabrizi, B., Mohammadi, Y., & Shamsizadeh, M. (2021). The effect of video-based educational program on satisfaction and comfort in patients undergoing transradial coronary angiography: A single-blinded, randomized controlled trial. *Journal of Vascular Nursing, 39*(2), 30–31. https://doi.org/10.1016/j.jvn.2021.01.001

Satisfaction and comfort

The mean scores of satisfaction and comfort in the two groups were examined at 2, 4, and 8 hours after the TCA (Tables 8.2 and 8.3). Before the intervention, there was no significant difference in the mean score of comfort between the two groups (Table 8-3). The mean scores of satisfaction and comfort in the intervention group were higher than in the control group. ... [Further analyses] indicated a significant difference in the level of satisfaction and comfort between the two groups ($p < 0.001$) (Tables 8-2 and 8-3)" (Oshvandi et al., 2021, pp. 29–30).

TABLE 8.2   SATISFACTION OF THE POPULATION IN THE INTERVENTION AND CONTROL GROUPS

Groups	2 Hours After		4 Hours After		8 Hours After	
Satisfaction	Intervention	Control	Intervention	Control	Intervention	Control
Mean (*SD*)	57.91 (1.951)	49.29 (2.262)	55.57 (2.86)	48.93 (3.41)	52.34 (2.42)	46.71 (2.85)
p-value	<.0001*					

SD = standard deviation.
* Repeated measures analysis of variance.
Oshvandi, K., Movaheditabar, E., Naghshtabrizi, B., Mohammadi, Y., & Shamsizadeh, M. (2021). The effect of video-based educational program on satisfaction and comfort in patients undergoing transradial coronary angiography: A single-blinded, randomized controlled trial. *Journal of Vascular Nursing, 39*(2), 30–31. https://doi.org/10.1016/j.jvn.2021.01.001

TABLE 8.3   COMFORT OF THE POPULATION IN THE INTERVENTION AND CONTROL GROUPS

Groups	Before		2 Hours After		4 Hours After		8 Hours After	
Comfort	Intervention	Control	Intervention	Control	Intervention	Control	Intervention	Control
Mean (*SD*)	3.64 (0.65)	3.49 (0.66)	1.97 (0.46)	2.18 (0.51)	1.48 (0.43)	2.09 (0.45)	1.10 (0.33)	1.83 (0.45)
p-value	<.29*, $t = -1.06$ <.0001†							

SD = standard deviation.
* Independent-samples *t*-test.
† Repeated measures analysis of variance.
Oshvandi, K., Movaheditabar, E., Naghshtabrizi, B., Mohammadi, Y., & Shamsizadeh, M. (2021). The effect of video-based educational program on satisfaction and comfort in patients undergoing transradial coronary angiography: A single-blinded, randomized controlled trial. *Journal of Vascular Nursing, 39*(2), 30–31. https://doi.org/10.1016/j.jvn.2021.01.001

STUDY QUESTIONS

1. Which measure of central tendency always represents an actual score in a distribution of sample data? Provide a rationale for your answer.

2. In the Oshvandi et al. (2021) study, what is the mode for the demographic variable of educational level for the sample? Might this educational level be a potential for error in this study? Provide a rationale for your answer.

3. In this study, what are the mean ages for the study participants in the intervention and control groups? Are these mean ages similar or different? Provide a rationale for your answer.

4. What is the mean systolic blood pressure (SBP) for the patients in the intervention group? Do these patients appear to have hypertension (HTN)? Provide a rationale for your answer.

5. Was smoking a contributor to cardiovascular disease (CVD) for the majority of patients in this study? Provide a rationale for your answer.

6. Were the intervention and control groups similar for the demographic characteristics in this study? Provide a rationale for your answer.

7. How did the mean satisfaction level for the intervention group change over time? What might this result indicate?

8. What is the effect of outliers on the mean? If the study data have extreme outliers (either high or low scores) in the data, what measure of central tendency should be reported in a study? Provide a rationale for your answer.

9. In the following hypothetical example, 10 patients in the emergency room were asked to rate their chest pain on a 0 to 10 scale and reported the following values: 1, 6, 7, 7, 8, 7, 6, 8, 7, 9. What are the mode, *MD*, and range for the pain scores? Provide a rationale for your answers.

10. Calculate the mean ($\bar{X}$) for the pain scores in Question 9. Does this distribution of scores appear to be normal or skewed? Provide a rationale for your answer.

Answers to Study Questions

1. The mode is the most frequently occurring score in a distribution of sample scores; thus it will always be an actual score in the distribution. Median is the middle score of the distribution, which, with an even number of items, may not be an actual score in the distribution. The mean is the average of all scores in the distribution of sample scores, so it is often not an actual score in the distribution (Grove & Gray, 2023; Kim et al., 2022).

2. Illiterate was the mode for the educational level of the entire sample ($N = 89$). Illiterate was the mode for the intervention group ($n = 20$) and for the control group ($n = 13$). A total of 33 (37%) of the study participants marked illiterate as their educational level. With many of the participants being illiterate, this might have affected their ability to complete the measurement methods in this study. The researchers would have strengthened their study by providing the reading levels for the scales used (Gray & Grove, 2021). The comprehension of the video-based educational program might have been altered for the intervention group. However, educational level was not identified as a limitation for this study.

3. The mean ages of the intervention ($\bar{X} = 56.34$) and control ($\bar{X} = 60.18$) groups were similar (see Table 8.1), because they varied by 3.84 years. In addition, the researchers conducted a t-test and determined the two groups were not significantly different for age.

4. No, the mean SBP for the intervention group was 119.61 mm Hg, which does not reflect HTN. This value reflects a normal SBP according to BP guidelines (Todkar et al., 2021; Whelton et al., 2018). You can calculate the range for the SBP for 68% of the study participants in the intervention group by adding and subtracting the standard deviation from the mean. For example, $119.61 \pm 17.12 =$ the SBP range of a high of 136.73 mm Hg to a low of 102.49 mm Hg (Grove & Gray, 2023). Thus 68% of the study participants had normal SBPs less than 140 mm Hg.

5. No, a majority of the patients in the sample did not smoke. A total of 62 participants (33 in the intervention group and 29 in the control group) did not smoke, which was 69.7% of the sample. Thus smoking is not a risk factor for CVD as experienced by most of the study participants.

6. Yes, Oshvandi et al. (2021, p. 30) reported "The two groups were homogenous in terms of demographic characteristics." In addition, Table 8.1 indicated that the intervention and control groups were not significantly different for any of the demographic characteristics examined in this study. The groups were similar or homogenous for the demographic characteristics at the start of the study. Homogenous groups reduce the potential for errors from extraneous variables (Gray & Grove, 2021; Kazdin, 2022).

7. The mean satisfaction score decreased over time from a high of 57.91 at 2 hours after the TCA to a low of 52.34 at 8 hours after TCA. This is a decline of 5.57 points on the PSQ used to measure satisfaction. The satisfaction level probably declined with the decreasing influence of the intervention over time.

8. An unusually low score(s) or outlier(s) decreases the value of the mean, and an unusually high score(s) increases the mean value (see Fig. 8.2). The mean in a study is most affected by outliers (Gray & Grove, 2021). If the outliers cause the interval- or ratio-level data to be skewed or not normally distributed, it is best to report the median in a study. If the data are normally distributed, then the mean is the best measure of central tendency to report.

9. Place the pain scores in order from the least to the greatest score: 1, 6, 6, 7, 7, 7, 7, 8, 8, 9. In this example, the mode or most frequently occurring score is 7, and the *MD* or middle score in the distribution is 7. The range for the pain scores is 1 to 9 or $9 - 1 = 8$.

10. $\bar{X} = (1 + 6 + 6 + 7 + 7 + 7 + 7 + 8 + 8 + 9) \div 10 = 66 \div 10 = 6.6$. The mode equals the median (see the answer to Question 9), which is different than the mean ($\bar{X} = 6.6$). In looking at the scores, the value of 1 might be an outlier in this small dataset. This outlier decreased the mean and potentially caused the distribution to be negatively skewed (see Fig. 8.2). In a negatively skewed distribution, the mode is equal to or similar to the *MD* and the mean is less than both. To determine whether this skewness is significant, the distribution of the data must be tested for normality. Exercise 27 provides the steps for determining the normality of a distribution of scores.

Follow your instructor's directions to submit your answers to the following questions for additional study. Your instructor may ask you to write your answers below and submit them as a hard copy for evaluation. Alternatively, your instructor may ask you to submit your answers online.

1. The number of patients enrolled in a cardiac rehabilitation program in Dallas, Texas for each month in 2023 included the following: 55, 63, 42, 75, 86, 66, 79, 75, 80, 72, 75, 56. Determine the mode, *MD,* and $\bar{X}$ for the number of patients enrolled in this rehabilitation program for 2023. Show your calculations.

2. In Oshvandi's et al. (2021) study, what is the mode for the demographic variable of job for the control group? What percentage of the patients in the control group had this job?

3. Was there a significant difference in the jobs held by the patients in the intervention group versus the control group? How might this result affect the study findings?

4. What is the mean diastolic blood pressure (DBP) for the patients in the intervention group? Do these patients appear to have HTN? Provide a rationale for your answer.

5. What is the design for the Oshvandi et al. (2021) study? What are the strengths of this design? How might the design influence the results obtained from this study?

6. How did the mean comfort level for the intervention group change over time? What might this result indicate?

7. Was there a significant difference between the intervention and control groups in this study for satisfaction level? What were the results and what do they mean?

8. What were the mean comfort levels for the intervention and control groups prior to the start of the study? Were the mean comfort levels significantly different for the two groups at that time? Provide a rationale for your answer. Discuss what these results mean.

9. Examine the information about insurance in Table 8.2. What is the mode for insurance in this sample? Should these results be generalized to people without insurance? Provide a rationale for your answer.

10. Are these findings from the study by Oshvandi et al. (2021) ready for use in clinical practice? Provide a rationale for your answer.

Measures of Dispersion: Range and Standard Deviation

STATISTICAL TECHNIQUE IN REVIEW

Measures of dispersion, or measures of variability, are descriptive statistical techniques conducted to identify individual differences of the scores or values in a sample. These techniques give some indication of how values in a sample are dispersed, or spread, around the mean. The measures of dispersion also indicate how different the scores on a particular scale are or the extent that individual scores deviate from one another. If the individual scores are similar, dispersion or variability values are small and the sample is relatively **homogeneous**, or similar, in terms of these scores. A **heterogeneous** sample has a wide variation in the scores, resulting in increased values for the measures of dispersion. Range and standard deviation are the most common measures of dispersion included in research reports (Grove & Gray, 2023).

The simplest measure of dispersion is the **range**. In published studies, range is presented in two ways: (1) the range includes the lowest and highest values obtained for a variable, or (2) the range is calculated by subtracting the lowest score from the highest score. For example, the range for the scores 8, 9, 9, 10, 11, 11, 19 might be reported as 8 to 19 (8–19). In this example, the range is used to identify the extremely high score, 19, in this distribution. Extremely high or low scores in a distribution are called **outliers**. The range can also be calculated as follows: $19 - 8 = 11$. In this form, the range is a difference score that uses only the two extreme values in a sample for the comparison. The range is sometimes reported in published studies but is not used in further analyses (Gray & Grove, 2021).

The **standard deviation** (*SD*) is a measure of dispersion that is the average number of points by which the scores or values of a distribution vary from the mean. It indicates the degree of error that would result if the mean alone were used to interpret the data for a variable in a study. Fig. 9.1 presents the normal curve with the *SD* values representing the variability of scores in the curve. In Fig. 9.1, you note that the mean is zero (0) and each $SD = 1$, with 68.3% of the scores between -1 and $+1$ *SD* from the mean. A total of 95% of the scores for a variable in a study are between -1.96 and $+1.96$ *SD* from the mean. Values that are greater than $+1.96$ or -1.96 *SD* from the mean are significantly different at $p = 0.05$ when alpha (α) is set at 0.05. In a normal curve, 99% of the participants' scores are between -2.58 and $+2.58$ *SD*s from the mean. Variable scores or values that are greater than $+2.58$ or -2.58 *SD*s are significant at $p = 0.01$ (Gray & Grove, 2021; Terrell, 2021).

The *SD* is an important statistic, both for understanding dispersion within a distribution and for interpreting the relationship of a particular value to the distribution. When the scores of a distribution deviate from the mean considerably, the *SD* or spread of scores is large. When the degree of deviation of scores from the mean is small, the *SD* or spread of the scores is small. The equation and steps for calculating the standard deviation are presented in Exercise 28, which is focused on calculating descriptive statistics.

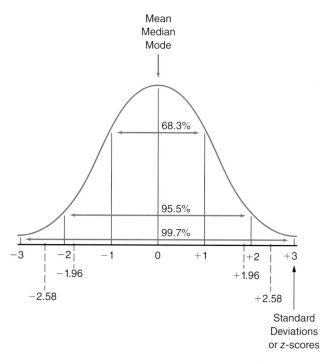

FIG. 9.1 ▪ NORMAL CURVE WITH THE STANDARD DEVIATION (*SD*) VALUES REPRESENTING THE VARIABILITY OF SCORES IN THE CURVE.

RESEARCH ARTICLE

Source

Brino, K. A. S., Derouin, A. L., & Silva, S. G. (2022). Problematic Internet use in adolescents and implementation of a social media hygiene protocol. *Journal of Pediatric Nursing, 63,* 84–89. https://doi.org/10.1016/j.pedn.2021.10.011

Introduction

Brino and colleagues (2022) conducted a quality improvement (QI) project to determine whether a social media hygiene education intervention designed for adolescents would improve their problematic Internet use (PIU) and their mental health status. The intervention was a 5-week educational program conducted via a telehealth system. PIU was measured using the Generalized Problematic Internet Use Scale (GPIUS-2). The GPIUS-2 is a 15-item Likert scale where adolescents self-reported their experiences on a scale ranging from 1, "Strongly Disagree," to 7, "Strongly Agree." The higher scores for GPIUS-2 indicated greater PIU and only the adolescents with a score of 52 or greater were offered the intervention in this study. Mental health outcomes were assessed using the Patient Health Questionnaire and Anxiety and Depression Scale (PHQ-ADS), which is a 16-item Likert scale. Brino and colleagues (2022, pp. 86–87) reported: "The PHQ-ADS combines the 16 items to derive a depression and anxiety total score, ranging from 0 to 48. Total scores from the PHQ-ADS are often used to categorize severity of depression and anxiety symptoms as minimal (0–9), mild (10–19), moderate (20–29) or severe (30–48)." The researchers concluded that the social media hygiene protocol could be used to reduce the severity of PIU and to improve mental health outcomes in adolescents.

Relevant Study Results

"Methods

Design

A within-adolescent pre-post design was used to evaluate changes in social media usage and mental health outcomes among adolescents with PIU seeking outpatient mental health care who received an ad hoc social media hygiene education intervention administered by their provider. . . . Outcomes were measured at the participant's initial clinical visit immediately preceding (pre-intervention) and immediately following completion of intervention (post-intervention). . . .

Setting

The setting for implementation was a nurse practitioner owned and fully staffed, pediatric outpatient behavioral health clinic in North Carolina. The clinic provides assessment and treatment for an average of 70–80 patients (aged 2–21 years) with mental and behavioral health conditions per week. Nearly half of the patients (46%) are adolescents between the age[s] of 12–18. . . .

Intervention

The intervention entailed a patient-centered education protocol using current screen time recommendations from the American Academy of Pediatrics as well as visual materials from internet blogs that focused on reducing internet-use and increasing social media awareness. The intervention for each participant was comprised of five, one-hour telehealth sessions completed over the course of five weeks" (Brino et al., 2022, p. 85).

"Results

A total of 125 adolescents age of 12 to 19 years seeking outpatient behavioral health care were invited to complete the GPIUS-2 during the three-month recruitment period, January through March 2020. Among the 125 approached, 75 completed the pre-intervention assessment. None of the 125 had an intellectual disability diagnosis. The GPIUS-2 total scores ranged from 26 to 122, and 50 of the 75 adolescents had a positive PIU screen as indicated by a total score of $\geq$52. Of the 50 who met the eligibility criteria, 22 did not receive the intervention due to scheduling conflicts. Therefore, the analysis sample included 28 adolescents with PIU. All 28 completed the pre- and post-intervention assessments.

The mean age of the 28 participants was 14.2 ($SD = 1.9$, range 12 to 17) years, consisting of primarily females (71.4%). The most common DSM-V [Diagnostic and Statistical Manual of Mental Disorders-5] mental health diagnoses among participants were anxiety (42.8%), depression (17.8%), ADHD [attention-deficit hyperactivity disorder] (28.5%), and adjustment disorder with mixed emotions (10.7%).

Table 9.1 summarizes the PIU and mental health results at the pre- and post-assessments as well the pre-minus-post difference scores. A significant improvement (reduction) was demonstrated for screen time as measured by average hours per day in the past 7-days ($t = 10.14$, $df = 27$, $p < 0.001$), severity of PIU as measured by the GPIUS-2 total scores ($t = 12.07$, $df = 27$, $p < 0.001$), and severity of depression and/or anxiety as indicated by the PHQ-ADS total scores ($t = 8.3$, $df = 27$, $p < 0.001$)" (Brino et al., 2022, p. 87).

TABLE 9.1   PREINTERVENTION AND POSTINTERVENTION PIU AND MENTAL HEALTH OUTCOMES (N = 28)

Variable	Pre Mean ± SD (min, max)	Post Mean ± SD (min, max)	Pre-Post Difference Mean ± SD (min, max)	Paired t-test p-value
Screen time, in hours per day	7.2 ± 3.7 (2.0, 16.0)	4.0 ± 2.8 (0.5, 11.0)	3.2 ± 1.7 (0.0, 7.0)	<0.001
GPIUS-2 total score	86.5 ± 15.1 (57.0, 122.0)	70.3 ± 14.8 (49.0, 99.0)	16.3 ± 7.1 (5.0, 29.0)	<0.001
PHQ-ADS total score	27.5 ± 9.2 (12.0, 42.0)	21.4 ± 8.7 (4.0, 38.0)	6.1 ± 3.9 (0.0, 15.0	<0.001

GPIUS-2 = Generalized Problematic Internet Use Scale; PHQ-ADS = Patient Health Questionnaire and Anxiety and Depression Scale; PIU = problematic Internet use; SD = Standard deviation. Screen time: Average hours per day during the past 7-days; GPIUS-2 total score: Severity of PIU; PHQ-ADS total score: Severity of depression or anxiety; preintervention and postintervention score: Higher scores indicate greater severity; pre-post difference: Greater positive difference scores indicate greater improvement (i.e., greater reduction in total scores). Pre-post difference skewness scores were less than 0.20.

Values abstracted from Table 2 in Brino, K. A. S., Derouin, A. L., & Silva, S. G. (2022). Problematic Internet use in adolescents and implementation of a social media hygiene protocol. *Journal of Pediatric Nursing, 63*, 87. https://doi.org/10.1016/j.pedn.2021.10.011

STUDY QUESTIONS

1. The mean ($\bar{X}$) is a measure of _____ _____ of a distribution, whereas the standard deviation (SD) is a measure of _____. Both the $\bar{X}$ and SD are _____ statistics.

2. What is the purpose of the range, and how is it determined in a distribution of scores? Provide an example of a range using hemoglobin A1c values for diabetics.

3. In the Brino et al. (2022) study, what were the $\bar{X}$, SD, and range for the demographic variable of age? Discuss the meaning of each of these descriptive statistics.

4. What was the range of ages for approximately 68% of the sample? Show your calculations and discuss the meaning of these results.

5. What measurement method was used to measure PIU in this study? What level of measurement was achieved with this instrument? Provide a rationale for your answer.

6. What was the $\bar{X}$, *SD*, and range for the adolescents' preintervention and postintervention screen time? How much did these values change after the social media hygiene protocol intervention?

7. Is there an outlier in the postintervention screen time data? Provide a rationale for your response.

8. Did the adolescents' screen time change significantly after the social media hygiene intervention? Provide a rationale for your response.

9. After the intervention, what was the range for screen time in hours per day for 95% of the study participants? Show your calculations.

10. What were the most common mental health diagnoses for this group of adolescents? What do these results indicate?

Answers to Study Questions

1. The $\bar{X}$ is a measure of central tendency of a distribution, whereas the standard deviation (SD) is a measure of dispersion. Both the $\bar{X}$ and SD are descriptive or summary statistics.

2. Range is the simplest measure of dispersion or variability, obtained by identifying the lowest and highest scores in a distribution or by subtracting the lowest score from the highest score in the distribution of scores (Grove & Gray, 2023). For example, five study participants' hemoglobin A1c (HbA1c) were 7.9, 7.4, 7.2, 7.8, and 7.6. The range for these scores would be 7.2 to 7.9 or $7.9 - 7.2 = 0.7$. The range identifies the lowest score and highest score in a distribution so it can be used to identify outliers, which are extremely high or low scores compared with the other scores in a distribution (Grove & Gray, 2023; Kim et al., 2022).

3. The mean age of the 28 study participants was 14.2, with an SD of 1.9 and a range of ages from 12 to 17 years. The study included only adolescents and the average age of 14.2 seems appropriate for the sample studied. The SD is small, indicating a homogeneous group with minimal variation in age. The range indicated that only adolescents were included in the sample, with no outliers for age (Gray & Grove, 2021).

4. Approximately 68% of the study participants were between 12.3 and 16.1 years of age, which is usually recorded as (12.3, 16.1). Calculations: 68.3% sample = $\bar{X} \pm SD$, which is $14.2 \pm 1.9 = (12.3, 16.1)$ in this sample. The participants are all adolescents with a narrow range of ages.

5. PIU was measured with the GPIUS-2 Likert scale that included self-reported ratings ranging from 1, "Strongly Disagree," to 7, "Strongly Agree." The total score for this 15-item scale was examined in this study (see Table 9.1). Likert scales include ordinal-level data; but if the scores from a multi-item scale are normally distributed, the data are analyzed as interval level (see Exercise 1; Bandalos, 2018; Waltz et al., 2017).

6. The adolescents' preintervention screen time, in hours per day, had a $\bar{X} = 7.2$, $SD = 3.7$, and a range of 2.0 to 16.0. The adolescents' postintervention screen time, in hours per day, had a $\bar{X} = 4.0$, $SD = 2.8$, and a range of 0.5 to 11.0. The preintervention and postintervention difference is presented in Table 9.1 as $\bar{X} = 3.2$, $SD = 1.7$, and a range of 0.0 to 7.0. After the social media hygiene intervention, the mean screen time declined by 3 hours per day. The SD and range also declined after the intervention, indicating less variability in the adolescents' screen time values.

7. In examining Table 9.1, the screen time minimal value postintervention was 0.5, which might be an outlier. Further examination of the data is needed to determine outliers for the dependent variables. However, if outliers were identified, they did not affect the distribution of scores because scores for all three dependent variables were normally distributed. Brino et al. (2022, p. 87) reported in the key for Table 9.1 that the "pre-post difference skewness scores were less than 0.20," so the data for all variables were normally distributed.

8. Yes, the adolescents' screen time in hours per day changed significantly from preintervention to postintervention as indicated by "$t = 10.14$, $df = 27$, $p < 0.001$" (Brino et al., 2022, p. 87). The p value is less than α, set at 0.05 for this study, indicating the results were significant for this variable (Gray & Grove, 2021).

9. In the Brino et al. (2022) study, the range for screen time hours per day for 95% of the adolescents after the intervention was from a low of -1.49 to a high of 9.49 (-1.49, 9.49). The negative number of screen time hours (-1.49) is confusing and would rarely be found in a study. When this kind of calculation happens, it is usually due to a nonnormal distribution and/or a small sample size (which is the case here with $N = 28$).

$$\text{Calculations: 95\% sample scores} = \bar{X} \pm (1.96 \times SD). \text{ In this study, } 4.00 \pm (1.96 \times 2.80)$$
$$= 4.00 \pm 5.49 = (-1.49, 9.49) \text{ in this sample.}$$

10. "The most common DSM-V [Diagnostic and Statistical Manual of Mental Disorders-5] mental health diagnoses among participants were anxiety (42.8%), depression (17.8%), ADHD [attention-deficit hyperactivity disorder] (28.5%), and adjustment disorder with mixed emotions (10.7%)" (Brino et al., 2022, p. 87). The percentages of adolescents with mental health diagnoses were high, especially for anxiety and ADHD. Mental health issues are a severe problem for adolescents that have a link to screen time. PIU and mental health issues require assessment and management by nurses in schools and clinical settings.

Questions for Additional Study

Name: _____ Class: _____

Date: _____

Follow your instructor's directions to submit your answers to the following questions for additional study. Your instructor may ask you to write your answers below and submit them as a hard copy for evaluation. Alternatively, your instructor may ask you to submit your answers online.

1. What type of design was implemented in the Brino et al. (2022) study? Were the groups in this study independent or dependent (i.e., paired)? Provide a rationale for your answer.

2. What were the dependent variables in this study (see Table 9.1)? Were these variables appropriate for this study? Provide a rationale for your response.

3. What analysis techniques were calculated to describe the dispersion or variability of the scores for the dependent variables identified in Question 2? Were these techniques appropriate? Provide a rationale for your response.

4. What measurement method was used to measure anxiety and depression in this study? What level of measurement was achieved with this instrument? Provide a rationale for your response.

5. What were the $\bar{X}$, *SD*, and range for the dependent variables of anxiety and depression for the preintervention scores? Discuss the meaning of each of these descriptive statistics.

6. What is the range of the preintervention PHQ-ADS total scores for approximately 68% of the adolescents in this sample? Show your calculations and discuss the meaning of these results.

7. What was the $\bar{X}$, *SD*, and range for the adolescents' postintervention PHQ-ADS total scores? How much did these values change from preintervention to after the social media hygiene protocol intervention? Discuss the meaning of these results.

8. Did the adolescents' PHQ-ADS total score change significantly after the social media hygiene intervention? Provide a rationale for your response.

9. Is PIU a severe issue for adolescents in this study? Provide a rationale for your response.

10. Are the findings from the Brino et al. (2022) study ready for use in practice? Provide a rationale for your response.

STATISTICAL TECHNIQUE IN REVIEW

Most research reports describe the participants who compose the study sample. This description of the sample is called the **sample characteristics.** These characteristics are often presented in a table and narrative within the research report. Data are collected for demographic and clinical variables to describe the sample. **Demographic variables** are attribute variables such as age, gender, and ethnicity collected to describe a sample and as a basis for comparison with the demographic characteristics in other studies. **Clinical variables** are selective physical, emotional, and cognitive variables collected and analyzed to describe the specific clinical characteristics of the study sample. The sample characteristics might be presented for the entire sample or for the different groups in a study (e.g., intervention and control groups) (Grove & Gray, 2023; Kazdin, 2022). If a study includes an intervention group and a comparison or control group, the demographic and clinical characteristics for these two groups are usually compared prior to the conduct of the study. The groups need to be similar at the start of the study to decrease the potential for extraneous variables altering the effect of the intervention on the dependent variables (Gray & Grove, 2021; Shadish et al., 2002).

The descriptive statistics conducted to generate the sample characteristics depend on the level of measurement of the demographic and clinical variables included in a study (see Exercise 1; Grove & Gray, 2023). For example, data collected on gender are nominal level and can be described using frequencies, percentages, and mode (see Exercises 6 and 8). Measuring an educational level usually produces ordinal data that can be described using frequencies, percentages, mode, median, and range. Obtaining each participant's specific age is an example of ratio data that can be described using mean, median, range, and standard deviation (see Exercise 9). Interval and ratio data are analyzed with the same statistical techniques and are sometimes referred to as interval- or ratio-level data in this text.

RESEARCH ARTICLE

Source

Riegel, B., Dickson, V. V., Lee, C. S., Daus, M., Hill, J., Irani, E., Lee, S., Wald, J. W., Moelter, S. T., Rathman, L., Streur, M., Baah, F. O., Ruppert, L., Schwartz, D. R., & Bove, A. (2018). A mixed methods study of symptom perception in patients with chronic heart failure. *Heart & Lung, 47*(2), 107–114. https://doi.org/10.1016/j.hrtlng.2017.11.002

Introduction

Riegel and colleagues (2018) conducted a longitudinal sequential explanatory mixed methods study to examine the symptom perceptions of patients with chronic heart failure (HF). A mixed methods study includes both quantitative and qualitative research methods. An exploratory sequential design begins with the collection and analysis of qualitative data, followed by the collection of quantitative data. Often, findings of the qualitative data analyses are used to design the quantitative phase (Creswell & Clark, 2018; Gray & Grove, 2021). Riegel et al. (2018) enrolled a small sample of 36 HF patients to allow depth rather than breadth of data collected (Creswell & Creswell, 2023; Creswell & Poth, 2018). "Maximum variability was sought in participant age, gender, HF duration and severity, and comorbidity" to promote understanding of HF patients' perceptions and management of their symptoms (Riegel et al., 2018, p. 108). The researchers collected demographic data such as age, gender, education, socioeconomic status, race, employment, marital status, and self-reported income. Likert scales were used to collect data on depression, decision-making, and self-care maintenance and management. "Clinical characteristics (e.g. such as HF duration, type, ejection fraction) were abstracted from the medical record" (Riegel et al., 2018, p. 109). Other clinical data such as cognitive function, comorbidity, and New York Heart Association (NYHA) class were also collected to describe the patients with HF.

Riegel et al. (2018) determined "that although some HF patients had systems in place for monitoring their symptoms, problems with symptom detection were evident, interpretation was poor, and problems in management delayed response. . . . Notably, even the most savvy patients in this sample were not able to avoid a HF hospitalization. Further research is greatly needed on this topic if we are to achieve the goal of rapid response to signs and symptoms and early medical intervention in patients with HF, thereby decreasing HF hospitalization" (Riegel et al., 2018, p. 113).

Relevant Study Results

"After obtaining Institutional Review Board approval, we enrolled a sample of community dwelling HF patients from outpatient settings affiliated with two university hospitals in Philadelphia, Pennsylvania. All participants gave written informed consent. We collected baseline and 3-month data during home visits. Biweekly, participants were telephoned to ask about their symptoms over the past week. Those who had experienced symptoms were interviewed in depth" (Riegel et al., 2018, p. 108).

"Results

The enrolled sample of 36 was predominately male (67%), older (64 ± 15.2 years), White (61%), and functionally compromised (56% NYHA class III), with a moderate level of comorbidity (42%). See Table 10.1. Seven participants withdrew or were lost to follow-up before the final home visit, but only one withdrew early, so a rich dataset was available on each of these participants.

At enrollment, self-care was poor overall. Self-care maintenance scores were barely adequate (mean 69.8 ± 13.5, range 33–93). Self-care management scores (64.4 ± 18.9, range 35–90) and self-care confidence were low (mean 68.4 ± 19.1, range 17–100) as well. The HFSPS [Heart Failure Somatic Perception Scale] total score was low (mean 8.1 ± 10.6, range 0–51), the HFSPS Dyspnea subscale score was also low (mean 1.8 ± 3.7, range 0–15), as was the daily diary fatigue score (mean 4.1 ± 6.6, range 0–24), indicating that few were symptomatic on enrollment. Within the 3-month follow-up period, four participants were admitted to the hospital for HF; two of these four were admitted twice" (Riegel et al., 2018, p. 109).

TABLE 10.1 DEMOGRAPHIC AND CLINICAL CHARACTERISTICS OF THE FULL SAMPLE ($N = 36$)		
	Mean ± *SD*	***n*, Percentage (%)**
Patient Characteristics		
Age (years)	63.8 ± 15.2	
Socioeconomic status (Barratt Simplified Measure of Social Status)	43.8 ± 11.1	
Depression (PHQ–9)	4.5 ± 4.1	
MoCA score	25.28 ± 3.1	
CCI score	3.36 ± 2.0	
Ejection fraction (%)	37.4 ± 16.8	
HF duration in months	135.4 ± 102.2	
Total number of medications	10.9 ± 4.8	
Male		24 (66.7)
Race		
African American		9 (25.0)
Caucasian		22 (61.1)
Mixed or other		5 (13.9)
Education		
High school or less		6 (16.7)
Some trade or college education (e.g., vocational, associate's degree)		16 (44.4)
College (bachelor's degree or higher)		14 (38.9)
Employment		
Employed full- or part-time		12 (33.3)
Unemployed (e.g., sick leave, disability, retired)		23 (63.9)
Other (e.g., student)		1 (2.8)
Marital Status		
Single		4 (11.1)
Married		24 (66.7)
Divorced or separated		6 (16.7)
Widowed		2 (5.6)
Self-Reported Income		
More than enough to make ends meet		20 (55.6)
Enough to make ends meet		13 (36.1)
Not enough to make ends meet		3 (8.3)
Quality of Support		
Satisfactory		2 (5.6)
Good		6 (16.7)
Very good		28 (77.8)

TABLE 10.1	DEMOGRAPHIC AND CLINICAL CHARACTERISTICS OF THE FULL SAMPLE (*N* = 36)—cont'd	
	Mean ± *SD*	*n*, Percentage (%)
Perceived Health		
Poor		5 (14.3)
Fair		16 (45.7)
Good		8 (22.9)
Very good		6 (17.1)
Abnormal MoCA Score (<26)		19 (52.8)
Categorized CCI Score		
Low level (CCI 1–2)		13 (36.1)
Moderate level (CCI 3–4)		15 (41.7)
High level (CCI ≥5)		8 (22.2)
Common Comorbid Conditions		
Atrial fibrillation		15 (41.7)*
Myocardial infarction		14 (38.9)
Sleep disordered breathing		14 (38.9)
Diabetes		13 (36.1)
Chronic pain		8 (22.2)
Chronic obstructive pulmonary disease		8 (22.2)
Cerebrovascular accident		7 (19.4)
Renal disease		6 (16.7)
NYHA Class		
I		3 (8.6)
II		11 (31.4)
III		20 (57.1)
IV		1 (2.9)

CCI = Charlson Comorbidity Index; HF = heart failure; PHQ-9 = Patient Health Questionnaire; MoCA = Montreal Cognitive Assessment; NYHA = New York Heart Association.

*Percentages were calculated by the formula: $n/36 \times 100$. (Each disease was treated individually, so the sum of percentages under "common comorbidity conditions" is not 100.)

From Riegel, B., Dickson, V. V., Lee, C. S., Daus, M., Hill, J., Irani, E., Lee, S., Wald, J. W., Moelter, S. T., Rathman, L., Streur, M., Baah, F. O., Ruppert, L., Schwartz, D. R., & Bove, A. (2018). A mixed methods study of symptom perception in patients with chronic heart failure. *Heart & Lung, 47*(2), 110. https://doi.org/10.1016/j.hrtlng.2017.11.002

STUDY QUESTIONS

1. What type of variables are age, gender, education, and socioeconomic status in the Riegel et al. (2018) study? Are these variables commonly described in nursing studies? Provide a rationale for your response.

2. What levels of measurement are the age and gender variables identified in Table 10.1? Provide a rationale for your response.

3. What analysis techniques were conducted to describe age and gender? Were these analysis techniques appropriate? Provide a rationale for your response.

4. What was the mode for marital status in this study? Provide a rationale for your response.

5. What level of measurement is the quality of support variable? Provide a rationale for your response.

6. What statistics were conducted to describe quality of support? Were these appropriate? Could additional statistics have been conducted? Provide a rationale for your response.

7. Was a mean calculated for the clinical variable of perceived health? Provide a rationale for your response.

8. Was the sample for the Riegel et al. (2018) study adequately described? Provide a rationale for your response.

9. Describe the dyspnea subscale score for this sample of patients with HF. Were there outliers in these data? Provide a rationale for your response.

10. Were the HF patients' self-care confidence scores strong in the study? Provide a rationale for your answer. What do these scores indicate clinically about this sample?

Answers to Study Questions

1. Age, gender, education, and socioeconomic status are demographic variables that were described in this study. Riegel et al. (2018) identified these as demographic variables in the study narrative and in Table 10.1. Yes, these are common demographic variables described by nurses and other health professionals in their studies. Researchers can compare their sample characteristics with those from other studies including these variables (Gray & Grove, 2021). Federal grant guidelines often encourage researchers to describe their sample with these common demographic variables (see National Institute of Nursing Research website at https://www.ninr.nih.gov/researchandfunding/desp/oep/fundingopportunities).

2. Age is measured at the ratio level because the specific age of each patient in years was obtained. Age in years is a continuous variable where each year equals 12 months or 365 days. Age has an absolute zero where 0 years old indicates the absence of age (see Exercise 1; Grove & Gray, 2023; Waltz et al., 2017). The data collected for gender in this study include two categories, male and female. These categories are basically exhaustive and mutually exclusive because all study participants fit into one category. Male and female gender cannot be ranked, so the data are nominal.

3. Mean ($\bar{X}$) and standard deviation (*SD*) were computed to describe the variable of age because it was measured at the ratio level. Ratio-level data are best analyzed with parametric statistics, such as $\bar{X}$ and *SD* (see Exercise 1; Grove & Gray, 2023; Kim et al., 2022). Frequencies and percentages were calculated to describe the variable of gender. The data for gender are nominal-level measurements, so frequencies and percentages are appropriate (see Exercise 6). The researchers might have also identified the mode, which was male (66.7% or 67%) for this sample (Waltz et al., 2017).

4. The mode for marital status was married, which included 24 participants (66.7%). The mode is the measure of central tendency for analyzing nominal-level data. Mode is defined as the numerical value or score that occurs with the greatest frequency in a dataset (see Exercise 8; Grove & Gray, 2023; Terrell, 2021).

5. The quality of support variable is measured at the ordinal level. The measurement of quality of support was achieved using four categories (i.e., poor, fair, good, and very good) that can be ranked from a low of poor to a high of very good. These categories can be ranked but do not have equal intervals between the categories as with interval-level data (see Exercise 1; Grove & Gray, 2023; Waltz et al., 2017).

6. The quality of support variable was described with frequencies and percentages. Frequencies and percentages are appropriate analyses, but the data for quality of support are at the ordinal level and additional analyses of median and range could have been calculated to expand the description of this variable (Grove & Gray, 2023).

7. Riegel et al. (2018) analyzed perceived health data as though at the ordinal level. Frequencies and percentages were calculated but not $\bar{X}$ or SD (Grove & Gray, 2023; Waltz et al., 2017). Perceived health was organized into four categories (i.e., poor, fair, good, and very good) that are exhaustive and exclusive. Perceived health levels can be ranked from a low of poor to a high of very good. However, perceived health was not considered a continuous variable in this study (Gray & Grove, 2021; Kim et al., 2022).

8. Yes, the sample was adequately described for common demographic variables such as age, socioeconomic status, gender, race, education, employment, marital status, and self-reported income. Clinical characteristics were also detailed for this group of patients with HF, including depression, HF duration, quality of support, perceived health, categorized Charlson Comorbidity Index, common comorbid conditions, and NYHA class (see Table 10.1). The descriptive data analyses were appropriate for the level of measurement of the demographic and clinical variables, including frequencies and percentages for nominal- and ordinal-level data and ($\bar{X}$) and SD for ratio-level data. The description of these demographic and clinical variables provided a detailed picture of the sample in Table 10.1 that was supplemented by the study narrative.

9. "The dyspnea subscale score was also low (mean 1.8 ± 3.7, range 0–15)" (Riegel et al., 2018, p. 109). Yes, the distribution of dyspnea data appeared to have an outlier because the mean was 1.8 and the top score in the range is 15 (see Exercise 9). The score of 15 is much higher than the mean and is probably an outlier. However, the distribution of scores needs to be examined further for outliers and normality of the distribution (see Exercise 27).

10. No, the self-care confidence scores in this study were not strong. Riegel et al. (2018, p. 109) stated the "self-care confidence scores were low (mean 68.4 ± 19.1, range 17–100)." Low self-confidence scores are clinically important because they indicate the uncertainty and probable problems these patients and family members are having in assessing and managing their HF symptoms. These patients need additional support and education to improve their self-confidence and possibly decrease their HF symptoms and reduce their need for hospitalization.

Questions for Additional Study

10

Name: _____ Class: _____

Date: _____

Follow your instructor's directions to submit your answers to the following questions for additional study. Your instructor may ask you to write your answers below and submit them as a hard copy for evaluation. Alternatively, your instructor may ask you to submit your answers online.

1. In the Riegel et al. (2018) study, what level of measurement is the employment variable? Provide a rationale for your response with documentation.

2. What statistics were conducted to describe heart failure (HF) duration in this study? Were these appropriate? Provide a rationale for your response.

3. What is the mode for the New York Heart Association (NYHA) class in the Riegel et al. (2018) study? Why is this clinically important?

4. What statistics were conducted to describe the NYHA class in this study? Were these appropriate? Provide a rationale for your response.

5. In the Riegel et al. (2018) study, depression was measured with the Patient Health Questionnaire (PHQ-9). What level of measurement is the depression variable? Provide a rationale for your response with documentation.

6. What statistics were conducted to describe depression in this study? Were these appropriate? Provide a rationale for your response.

7. Was the sample size adequate for this study? Provide a rationale for your response.

8. Describe the fatigue scores for this sample of patients with HF. Do these data appear to have an outlier(s)? Provide a rationale for your response.

9. Describe the HF patients' self-care maintenance and self-care management scores. Discuss the clinical importance of these scores.

10. Are the findings from the Riegel et al. (2018) study ready for use in practice? Provide a rationale for your response with documentation.

Interpreting Scatterplots

STATISTICAL TECHNIQUE IN REVIEW

Scatterplots or scattergrams are used to describe relationships between two variables and to provide a graphic representation of data from a study. Variables are illustrated on two axes, x and y. The x-axis is the horizontal axis, and the y-axis is the vertical axis (see Fig. 11.1). To provide a visual image of the data, each point on the graph is a participant's values for variables x and y, thus representing the relationship between these variables on the graph. Each participant's values on the two variables are plotted on the graph, and the number of points on the graph depends on the study sample size (Gray & Grove, 2021). In the example scatterplot in Fig. 11.1, there are 20 points, so this example includes a sample of 20 participants.

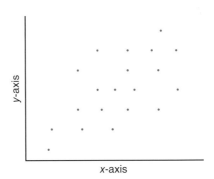

FIG. 11-1 ▬ **FORMAT FOR A SCATTERPLOT.**

Direction and Strength of Relationships in Scatterplots

The display of points on the scatterplot graph indicates the direction (i.e., positive or negative) and strength (i.e., weak, moderate, or strong) of the relationship between the two variables studied. Scatterplot points moving from the lower left corner to the upper right corner illustrate a **positive or direct linear relationship**. In a positive relationship the variables being correlated vary together in the same direction. When one variable value increases, the other variable value increases, or when one variable decreases, the other variable decreases. Fig. 11.2 identifies a positive relationship between the variables of low-density lipoprotein (LDL) cholesterol and grams of dietary fat consumed a day: as the grams of fat consumed increase, so does the LDL cholesterol value. The line through the points on the graph identifies the direction or nature of the relationship (Gray & Grove, 2021).

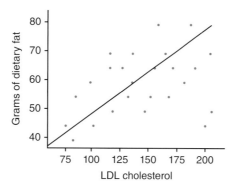

FIG. 11.2 ▪ **POSITIVE RELATIONSHIP BETWEEN LOW-DENSITY LIPOPROTEIN (LDL) CHOLESTEROL AND GRAMS OF DIETARY FAT CONSUMED (*N* = 24).**

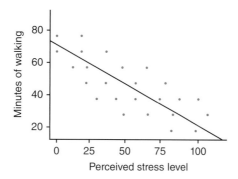

FIG. 11.3 ▪ **NEGATIVE RELATIONSHIP BETWEEN MINUTES OF WALKING AND PERCEIVED STRESS LEVEL (*N* = 25).**

In a **negative or inverse linear relationship,** the values for two variables vary in the opposite or inverse direction; as the values for one variable increase, the values for the other variable decrease. In a negative relationship the points on the scatterplot move from the upper left corner to the lower right corner. Fig. 11.3 demonstrates a negative relationship between the variables of perceived stress level and minutes of walking. An increase in minutes of walking is associated with a decrease in perceived stress level (Grove & Gray, 2023).

The strength or magnitude of the relationships shown in scatterplots range from −1 to +1, with −1 indicating a perfect negative relationship between two variables and +1 indicating a perfect positive relationship between two variables. Pearson *r* (see Exercises 13 and 29) is calculated to determine the strength of the relationship between two continuous variables or variables measured at the interval or ratio level (see Exercise 1). The strengths of relationships are determined using the absolute value of the *r*. A weak relationship is <0.30, a moderate relationship is 0.30 to 0.50, and a strong relationship is >0.50. (Cohen, 1988; Gray & Grove, 2021; Plichta & Kelvin, 2013). The closer the plotted points are to each other and the more they approximate a straight line, the stronger the linear relationship between the two variables (see Figs. 11.2 and 11.3). Conversely, if the plotted points are further away from each other and widespread across the graph, this indicates a weak relationship that is closer to 0. The widespread data points in Fig. 11.4 demonstrate a relationship approximately equal to 0, or no relationship (Grove & Gray, 2023). A scatterplot

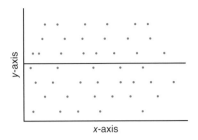

FIG. 11.4 ■ **SCATTERPLOT OF A RELATIONSHIP APPROXIMATELY EQUAL TO 0.0.**

visually represents a relationship between two variables, but Pearson r correlational analysis must be calculated to determine the specific value for the strength of the relationship and to determine statistical significance (Gray & Grove, 2021; Kim et al., 2022).

Identifying Outliers by Developing a Scatterplot

When looking at scatterplots, it is important to identify outliers. **Outliers** are extreme values in the dataset that occur with inherent variability, measurement error, sampling error, and errors in study implementation. Outliers are exceptions to the overall findings of a study that can affect the normality of the distribution and result in a skewed set of data (see Exercises 8 and 27; Grove & Gray, 2023). Fig. 11.2 has an example of two outliers in the lower right corner of the graph. These values represent participants with high LDL cholesterol values close to 200, whose consumption of dietary fat is 40 to 45 grams per day. Researchers use scatterplots to identify linear and nonlinear relationships, but the focus of this exercise is understanding linear relationships (Gray & Grove, 2021; Kim et al., 2022).

RESEARCH ARTICLE

Source

Faria, G., Santos, P. B., Marinho, R. S., Firmino, S. M., Rizzatti, F. P., Mendes, R. G., Borghi-Silva, A., & Roscani, M. G. (2022). Association of right ventricle diastolic diameter with pulmonary function, exercise tolerance and exacerbation period in patients with chronic obstructive pulmonary disease: A prospective study. *Heart & Lung, 55,* 11–15. https://doi.org/10.1016/j.hrtlng.2022.04.003

Introduction

Faria and colleagues (2022) conducted a prospective longitudinal study to examine the association of right ventricular diastolic diameter (RVDD) with exercise tolerance, pulmonary function, and exacerbation periods for individuals with chronic obstructive pulmonary disease (COPD). This observational study included 91 patients diagnosed with COPD who were stratified into two groups, those with RVDD greater than 35 mm and those with RVDD less than 35 mm. All participants were clinically assessed using echocardiography to determine RVDD, spirometry to measure pulmonary function of forced vital capacity (FVC), and the 6-minute walking test (6MWT) to determine exercise tolerance. These patients were followed for 12 months through telephone calls and medical consultation every 3 months. Faria et al. (2022) concluded that increased RVDD was associated with decreased pulmonary function and exercise tolerance and increased exacerbations in patients with COPD.

Relevant Study Results

"Statistical analysis

The required number of patients to be assessed is $n = 40$, being necessary 20 patients for each group evaluated, assuming a risk of α of 5%, effect size 0.6 and β of 0.95. The Shapiro-Wilk test was used to verify the normality of the data. Descriptive variables were listed as mean, standard deviation, and percentage (%). To test the hypothesis of our study, we applied: (1) The Student's t-test for comparison between patients with exacerbation vs no-exacerbation; (2) The Pearson correlation analysis was performed to investigate the correlations between variables, and (3) A linear regression model was used to determine the influence of RVDD on distance in 6MWT. A p value ≤ 0.05 was considered as statistically significant for all tests, and all tests were made in GraphPad Prism 7.0 (GraphPad Software, California, USA).

Results

This study included 91 eligible patients. In the one-year follow-up, 25 (17%) patients had exacerbation and hospitalization for COPD. . . . The patients were predominantly classified as GOLD [Global Initiative for Chronic Obstructive Lung Disease] II (40%) and III (36%) COPD severities. The included patients were also stratified according to RVDD greater and less than 35 mm. . . . It was found that patients with RVDD greater than 35 mm had worse FC [functional capacity] in the 6MWT ($p = 0.05$), with no significant difference in age. Additionally, these patients had more exacerbation during the one-year follow-up ($p = 0.05$).

There was a statistically significant correlation of the . . . predicted FVC and the RVDD ($r = -0.26$; $p = 0.02$) in patients with COPD exacerbation (Fig. 11.5, $p < 0.05$), demonstrating that the larger the RVDD, the worse the pulmonary function. Additionally, there was a statistically significant correlation between the 6MWT and the RVDD ($R = -0.55$; $p = 0.03$) in COPD patients with exacerbations, which means the larger the RVDD, the worse the FC in these individuals (Fig. 11.6)" (Faria et al., 2022, pp. 12–13).

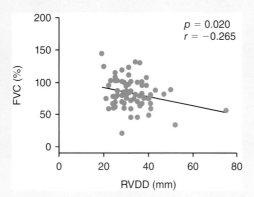

FIG. 11.5 ▪ **RELATIONSHIP OF FORCED VITAL CAPACITY (FVC) VS RIGHT VENTRICULAR DIASTOLIC DIAMETER (RVDD) IN CHRONIC OBSTRUCTIVE PULMONARY DISEASE (COPD) PATIENTS ($N = 76$).** Faria, G., Santos, P. B., Marinho, R. S., Firmino, S. M., Rizzatti, F. P., Mendes, R. G., Borghi-Silva, A., & Roscani, M. G. (2022). Association of right ventricle diastolic diameter with pulmonary function, exercise tolerance and exacerbation period in patients with chronic obstructive pulmonary disease: A prospective study. *Heart & Lung, 55,* 14. https://doi.org/10.1016/j.hrtlng.2022.04.003

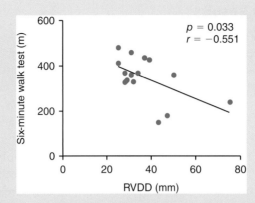

FIG. 11.6 ■ **RELATIONSHIP OF THE 6-MINUTE WALK TEST IN THE GROUP WITH EXACERBATION FOR THE DISEASE.** Faria, G., Santos, P. B., Marinho, R. S., Firmino, S. M., Rizzatti, F. P., Mendes, R. G., Borghi-Silva, A., & Roscani, M. G. (2022). Association of right ventricle diastolic diameter with pulmonary function, exercise tolerance and exacerbation period in patients with chronic obstructive pulmonary disease: A prospective study. *Heart & Lung, 55,* 14. https://doi.org/10.1016/j.hrtlng.2022.04.003

"Discussion

The main point observed in this study was that diameters of RVDD greater than 35 mm were associated with worse FC and more frequent exacerbation of the disease in the one-year follow-up. Patients with COPD, in addition to frequent exacerbations and hospitalizations, may progress to ventricular dysfunction and right heart failure. . . .

The main clinical implication for the future practice of this study is that the RVDD may be a good echocardiographic variable to monitor [in] COPD patients who need more aggressive therapeutic strategies as a way to prevent hospitalization for exacerbation, and to identify patients who may benefit from inclusion in a pulmonary rehabilitation program with the aim of improving FC.

Further studies are necessary to investigate prospectively echocardiographic variables, including the RVDD, as potential predictors of unfavorable outcomes in COPD patients" (Faria et al., pp. 13–14).

STUDY QUESTIONS

1. What is a scatterplot? What elements are included in a graph of a scatterplot?

2. In Fig. 11.2, what variable is on the *x*-axis and what variable is on the *y*-axis? What type of relationship is shown in Fig. 11.2? Provide a rationale for your response.

3. What is an outlier? What are the potential reasons for outliers occurring in a study?

4. Does the scatterplot in Fig. 11.2 include any outliers? Provide a rationale for your response.

5. What type of relationship (i.e., positive or negative) does Fig. 11.3 illustrate? Provide a rationale for your answer. What is the meaning of this relationship?

6. By looking at the scatterplot shown in Fig. 11.3, can you tell approximately what the magnitude of the relationship might be? Provide a rationale for your response.

7. What is the strength of the relationship presented in Fig. 11.4? Provide a rationale for your response.

8. Review Fig. 11.5 from the Faria et al. (2022) study and identify how many data points are on this scatterplot. What does each point represent?

9. What variables were graphed in Fig. 11.5? What type of relationship is presented in this figure? Provide a rationale for your response.

10. What is the strength or magnitude of the relationship in Fig. 11.5? Is this relationship significant? Provide a rationale for your response. What are the clinical implications of this result for patients with COPD?

Answers to Study Questions

1. A scatterplot is used to describe a relationship between two variables and provides a graphic representation of the data collected on these two variables from study participants. The elements included in a scatterplot are presented in Fig. 11.1. These elements include an *x*-axis with the name of one variable and a *y*-axis with the name of the other variable examined for association. The points that represent the participants' values for two study variables are plotted on the scatterplot (Gray & Grove, 2021; Terrell, 2021).

2. Fig. 11.2 shows a positive or direct relationship between the LDL cholesterol and grams of dietary fat. The plotted points move from the lower left corner to the upper right corner, indicating a positive relationship where the two variables change in the same direction. Therefore a decrease in LDL cholesterol is associated with a decrease in grams of dietary fat, or vice versa, an increase in grams of dietary fat is associated with an increase in LDL cholesterol. Normally, individuals consume about 55 to 70 grams of dietary fat a day.

3. Outliers are extreme values in the dataset that occur with inherent variability, measurement error, sampling error, and errors in study implementation. Outliers are exceptions to the overall study results that can affect the normality of a distribution (Gray & Grove, 2021; Kazdin, 2022; Kim et al., 2022).

4. Yes, Fig. 11.2 has two outliers in the right lower corner above the LDL cholesterol value of 200. These participants' values are very different than the others on the scatterplot because they consume diets low in fat and have high LDL cholesterol values. The distribution of data in a study should be tested for normality before implementing inferential statistics. LDL cholesterol and grams of dietary fat are measured at the ratio level; so, if the scores are normally distributed, parametric analyses can be conducted (Gray & Grove, 2021).

5. Fig. 11.3 illustrates a negative relationship. The points in this scatterplot extend from the left upper corner to the right lower corner, which is typical of a negative relationship. In this graph, minutes of walking is negatively associated with perceived stress level. Thus as the minutes of walking increase, the participants' perceived stress levels decrease.

6. Yes, by looking at a scatterplot you can know the approximate strength of a relationship. With strong relationships, the plotted points are close together and located on or close to the line drawn through the points. A moderate relationship has increased spacing among the points and varying distance of the points from the line drawn through them. Weak relationships have varied spacing of the points with no clear direction as the *r* value approaches 0.0 (see Fig. 11.4). Thus Fig. 11.3 approximates a strong relationship based on the placement of the points to each other and the line. However, the specific strength of the relationship between two variables is determined with Pearson *r* correlational analysis and is what is presented in a research report (Terrell, 2021).

7. Fig. 11.4 approximates a very weak or no relationship because the plotted points are widespread and do not form a direction for the relationship. For example, a person's cognitive score would not be expected to have an association with their number of siblings. Thus the relationship would be weak and close to 0.0.

8. In the Faria et al. (2022) study, the note under Fig. 11.5 identified that the graph included the scores from 76 patients with COPD. Thus the plotted points are the scores or values for each participant's RVDD in mm and FVC in percentages.

9. In Fig. 11.5 of the Faria et al. (2022) study, the variable on the x-axis is RVDD in mm, and the variable on the y-axis is FVC in percentage (%). These might also be referred to as the x-variable and y-variable. Fig. 11.5 is a negative relationship because the data points extend from the left upper corner of the graph to the right lower corner of the graph and the reported $r = -0.265$.

10. The strength of the relationship in Fig. 11.5 is $r = -0.265$, which is a weak relationship (<0.30 in absolute value) (Cohen, 1988; Grove & Gray, 2023). The r value is significant because $p = 0.020$ is less than the alpha $= 0.05$ set for this study. The study results identified a weak, negative association of the participants' RVDD with their FVC. When the participants' RVDD values got higher (>35 mm), their FVCs were reduced.

Questions for Additional Study

Name: _____ Class: _____

Date: _____

Follow your instructor's directions to submit your answers to the following questions for additional study. Your instructor may ask you to write your answers below and submit them as a hard copy for evaluation. Alternatively, your instructor may ask you to submit your answers online.

1. Why might researchers choose to include a scatterplot in the publication of their study?

2. Examine the direction and magnitude of the scatterplots in this exercise. Then develop your own scatterplot that presents a moderate, positive relationship between two variables for a sample of 30 individuals with heart failure (HF).

3. Identify the *x*-variable and the *y*-variable presented in Fig. 11.6 of the Faria et al. (2022) study. What is the importance of examining these variables in this study?

4. Describe the pattern of plotted points in Fig. 11.6 from the Faria et al. (2022) study. What type of relationship (i.e., positive or negative) does this figure illustrate? Provide a rationale for your response.

5. Did Fig. 11.6 include any outliers? Provide a rationale for your response. If an outlier was identified, did it affect the distribution of the data presented in this figure? Provide a rationale for your response.

6. What is the strength of the relationship shown in Fig. 11.6? Is this relationship significant? Provide a rationale for your response.

7. State the null hypothesis for the two variables presented in Fig. 11.6. Was the hypothesis accepted or rejected? Provide a rationale for your response.

8. What is the meaning of the relationship presented in Fig. 11.6?

9. Did this study have an adequate sample size? Provide a rationale for your response.

10. Discuss the clinical importance of the findings from the Faria et al. (2022) study.

Algorithm for Determining the Appropriateness of Inferential Statistical Techniques Included in Research Reports

STATISTICAL TECHNIQUE IN REVIEW

Multiple factors are involved in determining the appropriateness of the inferential statistical techniques reported in nursing studies. **Inferential statistics** are conducted to examine relationships, make predictions, and determine differences among groups or variables in studies. When conducting data analyses for their studies, researchers consider many aspects of the study, including the study purpose, hypotheses or questions, level of measurement of the variables, design, and number of groups studied. Determining the appropriateness of the various inferential statistics reported for a particular study is not straightforward. Often, there is not necessarily one right statistical technique for a study.

One approach for judging the appropriateness of a statistical technique in a study is to use an **algorithm** or decision tree. The algorithm directs you by gradually narrowing the number of statistical techniques as you make judgments about the nature of the study and the data. An algorithm for judging the suitability of statistical procedures in studies is presented in Fig. 12.1. This algorithm was developed by the coauthor of this text, Daisha Cipher. Fig. 12.1 includes the four key factors related to the appropriateness of a statistical technique:

1. Nature of the research question or hypothesis (focus on differences or associations/relationships) for a study
2. Level of measurement (i.e., nominal, ordinal, or interval/ratio) of the dependent or research variables
3. Number of groups studied
4. Research design element (i.e., independent or paired samples)

Evaluating the statistical techniques reported in a study requires you to make several judgments about the nature of the data and what the researchers wanted to know. The study purpose and research questions or hypotheses need to be examined to determine whether the focus of the study was examining associations or relationships, making predictions, or determining group differences. Research questions are often used to direct descriptive and correlational studies. However, quasi-experimental and experimental studies focused on determining the effectiveness of an intervention or treatment are best directed by hypotheses (Grove & Gray, 2023; Kazdin, 2022; Shadish et al., 2002).

You also need to determine whether the study variables were measured at the nominal, ordinal, interval, or ratio level (see Fig. 12.1; review Exercise 1). You might see statistical techniques identified as parametric or nonparametric, depending on the level of measurement of the study variables. **Nonparametric statistics** are usually conducted for variables measured at the nominal or ordinal levels (Pett, 2016). If the study variables are measured at either the interval or ratio levels and the values of the variables for the study participants are normally

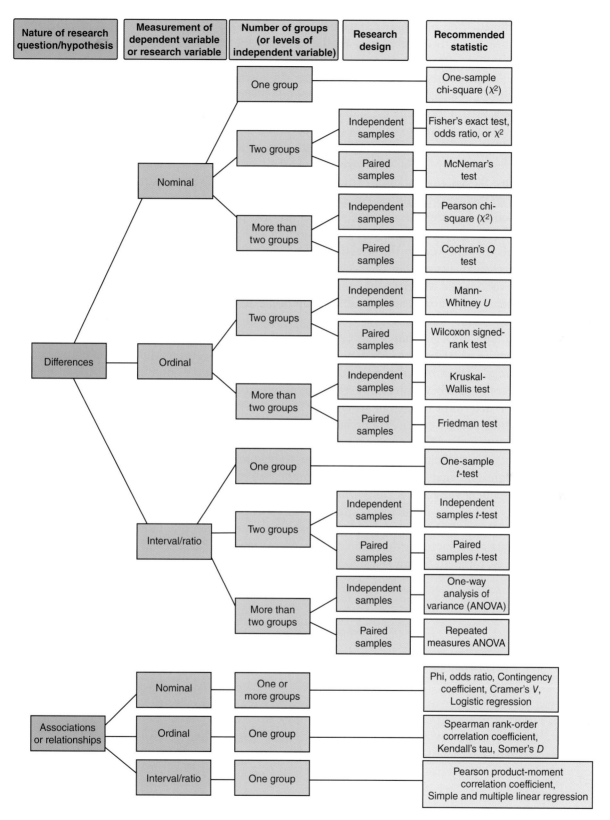

FIG. 12.1 ■ **ALGORITHM OR DECISION TREE FOR DETERMINING APPRO-PRIATE STATISTICAL TECHNIQUES FOR NURSING STUDIES.** Redrawn from Gray, J. R., & Grove, S. K. (2021). *The practice of nursing research: Appraisal, synthesis, and generation of evidence* (9th ed., p. 532). St. Louis, MO: Elsevier.

distributed, then **parametric statistics** are conducted (see Exercise 1; Kim et al., 2022). Remember the analysis techniques are the same whether the data use interval or ratio levels of measurement. Researchers run a computer program to determine whether the dependent variables' frequency distributions are normally distributed (see Exercise 27). If the distribution of values or scores collected for a dependent variable are not normally distributed or are skewed, then nonparametric statistics are conducted even though the variables were measured at the interval or ratio level (Gray & Grove, 2021; Kim et al., 2022).

In Fig. 12.1, examination of the research design element involves determining whether the samples or groups in a study are independent or paired. With **independent samples or groups**, the assignment of one study participant to a group is unrelated to the assignment of other participants to groups. For example, if participants are randomly assigned to the intervention and control groups, the samples are independent. In **paired samples** (also called dependent samples or groups), participants or observations selected for data collection are related in some way to the selection of other participants or observations. For example, if study participants serve as their own control by using their pretest data as a control group, the observations and therefore the groups are paired. Some studies require repeated measures of the dependent variable on the same group of participants, resulting in paired samples (Gray & Grove, 2021; Kazdin, 2022).

To apply the algorithm in Fig. 12.1, you would perform the steps previously introduced: (1) determine whether the research question or hypothesis focuses on differences or associations (i.e., relationships); (2) determine the level of measurement (i.e., nominal, ordinal, or interval/ratio) of the study variables; (3) select the number of groups that were included in the study; and (4) determine the design, with either independent or paired samples, that most closely fits the study you are critically appraising. The lines on the algorithm are followed through each selection to identify an appropriate statistical technique for the data being analyzed. The recommended statistic is identified in the far-right column in Fig. 12.1.

Regression analysis is focused on the prediction of a dependent variable using one or more independent variables. A study with one dependent variable (i.e., outcome) and one independent variable (i.e., predictor) is analyzed using simple linear regression (see Exercises 14 and 30). If the study has one dependent variable and more than one independent variable, then the data are analyzed with multiple linear regression (see Exercises 15 and 31; Gray & Grove, 2021; Kazdin, 2022; Kim et al., 2022; Terrell, 2021).

STUDY QUESTIONS

Directions: Answer the following questions by reviewing the statistical content and applying the algorithm in Fig. 12.1 of this exercise.

1. What are the reasons for conducting inferential statistics in nursing research?

2. Discuss the independent and paired samples or groups reported in studies. Why is knowing the type of group important in critically appraising the statistical technique in a research report?

3. Which statistic would be conducted for a hypothetical study focused on examining differences in reported lower extremity neuropathy, measured at the ordinal level, for two independent groups of patients with type 2 diabetes? Provide a rationale for your answer.

4. Which statistic would be conducted for a hypothetical study focused on examining differences for variables measured at the nominal level in one group? Provide a rationale for your answer.

5. Which statistic would be conducted for a hypothetical study focused on examining the relationship between the variables body mass index (BMI) and blood pressure (BP) in a group of patients with cardiovascular disease (CVD)? Provide a rationale for your answer.

6. Which statistic would be conducted for a hypothetical study focused on examining differences in weight loss for overweight individuals assigned to a control, placebo, or intervention group? The study design included repeated measures of weight at 3 months, 6 months, and 9 months. Provide a rationale for your answer.

7. Study hypothesis: *Menopausal women taking calcium 1000 mg plus vitamin D$_3$ 2000 International Units (IU) have higher bone density scores than women taking only calcium 1000 mg.* The women were randomly selected and assigned to the intervention and standard care groups. What statistical technique would researchers conduct to test this hypothesis? Provide a rationale for your answer.

8. Kozel et al. (2022) conducted a study to examine the association between optimism and social support for women at risk for premature birth. The variables of optimism and social support were measured using Likert scales. What analysis technique was conducted to address the study purpose? Provide a rationale for your answer.
Source: Kozel, E., Barnoy, S., & Itzhaki, M. (2022). Emotion management of women at risk for premature birth: The association with optimism and social support. *Applied Nursing Research, 64,* 151568. https://doi.org/10.1016/j.apnr.2022.151568

9. Robinson et al. (2018) examined the effectiveness of a coloring intervention on the anxiety levels of parents at two points in time: before and after surgery for their child. Anxiety was measured with the Spielberger State Trait Anxiety Inventory (STAI), which is a Likert scale that produces a total anxiety score for each study participant. What statistical technique did these researchers use to address their study purpose? Provide a rationale for your answer.

   Source: Robinson, E. M., Baker, R., & Hossain, M. (2018). Randomized trial evaluating the effectiveness of coloring on decreasing anxiety among parents in a pediatric surgical waiting area. *Journal of Pediatric Nursing, 41*(1), 80–83. https://doi.org/10.1016/j.pedn.2018.02.001

10. Al-Rawajfah et al. (2022) conducted a study to determine the predictors of effective clinical teaching (ECT) from the perspective of nursing educators. The results revealed that gender, age, and attending infection control training were significant predictors of ECT. What analysis technique was conducted to determine this result? Provide a rationale for your answer.

    Source: Al-Rawajfah, O. M., Al Hadid, L., Madhavanprabhakaran, G. K., Francis, F. & Khalaf, A. (2022). Predictors of effective clinical teaching—nursing educators' perspective. *BMC Nursing, 21*(1), 1–9. https://doi.org/10.1186/s12912-022-00836-y

Answers to Study Questions

1. Inferential statistics are conducted to analyze data in nursing studies for these purposes: (1) to examine relationships (i.e., associations); (2) to make predictions; and (3) to determine differences between groups. Inferential statistics are usually conducted to analyze data in quantitative, mixed methods, and outcomes studies (Gray & Grove, 2021; Kim et al., 2022; Terrell, 2021).

2. Independent samples or groups exist when the assignment of a study participant to a group is unrelated to the assignment of other participants to groups. For example, samples are independent when participants are randomly assigned to the intervention or control groups. With paired samples, the participants or observations selected for data collection are related in some way, such as participants serving as their own control in a pretest-posttest design or repeated measures design (Gray & Grove, 2021; Kazdin, 2022; Terrell, 2021). The analysis techniques conducted vary based on whether the groups are independent or paired in a study (see Fig. 12.1).

3. The Mann-Whitney U (see Exercises 21 and 34 for more details) is the statistical technique conducted for this hypothetical study (Kim et al., 2022; Pett, 2016). Applying the algorithm in Fig. 12.1, you note: the study is focused on differences; the variable reported, neuropathy, is measured at the ordinal level; and the design includes two independent groups of patients with type 2 diabetes. This information assists you in identifying the Mann-Whitney U as an appropriate analysis technique.

4. The one-sample chi-square test would be conducted in this hypothetical study. Using the algorithm in Fig. 12.1, you note: the research question is focused on differences; the variables are measured at the nominal level; and the study included one group. This information assists you in identifying the one-sample chi-square test as the appropriate analysis technique (Kim et al., 2022; Pett, 2016; Terrell, 2021).

5. The Pearson product-moment correlation coefficient (see Exercises 13 and 29 for more details) would be the statistical technique conducted to analyze data in this hypothetical study. Applying the algorithm in Fig. 12.1, you note: the research question is focused on relationships or associations; and the variables BMI and BP are measured at the ratio level. This information assists you in identifying the Pearson product-moment correlation coefficient as the appropriate analysis technique (Gray & Grove, 2021; Terrell, 2021).

6. The repeated measures analysis of variance (ANOVA) would be conducted for this hypothetical study. Applying the algorithm in Fig. 12.1, you note: the study was focused on differences; weight is measured at the ratio level; and the design included three groups with repeated measures of weight. This information assists you in identifying the repeated measures ANOVA as an appropriate analysis technique to determine differences in the groups over time (Kim et al., 2022; Terrell, 2021).

7. The independent samples *t*-test (see Exercises 16 and 32 for more details) would be the statistical technique conducted for this hypothetical study. Applying the algorithm in Fig. 12.1, you note: the hypothesis is focused on differences; the dependent variable, bone density value, is measured at the ratio level; and the study included two independent groups (study participants randomly assigned to either the intervention or standard care group). This information assists you in identifying the independent samples *t*-test as an appropriate analysis technique to test this hypothesis (Grove & Gray, 2023; Kim et al., 2022).

8. The Pearson product-moment correlational coefficient was conducted to examine the relationship or association between optimism and social support in the Kozel et al. (2022) study (see Exercises 13 and 29 for more details). Applying the algorithm in Fig. 12.1, you note the study is focused on examining a relationship between two variables in a sample of women at risk for premature birth. The variables of optimism and social support were measured with Likert scales, and the data from these scales are analyzed with parametric statistics, providing the assumptions outlined in this exercise are met. This information supports conducting the Pearson correlation to analyze study data (Gray & Grove, 2021; Kim et al., 2022; Waltz et al., 2017).

9. The paired samples *t*-test was conducted in the Robinson et al. (2018) study (see Exercises 17 and 33 for more information). Applying the algorithm in Fig. 12.1, you note: the study was focused on determining differences; the anxiety scores produce data that are usually analyzed as though at the interval level; and the study included dependent groups with anxiety measure presurgery and postsurgery. This information supports the researchers analyzing their data with a paired samples *t*-test (Gray & Grove, 2021; Kim et al., 2022).

10. Multiple linear regression was conducted in the Al-Rawajfah et al. (2022) study to predict effective ECT from the perspective of nursing educators (Kim et al., 2022; Terrell, 2021). The independent variables of gender, age, and attending infection control training were significant predictors of the dependent variable ECT. Multiple regression is required when more than one independent variable is used to predict a dependent variable (see Exercises 15 and 31 for more information).

Questions for Additional Study

Name: _____ Class: _____

Date: _____

Follow your instructor's directions to submit your answers to the following questions for additional study. Your instructor may ask you to write your answers below and submit them as a hard copy for evaluation. Alternatively, your instructor may ask you to submit your answers online.

Directions: Answer the following questions by reviewing the statistical content and applying the algorithm in Fig. 12.1 of this exercise.

1. Discuss the differences between parametric and nonparametric statistical techniques. Provide an example of a parametric statistical technique and a nonparametric statistical technique using the algorithm in Fig. 12.1.

2. A hypothetical study focused on examining differences among the randomly assigned intervention, placebo, and standard care groups. The dependent variable perception of pain was measured using a Likert perception of pain scale; however, the data for pain perception were not normally distributed (i.e., they were skewed) (Gray & Grove, 2021). What statistic was conducted to analyze the pain perception data? Provide a rationale for your answer.

3. What statistic would be conducted for a hypothetical study focused on predicting a dependent variable using one independent variable that was measured at the ratio level in a sample of patients with heart failure? Provide a rationale for your answer.

4. Hypothetical study hypothesis: *Nurses working in healthcare organizations with magnet status have higher job satisfaction than nurses working in organizations without magnet status.* Job satisfaction was measured with a multi-item Likert scale. What statistical technique would researchers use to test this hypothesis? Provide a rationale for your answer.

5. What statistical technique would be conducted for a hypothetical study focused on examining differences among three paired groups with the dependent variable of reported functional status measured at the ordinal level? Provide a rationale for your answer.

6. Lee et al. (2018) examined selective symptoms (dyspnea, anxiety, depression, and fatigue) to predict their contribution to impaired physical performance in patients with chronic obstructive pulmonary disease (COPD). Dyspnea was measured with FEV1 (forced expiratory volume in one second); anxiety, depression, and fatigue were measured with multi-item Likert scales. Physical performance was measured with the 6-minute walk test (6MWT), which was the distance patients could walk in 6 minutes. What is the level of measurement for each of the study variables? Provide a rationale for your answer.
Source: Lee, H., Nguyen, H. Q., Jarrett, M. E., Mitchell, P. H., Pike, K. C., & Fan, V. S. (2018). Effect of symptoms on physical performance in COPD. *Heart & Lung, 47*(2), 149–156. https://doi.org/10.1016/j.hrtlng.2017.12.007

7. The focus of the Lee et al. study was presented in Question 6. What type of inferential statistical technique did Lee et al. (2018) conduct to analyze the data in their study? Provide a rationale for your answer.

8. Hersch et al. (2016) conducted a randomized controlled trial (RCT) that examined the effect of a web-based stress management intervention on nurses' stress. The study included 104 participants that were randomized into an intervention or control group. Nurses' stress was measured with the Nursing Stress Scale, a multi-item Likert scale that provided a total stress score. What inferential statistical technique was conducted to examine the effect of the web-based intervention? Provide a rationale for your answer.
Source: Hersch, R. K., Cook, R. F., Deitz, D. K., Kaplan, S., Hughes, D., Friesen, M. A., & Vezina, M. (2016). Reducing nurses' stress: A randomized controlled trial of a web-based stress management program for nurses. *Applied Nursing Research, 32*(1), 18–25. https://doi.org/10.1016/j.apnr.2016.04.003

9. Caceres et al. (2022) conducted a study to examine the associations of lifetime trauma with cardiovascular health (CVH) among older and middle-aged Latina women. Relationships among the variables CVH scores, count of lifetime trauma, age, and emotional support were examined. CVH was measured with the LS7 scale, lifetime trauma was measured with the Trauma History Questionnaire, and emotional support was measured with the Patient-Reported Outcomes Measurement System (PROMIS) Likert scale. The study included one group and the measurement methods provided interval/ratio-level data. What inferential statistical technique was conducted to examine the relationships among these variables? Provide a rationale for your answer.
Source: Caceres, B. A., Doan, D., Barcelona, V., & Suero-Tejeda, N. (2022). Lifetime trauma and cardiovascular health in Latinas. *Nursing Research,* 71(1), 66–74. https://doi.org/10.1097/NNR.0000000000000560

10. Faith et al. (2021) examined the psychosocial outcomes after a summer camp for youth with bleeding disorders. The youths' attitude toward illness and hope were measured with Likert scales before and after their camp experience (pretest-posttest design). What inferential statistical technique was conducted to examine the change that occurred from the camp experience? Provide a rationale for your answer.
Source: Faith, M. A., Boone, D. M., Kalin, J. A., Healy, A. S., Rawlins, J. & Mayes, S. (2021). Improvements of psychosocial outcomes following a summer camp for youth with bleeding disorders and their siblings. *Journal of Pediatric Nursing, 61,* 144–150. https://doi.org/10.1016/j.pedn.2021.05.001

Understanding Pearson Product-Moment Correlation Coefficient

STATISTICAL TECHNIQUE IN REVIEW

Many studies are conducted to identify relationships between two or more variables. The correlational coefficient is the mathematical expression of the relationship or association studied. Two common analysis techniques used to examine relationships in healthcare studies are the Pearson product-moment correlation coefficient (r) and the Spearman rank-order correlation coefficient (rho) (see the algorithm Fig. 12.1 in Exercise 12). The **Pearson correlation coefficient** is a parametric analysis technique conducted to examine bivariate correlations between continuous variables measured at the interval and ratio levels (Gray & Grove, 2021; Kim et al., 2022). **Bivariate correlation** measures the extent of the relationship between two variables at a time in a study. Pearson r is calculated to determine the strength and direction of relationships in correlational studies. Therefore the purpose of correlational research is to examine relationships and *not to determine cause and effect* between independent and dependent variables (Grove & Gray, 2023). Cause and effect are the focus of quasi-experimental and experimental studies conducted to determine the effect of an intervention on an outcome (Kazdin, 2022; Shadish et al., 2002).

The Spearman rank-order correlation coefficient is a nonparametric analysis technique conducted to examine relationships when variables are measured at the ordinal level (see Exercise 20; Pett, 2016). This analysis technique is also calculated when the data collected do not meet the normality assumption of the Pearson r correlation coefficient (Gray & Grove, 2021).

Types of Relationships

Relationships are interpreted in terms of direction and strength. The direction of the relationship is expressed as either positive or negative. A **positive or direct relationship** exists when one variable increases as the other variable increases or when one variable decreases as the other decreases. The variables change in the same direction (see Exercise 11). For example, a moderate increase in calorie intake per day is related to an increase in weight gain. Conversely, a **negative or inverse relationship** exists when one variable increases as the other variable decreases. For example, an increase in minutes of exercise per day is related to a decrease in weight (Grove & Gray, 2023; Heavy, 2019).

The strength or magnitude of a relationship is described as weak, moderate, or strong. Pearson r is never less than -1.00 or greater than $+1.00$, so an r value of -1.00 or $+1.00$ indicates the strongest possible relationship, either negative or positive, respectively. An r value of 0.00 indicates no relationship or association between two variables. To describe a relationship, the labels *weak* ($r < 0.30$), moderate ($r = 0.30-0.50$), and strong ($r > 0.50$) are used in conjunction with both positive and negative values of *r* (Cohen, 1988; Gray & Grove, 2021; Plichta & Kelvin, 2013).

The significance of *r* values can be determined by examining the Table of Critical Values for *r* for the Pearson product-moment correlation coefficient in Appendix B at the back of this text. To use this table, you need to know the level of significance or alpha for the study, which is usually set at 0.05. The degrees of freedom (*df*) for a Pearson *r* value is the sample size minus 2 ($N - 2$). For example, if a study had $r = 0.36$, a sample size of 50, and alpha set at 0.05, is the *r* value statistically significant? The answer is yes because the $r = 0.36$ with a $df = 48$ is larger than the critical table value 0.2787 for alpha = 0.05 for a two-tailed test (see Exercise 29 for calculating and determining the significance of Pearson *r* correlation coefficients).

Mirror-Image Table of Pearson *r* Results

A **mirror-image table**, as the name implies, has the same labels for variables in the same order for both the *x*- and *y*-axes (see Exercise 7 for a discussion of *x*- and *y*-axes). Frequently, numbers or letters are assigned to each variable, and only the letter or number designator is used to label one of the axes. To find the *r* value for a pair of variables, look along the labeled or *y*-axis in Table 13.1 and then along the *x*-axis, using the number designator assigned to the variable to identify a selected relationship, and find the cell in the table with the *r* value. Table 13.1 is an example of a mirror-image table that displays the relationships among the variables of hours of class attended per week, hours studying per week, and final grade as a percentage. The results in the table are intended as an example of a mirror-image table and are not based on research. If you were asked to identify the *r* value for the relationship between hours of class attended per week and the final grade as a percentage, the answer would be $r = 0.52$; for between hours studying per week and final grade as a percentage, the answer would be $r = 0.58$. The dash (–) marks located on the diagonal line of the table represent the variable's correlation with itself, which is always a perfect positive correlation or $r = +1.00$. Because the results are the same in both sides of the mirror-image table, most researchers only include half of the table in their final report (Gray & Grove, 2021; Terrell, 2021).

Effect Size of an *r* Value

The Pearson *r* (in absolute value) is equal to the effect size (*ES*) or the strength of a relationship between two continuous variables. In Table 13.1, the association between hours of class attended per week and hours of studying per week is $r = 0.34$; thus the $r = ES = 0.34$ for this relationship. The *ES* is used in power analysis to determine sample size and examine the power of study results (Aberson, 2019; Cohn, 1988). Exercise 24 describes the elements of power analysis, and Exercise 25 includes the steps for conducting a power analysis for different statistical techniques.

The strength of the *ES* is the same as that for the *r* values, with a weak *ES* as <0.30, a moderate *ES* 0.30 to 0.50, and a strong *ES* >0.50. The smaller the *ES*, the greater the sample size needed to detect significant relationships in studies (Aberson, 2019; Lohr, 2022). A large *ES* or association between two variables requires a smaller sample size to identify a significant

TABLE 13.1   MIRROR-IMAGE PEARSON *r* CORRELATION TABLE

Variables	1	2	3
1. Hours of class attended per week	–	0.34	0.52
2. Hours studying per week	0.34	–	0.58
3. Final grade as a percentage	0.52	0.58	–

relationship. The sample size needed for correlational studies increases as the number of variables studied increases. Correlational studies usually involve examining relationships among multiple variables, so a large sample size is important (Cohen, 1988; Gray & Grove, 2021; Kazdin, 2022; Lohr, 2022).

Percentage of Variance Explained in a Relationship

There is some variation in the relationship between the values of two variables for individual participants. Some of the variation in values is explained by the relationship between the two variables and is called **explained variance**, which is calculated by r^2 and is expressed as a percentage. To calculate the percentage of variance explained, square the r value and multiply by 100% to determine a percentage (Cohen, 1988; Grove & Gray, 2023).

Formula: % variance explained = r^2 × 100%

Example: r = 0.58 (correlation between hours studying and final grade as a percentage)
$(0.58)^2$ × 100% = 0.3364 × 100% = 33.64% variance explained

In this example, the hours studying per week explains 33.64% of the variance in the final course grade. However, part of the variation is the result of factors other than the relationship and is called **unexplained variance**. In the example provided, 100% − 33.64% (explained variance) = 66.36% (unexplained variance). Fig. 13.1 demonstrates the concepts of explained and unexplained variance in this example.

Calculating the percentage of variance explained helps researchers and nurses understand the practical implications of reported results. The stronger the r value, the greater the percentage of variance explained. For example, if r = 0.50, then 25% of the variance in one variable is explained by another variable; if r = 0.60, then 36% of the variance is explained. All Pearson r values need to be examined for clinical importance; the potential for clinical importance increases with moderate and strong relationships, where r ≥ 0.30 and yields a 9% or higher percentage of variance explained. Keep in mind that a result may be statistically significant (p ≤ 0.05), but it may not represent a clinically important finding. For example,

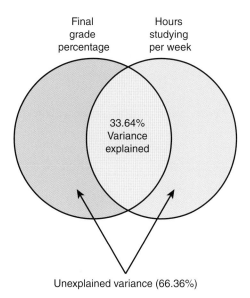

FIG. 13.1 ■ **PERCENTAGES OF EXPLAINED AND UNEXPLAINED VARIANCES IN A RELATIONSHIP.**

the correlation between hours of computer time and minutes of exercise is $r = 0.195$, $df = 100$. This r (0.195) value is greater than the critical value of r (0.1946) for alpha = 0.05 for a two-tailed Pearson correlation test (see Appendix B). This result is statistically significant, but the percentage of variance explained is 3.80%, which has limited clinical importance. Thus the r values in a study need to be examined for statistical significance and clinical importance (Grove & Gray, 2023; Terrell, 2021).

RESEARCH ARTICLE

Source

Hartson, K. R., Gance-Cleveland, B., Amura, C. R., & Schmiege, S. (2018). Correlates of physical activity and sedentary behaviors among overweight Hispanic school-aged children. *Journal of Pediatric Nursing, 40*(1), 1–6. https://doi.org/10.1016/j.pedn.2018.01.019

Introduction

Hartson and colleagues (2018) examined the correlates of physical activity (PA) and sedentary screen time behaviors among overweight Hispanic children ages 7 to 14 years. The PA (in days/week moderate PA $\geq$ 60 minutes), sedentary screen time behavior (in hours/week), body mass index (BMI) percentile (%), body esteem, and self-esteem were examined for the child. Body esteem was measured with the Body Esteem Scale, which included 24 items. Self-esteem was measured with the Rosenberg Self-Esteem Scale, which was considered reliable and valid and had been used with many populations. Both of these scales were multi-item Likert scales (Waltz et al., 2017). The fruit intake (in servings/day) and vegetable intake (in servings/day) were examined for both the child and parent.

Hartson et al. (2018, p. 1) concluded: "Understanding the correlates of physical activity and sedentary screen time behaviors in this underrepresented population allows nurses to better understand the connections between physical activity and other aspect of well-being in children. Further investigation is needed to determine how these relationships can be incorporated into physical activity interventions that improve the health of overweight Hispanic school-aged children."

Relevant Study Results

"Methods

Study Design

This was an exploratory correlation analysis of secondary data from the Mind Exercise Nutrition Do It! (MEND) 7–13 program conducted in a school district in the Western U.S. . . . The MEND 7– 13 program is a multi-component, community-based, family-focused health intervention developed . . . for overweight or obese children and their families. . . .

Analysis

SPSS Statistical Software, version 23, was used to conduct the analysis. Missing data analysis revealed large amounts of missing data for parental PA (45% missing), parental sedentary behavior (40% missing), and parental BMI (35% missing). Therefore, these variables were excluded from further analysis. For the variables of interest, no answers were outside of the range of potential answers, and in order to maximize sample size, no outliers were excluded. Pearson's correlations (r) were calculated to assess for correlations among child PA and sedentary behavior with potential child- and parent-correlates. Spearman's correlations (*rho*) were calculated to explore correlations among PA, sedentary behavior, and potential correlates stratified by gender, due to the small sample sizes" (Harton et al. (2018, pp. 2–3).

"Results

Participant Characteristics

The sample consisted of 40 child – parent dyads. The parental education of the sample was largely high school level or lower (80%), and most of the sample was from lower income households (75%). All of the children were Hispanic and of ages 7 to 14 years old. The sample of children was 50% male and 50% female. The parents were 80% mothers, 10% fathers, and 10% grandparents or other. . . .

On average, the children participated in at least 60 min of moderate PA on 3.19 ($SD = 2.40$) days per week and reported 7.09 ($SD = 6.30$) hours per week of sedentary screen time behaviors. Mean fruit intakes for children (mean = 2.24, $SD = 1.47$) and parents (mean = 2.26, $SD = 1.31$) were slightly above the recommended 2 cup-equivalents per day, while the mean vegetable intakes for children (mean = 1.56, $SD = 1.00$) and parents (mean = 1.91, $SD = 1.60$) were below the recommended 2.5 cup-equivalents per day, based on recommended amounts of fruits and vegetables required for a healthy nutrient-rich pattern of eating (U.S. Health and Human Services & U.S. Department of Agriculture, 2015). The mean child BMI percentile of the sample was 95.23% ($SD = 5.78$), which placed the sample mean BMI in the obese category, based on the Centers for Disease Control (CDC, 2015) growth reference curves. See Table 13.2 for additional baseline characteristics of the sample.

Correlations with Physical Activity and Sedentary Behavior

Child self-esteem ($r = 0.34$, $p < 0.05$) and parental vegetable intake ($r = 0.36$, $p < 0.05$) had a positive association of moderate size with PA in this coed sample of overweight Hispanic school-aged children. . . . Interestingly, BMI percentile, sedentary screen time behaviors, and body esteem were not associated with child PA. None of the potential correlates were associated with sedentary screen time behavior, except for body esteem which was negatively associated with sedentary screen time behavior in males. . . . See Table 13.3 for Pearson's correlations" (Hartson et al., 2018, p. 3).

TABLE 13.2 BASELINE CHARACTERISTICS

	n (%)	Mean	SD
Child Variable			
PA (days/week moderate PA ≥60 min)	37 (92.5)	3.19	2.40
Sedentary screen time behavior (h/wk)	38 (95.0)	7.09	6.30
BMI%	40 (100.0)	95.23	5.78
Fruit intake (servings/day)	39 (97.5)	2.24	1.47
Vegetable intake (servings/day)	37 (92.5)	1.54	1.00
Body esteem	38 (95.0)	13.00	4.92
Self-esteem	39 (97.5)	21.64	5.93
Parental Variable			
Fruit intake (servings/day)	39 (97.5)	2.26	1.31
Vegetable intake (servings/day)	37 (92.5)	1.91	1.60

BMI, Body mass index; PA, physical activity; SD, standard deviation.
From Hartson, K. R., Gance-Cleveland, B., Amura, C. R., & Schmiege, S. (2018). Correlates of physical activity and sedentary behaviors among overweight Hispanic school-aged children. *Journal of Pediatric Nursing, 40*, 3.

"Limitations

The sample size was small for a correlational analysis, which limited the robustness of the results; however, it allowed for the collection of data from a population that is commonly underrepresented in research, and yet, has high needs for healthcare resources. . . . Other limitations include that only one parent was surveyed, rather than two when available, and the use of non-validated single item measures for PA and sedentary behavior. Single item measures increased feasibility, but limited the depth of the constructs and could potentially affect the validity of the conclusions. . . . Also, the sedentary activity questions did not explicitly include sedentary time while texting, playing smartphone games, or using social media, all of which could increase hours of sedentary time per week. Future research will need to incorporate trends in sedentary use of technology in order to obtain accurate measures of sedentary screen time behaviors" (Hartson et al., 2018, pp. 4–5).

TABLE 13.3   PARENT- AND CHILD-CORRELATES OF CHILD PHYSICAL ACTIVITY AND SEDENTARY BEHAVIOR (PEARSON'S CORRELATIONS, *r*)

	PA	Sedentary Behavior	BMI%	Fruit intake	Veg intake	Body esteem	Self-esteem	Parent Fruit	Parent veg
PA	–								
Sedentary behavior	0.05	–							
BMI%	0.08	0.13	–						
Fruit intake	0.31	−0.08	−0.12	–					
Vegetable intake	0.05	−0.26	0.16	**0.55****	–				
Body esteem	0.06	−0.04	**−0.40***	0.22	−0.04	–			
Self-esteem	**0.34***	0.06	−0.14	**0.34***	0.12	**0.44****	–		
Parent fruit intake	0.19	0.09	0.14	**0.53****	0.25	0.06	0.10	–	
Parent vegetable intake	**0.36***	0.05	0.15	**0.60****	0.15	−0.08	0.09	**0.78****	–

BMI, Body mass index; PA, physical activity.
Note: **p < 0.05, **p < 0.01*, two-tailed.
From Hartson, K. R., Gance-Cleveland, B., Amura, C. R., & Schmiege, S. (2018). Correlates of physical activity and sedentary behaviors among overweight Hispanic school-aged children. *Journal of Pediatric Nursing, 40*, 4.

STUDY QUESTIONS

1. What design was used to conduct the Hartson et al. (2018) study? Did the design address the purpose of this study? Provide a rationale for your response.

2. Identify the descriptive results for the BMI percentile in this sample. What do these results indicate clinically for these children?

3. In the Hartson et al. (2018) study, Table 13.3 is what type of table? What values are presented in this table? What do the dashes (–) along the diagonal of this table indicate?

4. What is the value of the Pearson *r* for the relationship between child PA and sedentary behavior? Is this relationship positive or negative? What is the strength of this relationship? Provide a rationale for your response.

5. Is the relationship between child PA and self-esteem statistically significant? Provide a rationale for your response.

6. State the null hypothesis for the relationship between child PA and self-esteem. Was the null hypothesis accepted or rejected? Provide a rationale for your response.

7. What is the Pearson *r* and *ES* for the association between parent fruit intake and child fruit intake? Describe this relationship using words rather than numbers.

8. What percentage of variance is explained by the relationship between the variables of parent fruit intake and child fruit intake? Show your calculations and round your answer to two decimal places.

9. Is the relationship in Question 8 clinically important? Provide a rationale for your response.

10. Do the results in Table 13.3 support the statement that the child BMI percentile causes reduced body esteem? Provide a rationale for your response.

Answers to Study Questions

1. Hartson et al. (2018) conducted an exploratory correlational study with a correlational descriptive design (Kazdin, 2022). The study involved secondary analysis of data from the MEND 7 to 13 program. Yes, this correlational design addressed the correlates of PA and sedentary behaviors among overweight Hispanic school-age children identified in the study title (Grove & Gray, 2023; Kazdin, 2022; Shadish et al., 2002).

2. The BMI percentile, based on all 40 children in the sample, had a mean of 95.23% and an *SD* of 5.78 (see Table 13.2). As indicated in the study narrative, the 95.23% BMI placed these children in the obese category based on the CDC (2015) growth reference curve. The baseline characteristics reported a serious weight problem for these Hispanic children (see Table 13.2). In addition, understanding of the correlates of PA is important for the development of future interventions to increase PA in Hispanic children and decrease their sedentary behaviors to promote weight loss and improve their health.

3. Table 13.3 is a mirror-image correlational table used to present the Pearson *r* results in research reports (Gray & Grove, 2021). The dashes along the diagonal of Table 13.3 indicate that each variable is correlated with itself, such as the dash for the relationship of PA with PA. When a variable is correlated with itself, the $r = +1.00$ (a perfect positive relationship); and researchers put either the dashes or 1.00 along the table diagonal.

4. $r = 0.05$. The *r* value is listed in Table 13.3 and can be identified by locating where the variable of PA intersects with the variable of sedentary behavior. This *r* value is positive (no minus sign) but is so close to zero that the results indicate no relationship between PA and sedentary behavior (Grove & Gray, 2023; Terrell, 2021).

5. $r = 0.34^*$ is a statistically significant, moderate, positive relationship between child PA and self-esteem. The * indicates that the *r* value is statistically significant because its probability is $p < 0.05$ as identified in the footnote for Table 13.3. Most nurse researchers set their level of significance or alpha = 0.05. Because $p < 0.05$ is smaller than the alpha set at 0.05 for this study, the relationship is statistically significant (Grove & Gray, 2023; Kim et al., 2022).

6. Null hypothesis: *There is no relationship between PA and self-esteem in overweight school-aged Hispanic children.* This null hypothesis was rejected because there is a significant relationship (0.34*) between PA and self-esteem in this study (see the answer to Question 5). When a result is statistically significant, the null hypothesis is rejected (Gray & Grove, 2021; Shadish et al., 2002).

7. Pearson $r = 0.53^{**} = ES$. The *r* value is the *ES* in correlational studies (see Exercise 24; Cohen, 1988; Gray & Grove, 2021; Lohr, 2022). There is a statistically significant, large, positive relationship between parent fruit intake and child fruit intake, where an increase in parent fruit intake is associated with an increase in child fruit intake. The relationship also indicates that a decrease in parent fruit intake is associated with a decrease in child fruit intake.

8. The percentage of variance = 28.09%. The percentage of variance = $r^2 \times 100\% = 0.53^2 \times 100\% = 0.2809 \times 100\% = 28.09\%$.

9. Yes, the strong, positive relationship between parent and child fruit intake is clinically important because this relationship explains 28.09% of the variance between these two variables (Grove & Gray, 2023). In addition, it is clinically important for nurses to encourage parents to increase their fruit intake because it is positively associated with their child's fruit intake (Hartson et al., 2018). This is an expected relationship because parents provide their children's food and are role models for them in what they eat.

10. No, Pearson r is calculated to examine a relationship or association between two variables and does not determine causality (Gray & Grove, 2021; Shadish et al., 2002). A relationship indicates that two variables are linked to each other but not that an intervention causes an outcome. Causality indicates a strong relationship between two variables, but one of the variables must precede the other in time and be present when the effect occurs, which is not evident in this study (Shadish et al., 2002).

Name: _____ Class: _____

Date: _____

Follow your instructor's directions to submit your answers to the following questions for additional study. Your instructor may ask you to write your answers below and submit them as a hard copy for evaluation. Alternatively, your instructor may ask you to submit your answers online.

1. Were the vegetable intakes for both the parents and children in this study adequate? Provide a rationale for your answer.

2. Is the sample size in this study adequate? Provide a rationale for your response.

3. What is the value of the Pearson r for the relationship between child self-esteem and body esteem? Describe this relationship and discuss its statistical significance.

4. Describe the correlation $r = -0.40^*$ using words. Is this a statistically significant correlation? Provide a rationale for your response.

5. What is the largest relationship in Table 13.3? What percentage of variance was explained by this relationship? Show your calculations and round your answer to two decimal places.

6. Is the relationship in Question 5 clinically important? Is the relationship statistically significant? Provide rationales for your responses.

7. State the null hypothesis for the relationship between sedentary behavior and BMI%. Was the hypothesis accepted or rejected? Provide a rationale for your response.

8. What Pearson *r* value was calculated for the relationship between PA and BMI%? What were the *ES* and the strength of this relationship? Was the relationship statistically significant? Provide a rationale for your responses.

9. In a hypothetical study, BMI and perceived quality of life were correlated at Pearson $r = 0.32$. The sample size was $N = 92$, alpha $= 0.05$, and the data were examined with a two-tailed test. Using the Table of Critical Values for Pearson *r* in Appendix B, determine whether $r = 0.32$ is statistically significant. Provide a rationale for your response.

10. Are the findings from the Hartson et al. (2018) study ready for use in practice? Provide a rationale for your response.

Understanding Simple Linear Regression

STATISTICAL TECHNIQUE IN REVIEW

In nursing practice, the ability to predict future events or outcomes is extremely important in providing quality, cost-effective, safe health care (Straus et al., 2019). Nurse researchers calculate and report linear regression results in their studies as a basis for making these predictions. **Linear regression** provides a means to estimate or predict the value of a dependent variable based on the value of one or more independent variables or predictors (Gray & Grove, 2021; Kim et al., 2022). The regression equation is a mathematical expression of the theorized influential association between a predictor and an outcome. The link between the theoretical statement and the equation is made prior to data collection and analysis. **Simple linear regression** is a statistical technique conducted to determine the relationship between one predictor variable (x) and a dependent variable (y) (Prion & Haerling, 2020). The assumptions for simple linear regression include normal distribution of the dependent (y) variable, linear relationship between x and y, and independent observations (see Exercise 30 for a detailed discussion of assumptions).

The regression line developed from simple linear regression is usually plotted on a graph, with the horizontal axis representing x (the predictor variable) and the vertical axis representing the y (the dependent or predicted variable; Fig. 14.1). The value represented by the letter a is referred to as the y-intercept, or the point where the regression line crosses or intercepts the y-axis. At this point on the regression line, $x = 0$. The value represented by the letter b is referred to as the slope, or the coefficient of x. The slope determines the direction and angle of the regression line within the graph, which expresses the extent to which y changes for every one-unit change in x. The score on variable y (dependent variable) is predicted from the

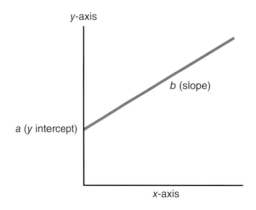

FIG. 14.1 ■ GRAPH OF A SIMPLE LINEAR REGRESSION LINE.

study participant's known score on variable *x*. The predicted score or estimate is referred to as *ŷ* (expressed as *y*-hat) (King & Eckersley, 2019; Tarrell, 2021).

Simple linear regression is an effort to explain the dynamics within a scatterplot (see Exercise 11) by drawing a straight line through the plotted scores or values. No single regression line can be used to predict, with complete accuracy, every *y* value from every *x* value. However, the purpose of the regression equation is to develop the line to allow the highest degree of prediction possible: the **line of best fit**. The procedure for developing the line of best fit is the **method of least squares**. If the data were perfectly correlated, all data points would fall along the straight line or line of best fit. However, not all data points fall on the line of best fit in studies, but the line of best fit provides the best equation for the values of *y* to be predicted by locating the intersection of points on the line for any given value of *x*.

The algebraic equation for the regression line of best fit is *y = bx+a,* where:

y = dependent variable (outcome)

x = predictor (independent variable)

b = **slope of the line** (beta, or what the increase in the value is along the *x*-axis for every unit of increase in the *y* value), also called the regression coefficient.

a = y-intercept (the point where the regression line intersects the *x*-axis), also called the regression constant.

Research reports present linear regression results in figures, tables, and/or narrative format (American Psychological Association [APA], 2020). The equation or formula developed from the regression results and a figure of the line of best fit for the study data might also be included. In Fig. 14.2, the *x*-axis represents gestational age in weeks and the *y*-axis represents birth weight in grams. As gestational age increases from 20 weeks to 34 weeks, birth weight also increases. In other words, the slope of the line is positive. This line of best fit can be used to predict the birth weight (dependent variable) for an infant based on his or her gestational age in weeks (predictor). Fig. 14.2 is an example of a line of best fit that was developed from hypothetical data. In addition, the *x*-axis starts at 22 weeks rather than 0, which is the usual

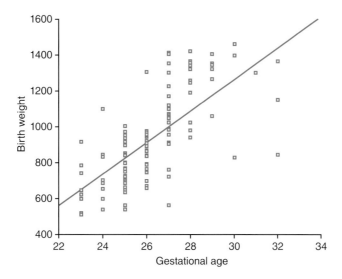

FIG. 14.2 ■ **EXAMPLE LINE OF BEST FIT FOR GESTATIONAL AGE AND BIRTH WEIGHT.**

start in a regression figure focused on gestational age. Using the equation $y = bx + a$, the birth weight of a baby born at 28 weeks of gestation is calculated as follows:

Equation: $y = bx + a$

In this example, $a = 500$, $b = 20$, and $x = 28$ weeks

$y = 20(28) + 500 = 560 + 500 = 1060$ grams

The regression line represents y for any given value of x. As you can see, some data points fall above the line and some fall below the line. If we substitute any x value in the regression equation and solve for y, we will obtain a $\hat{y}$ that will be somewhat different from the actual value. The distance between the $\hat{y}$ and the actual value of y is called **residual**, and this represents the degree of error in the regression line, as well as error of prediction. The regression line or the line of best fit for the data points is the unique line that will minimize error and yield the smallest residual (Kim et al., 2022; Zar, 2010). The step-by-step process for calculating simple linear regression in a study is presented in Exercise 30.

RESEARCH ARTICLE

Source

Kuroki, M. (2022). Healthcare coverage and out-of-pocket medical expenses: Evidence from the 2017 Tax Cuts and Jobs Act and the medical expense deduction. *Public Health, 205,* 58–62. https://doi.org/10.1016/j.puhe.2022.01.022

Introduction

Healthcare costs in the United States (U.S.) have been rising each year, creating a burden for both insured and uninsured individuals. The deduction of medical expenses provides an important tax relief for a small percentage of taxpayers. "Taxpayers can deduct out-of-pocket health insurance premiums and a wide range of medical expenses, such as preventative care, treatment, surgeries, dental and vision care, visits to psychologists and psychiatrists, as well as prescription medications and appliances, such as glasses, contacts, false teeth, and hearing aids. In 2016, approximately 8.8 million tax returns, or 5.9% of all tax returns, were filed with a medical expense deduction, whereas the number was 10.2 million, or 6.6% of all tax returns, in 2017, which is probably due to the lower threshold for the medical expense deduction in 2017" (Kuroki, 2022, p. 59). This study focused on two outcomes: (1) to determine the change in state-level tax returns with medical expense deductions and (2) to examine the annual percent change in the total medical expense deduction amount at the state level. The data for this study were obtained from the Internal Revenue Service (IRS).

Relevant Study Results

"Results

We present graphical evidence that shows the correlations between the uninsurance rate and outcomes of interest. Fig. 14.3 plots the percentage point change in the share of tax returns with medical expense deductions during 2016–2017 against the uninsurance rate in the same period. The ordinary least squares (OLS) regression line is inserted in the figure.... The likelihood of using the medical expense deduction increased in all states in 2017, but the increase was larger in states where the uninsurance rate was higher ($\beta = 0.06$, $p = 0.022$), suggesting that many uninsured people benefited from the lower threshold for the medical expense deduction in 2017.

Similarly, Fig. 14.4 plots percent change in the total medical expense deduction amount against the uninsurance rate. In line with the finding on the share of tax returns with a medical expense deduction, the percent increase in the medical expense deduction was also larger on average in states where the uninsurance rate was higher ($\beta = 0.9$, $p = 0.0003$)" (Kuroki, 2022, p. 62).

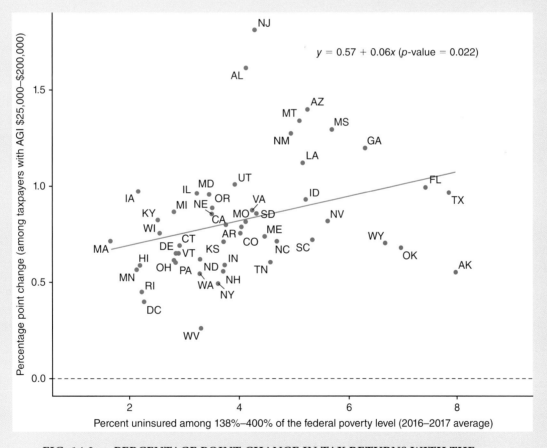

FIG. 14.3 ■ PERCENTAGE POINT CHANGE IN TAX RETURNS WITH THE MEDICAL DEDUCTION (2016−2017). *AGI,* Adjusted gross income. Kuroki, M. (2022). Healthcare coverage and out-of-pocket medical expenses: Evidence from the 2017 Tax Cuts and Jobs Act and the medical expense deduction. *Public Health, 205,* 61. https://doi.org/10.1016/j.puhe.2022.01.022

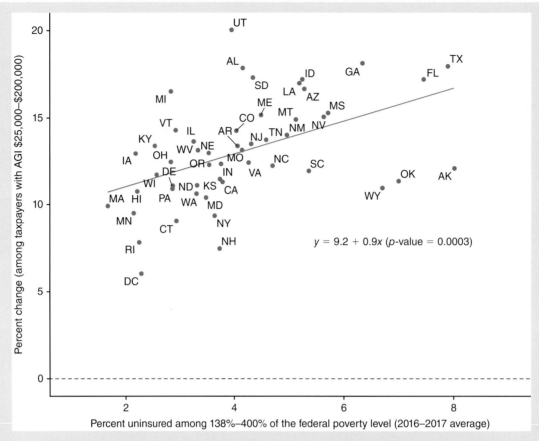

FIG. 14.4 ■ **PERCENTAGE CHANGE IN TOTAL MEDICAL EXPENSE DEDUC-TION (2016–2017).** *AGI,* Adjusted gross income. Kuroki, M. (2022). Healthcare coverage and out-of-pocket medical expenses: Evidence from the 2017 Tax Cuts and Jobs Act and the medical expense deduction. *Public Health, 205,* 61. https://doi.org/10.1016/j.puhe.2022.01.022

"Discussion and Conclusions

Given that the health insurance premiums and the costs of healthcare service have been increasing for many Americans, the effect of health insurance on out-of-pocket medical expenses is an important topic in public health. . . . However, the primary finding of this study is that states with higher shares of uninsured populations experienced a larger increase in the share of tax returns with a medical expense deduction, presumably because of unexpected and possibly catastrophic out-of-pocket medical expenses among the uninsured, after the threshold for the medical expense deduction was lowered in 2017. Also, the total medical expenditure deduction amounts increased more in states where the uninsurance rate was higher, consistent with the finding on the share of tax returns with a medical expense deduction" (Kuroki, 2022, p. 62).

STUDY QUESTIONS

1. What is the purpose of simple linear regression analysis and the regression equation?

2. What is the point where the regression line meets the y-axis called? Is there more than one term for this point and what is the value of x at that point?

3. In the formula $y = bx + a$, is a or b the slope? What does the slope represent in regression analysis?

4. What are the variables on the x- and y-axes in Fig. 14.2? Identify which variable is the predictor variable and which is the dependent variable.

5. What equation, developed from simple linear regression analysis, is presented in Fig. 14.2? Using this equation, what is the birth weight in grams (y) of an infant born at 30 weeks? Show your calculations.

6. What is the predictor variable in Fig. 14.3 and what is the dependent variable?

7. Does Fig. 14.3 have a positive or negative slope? Provide a rationale for your answer. Discuss the meaning of the slope of Fig. 14.3.

8. What regression equation was presented in Fig. 14.3? Was this equation significant? Provide a rationale for your response.

9. What is the y-intercept in Fig. 14.3? Show your calculations.

10. Calculate the percentage point change in tax returns with medical deductions (y) for 6% of uninsured taxpayers. Show your calculations.

Answers to Study Questions

1. Simple linear regression is a statistical technique conducted to estimate or predict the values of a dependent variable based on the values of one independent or predictor variable. Regression analysis is used to calculate a line of best fit based on the relationship between the predictor variable x and the dependent variable y. The equation developed with regression analysis can be used to predict the dependent variable (y) values based on values of the predictor variable (x) (Gray & Grove, 2021; Kim et al., 2022; Plichta & Kelvin, 2013).

2. The point where the regression line meets the y-axis is called the y-intercept and is also represented by a (see Fig. 14.1). In regression analysis, a is also called the regression constant. At the y intercept, $x = 0$.

3. In the equation $y = bx + a$, b is the slope of the line of best fit (see Fig. 14.1). The slope of the line indicates the amount of change in y for each one unit of change in x; b is also called the regression coefficient (Gray & Grove, 2021; Kim et al., 2022).

4. The predictor variable is gestational age, which is on the horizontal or x-axis. The dependent variable is birth weight in grams, which is on the vertical or y-axis.

5. The equation developed by simple linear regression in Fig. 14.2 was $y = 20x + 500$, where $a = 500$ and $b = 20$. The calculation of the birth weight for the gestational age of 30 weeks is: $y = 20(30) + 500 = 600 + 500 = 1100$ grams.

6. In Fig. 14.3, the predictor variable is the percent uninsured by state (2016–2017 average), which is on the x-axis. The dependent variable is the percentage point change in tax returns with medical deductions (2016–2017), represented on the y-axis.

7. Fig. 14.3 has a positive slope. The slope is represented by b in the equation on Fig. 14.3 and is a positive value ($b = 0.06$). In addition, the line of best fit extends from the lower left corner to the upper right corner, indicating a positive slope (Kim et al., 2022; Prion & Haerling, 2020). The line of best fit demonstrates that an increase in x (predictor) is associated with an increase in y (dependent variable). In Fig. 14.3, as the percentage of uninsured individuals in different U.S. states increases, the percentage of tax returns with medical deductions increases.

8. A regression equation might be expressed as $y = bx + a$ or $y = a + bx$. In Fig. 14.3, the equation is $y = a + bx = 0.57 + 0.06x$. This equation was significant at $p = 0.022$ as indicated in Fig. 14.3 and in the narrative of the article (Kuroki, 2022). The $p = 0.022$ is significant because it is less than the alpha $= 0.05$ set for this study (Grove & Gray, 2023; Terrell, 2021).

9. At the y-intercept, $x = 0$. Using the equation in Fig. 14.3, $y = 0.57 + 0.06(0) = 0.57 + 0 = 0.57$ (Gray & Grove, 2021; Kim et al., 2022).

10. In Fig. 14.3, the equation is $y = 0.57 + 0.06(x)$. If $x = 6\%$, the equation is $y = 0.57 + 0.06 (6\%) = 0.57 + 0.36\% = 0.93\%$ change in tax returns with medical deductions.

Follow your instructor's directions to submit your answers to the following questions for additional study. Your instructor may ask you to write your answers below and submit them as a hard copy for evaluation. Alternatively, your instructor may ask you to submit your answers online.

1. What is the line of best fit and how is it developed?

2. Is there error in the line of best fit developed through simple linear regression? Provide a rationale for your response.

3. In the study by Kuroki (2022), what are the variables on the *x*-axis and the *y*-axis in Fig. 14.4? What analysis was conducted to determine the results presented in Fig. 14.4? Provide a rationale for your response.

4. In Fig. 14.4, what equation was developed to predict the percent change in total medical expense deductions using the predictor variable percent uninsured in U.S. states. What were the values for *a* and *b* in the equation?

5. Was the equation presented in Fig. 14.4 significant? Provide a rationale for your response with documentation.

6. Calculate the percent change for the amount of total medical expense deductions (y) when 4% of the taxpayers are uninsured. Show your calculations. What does this result mean?

7. What is the y-intercept in Fig. 14.4? Show your calculations.

8. Calculate the percent change in the amount for total medical expense deductions (y) when 7% of the taxpayers are uninsured. Show your calculations. What does this result mean?

9. Was the sample size of Kuroki's (2022) study adequate? Provide a rationale for your response with documentation.

10. What conclusions were reached in Kuroki's (2022) study? Did these findings indicate a causal relationship? Provide a rationale for your response.

Understanding Multiple Linear Regression

STATISTICAL TECHNIQUE IN REVIEW

Simple linear regression was introduced in Exercise 14 and provides a means to estimate or predict the value of one dependent variable based on the value of an independent variable. However, when studying people with a focus on evidence-based practice, researchers usually examine two or more independent variables or predictors affecting the dependent variable of interest (Gray & Grove, 2021). Thus **multiple linear regression,** an extension of simple linear regression, is conducted when more than one independent variable or predictor is entered into the analysis to predict a dependent variable. The main advantage of a multiple linear regression model is the ability to examine the effects of several predictors on a dependent variable (Kim et al., 2022; Terrell, 2021).

Assumptions of Multiple Linear Regression

The assumptions of multiple linear regression are as follows:

1. Normal distribution of the dependent variable (see Exercise 27)
2. Linear relationship between x and y
3. Independent observations
4. Interval or ratio measurement of the dependent variable; however, if the dependent variable is measured with a Likert scale, and the frequency distribution is approximately normally distributed, these data are usually considered interval-level measurements and are appropriate to serve as the outcome in a linear regression model (Rasmussen, 1989; Waltz et al., 2017).
5. Values for the dependent variable are **homoscedastic**, or equally dispersed about the line of best fit (see Exercise 14; Gray & Grove, 2021; Kim et al., 2022).

Multicollinearity

With multiple predictors, researchers often correlate these predictors with the dependent variable to determine which are most highly correlated with the dependent variable. Pearson r analysis is typically computed to determine correlations for interval- and ratio-level data. Scores obtained with Likert scales that are normally distributed are analyzed as interval-level data (Grove & Gray, 2023; Waltz et al., 2017). To be effective, predictors need to have strong correlations with the dependent variable, but only weak correlations with the other predictor variables in the equation. **Multicollinearity** occurs when the predictors in the multiple regression equation are strongly correlated (over 0.85) with each other (Kim et al., 2022). Collinearity diagnostics are conducted to determine multicollinearity (see Exercise 31). Multicollinearity occurs in nursing studies, but it can be minimized by careful selection of predictor variables that have minimal or no correlation with each other. The ultimate goal of multiple linear regression is to find the best prediction model that has the least number of predictors with maximum explanation of the data (Gray & Grove, 2021; Terrell, 2021).

Multiple Linear Regression Results

The main result from multiple regression analysis is an R^2 value. For the addition of each predictor variable to the regression formula, the change in R^2 is reported. The R^2 is used to calculate the percentage of variance that is predicted by the regression formula. In the following hypothetical example, the predictors of number of pack-years of smoking (i.e., number of packs of cigarettes smoked per day times number of years of smoking), systolic blood pressure (SBP), and body mass index (BMI) were used to predict the incidence of myocardial infarction (MI) in older adults. The $R^2 = 0.387$, and the percentage of variance predicted is calculated by $R^2 \times 100\%$. In this example, the percentage of the variance in the dependent variable that is explained by the predictors is calculated as $0.387 \times 100\% = 38.7\%$. This means that 38.7% of the variance in the incidence of MIs in older adults is predicted by the pack-years of smoking, SBP, and BMI. The significance of an R^2 value is tested with an analysis of variance (ANOVA; see Exercises 18 and 35). The statistic for ANOVA is F, and a significant F value indicates that the regression equation has significantly predicted the variation in the dependent variable and that the R^2 value is not a random variation (Gray & Grove, 2021; Kim et al., 2022). The step-by-step process for calculating multiple linear regression is presented in Exercise 31.

RESEARCH ARTICLE

Source

Inayati, A., Lee, B., Wang, R., Chen, S., Hsu, H., Lu, C., & Head, Y. L. (2022). Determinants of fear of falling in older adults with diabetes. *Geriatric Nursing, 46,* 7–12. https://doi.org/10.1016/j.gerinurse.2022.04.017

Introduction

Fear of falling (FoF) is a critical factor that contributes to falls in older adults with diabetes. FoF often causes the elderly to avoid performance of essential, nonhazardous activities, which accelerates their physical and cognitive decline. Previous research was insufficient in predicting FoF in older adults. "Consequently, this study aimed to examine the important determinants of FoF in older adults with diabetes. . . . This study hypothesized that demographic and illness characteristics, physical function and capability, psychosocial and cognitive factors were important determinants of FoF among older adults with diabetes" (Inayati et al., 2022, p. 8). These researchers conducted a secondary data analysis of a previous study by Wang et al. (2021). Convenience sampling was used to obtain a sample of 240 elderly adults with diabetes. A power analysis was conducted that indicated 143 participants were needed for a study with an alpha = 0.05, power of 0.80, and effect size of 0.15 involving 16 independent variables for a multiple regression analysis.

The dependent variable FoF was measured with a 16-item, 4-point Likert scale. The scores range from 16 to 64 on this scale, with the higher scores indicating higher FoF. Diabetes distress was measured with an eight-item, 5-point Likert scale. Each item on the scale focused on a diabetic problem that was rated as not a problem (0 points) to a serious problem (4 points). The total scores of this scale ranged from 0 to 32 points, with higher scores indicating more severe diabetic-related problems. Handgrip was measured with a hand dynamometer, with higher values indicating greater muscle strength. The time up and go (TUG) variable was a balance test of standing, walking, turning around, and taking a seat. The more seconds taken to complete the TUG test, the worse the participant's performance. One-leg standing was a balance test on one leg measured in seconds. Cognitive function was measured with the Mini-Mental Status Examination (MMSE) that has scores ranging from 1 to 30, with 30 being a perfect score. Sarcopenia levels were measured with a scale that assessed sluggishness, assistance with walking, rising from a chair, climbing stairs, and fall history. Each item was assessed from 0 to 2, with the total score ranging from 0 to 10. The higher scores indicate greater problems with physical function and capacity. The following study excerpts present data analyses, results, and conclusions.

Relevant Study Results

"Data Analysis

SPSS* software version 26.0 was used for data analyses in this study. Independent *t*-tests and Pearson's correlation analyses were performed to test bivariate associations among variables. Multiple linear regression analysis . . . was conducted to identify the significant determinants of FoF. . . . Variables significantly associating with FoF (p-value < 0.10) in bivariate association analysis were simultaneously entered into multiple linear regression analysis. Variables with p-value < 0.05 were considered important determinants of FoF in multiple linear regression.

Results

. . . Participants included 147 women (61.41%) and 93 men (38.59%) with a mean age of 70.85 (4.24) years. The comorbidity of chronic diseases was not significantly associated with FoF; however, sex, age, education level, duration of diabetes, insulin treatment, HbA1c [hemoglobin A1c] levels, experiencing a hypoglycemia episode during the past year and fall history for the past year were significantly associated with FoF. As shown in Table 15.1, cognitive function, handgrip strength and one-leg standing test outcomes were significantly and negatively associated with FoF, whereas sarcopenia levels, TUG test outcomes and diabetes distress were significantly and positively associated with FoF.

Multiple Linear Regression for Important Determinants of FoF

The variance inflation factors ranged between 1.143 and 2.584 while tolerance scores ranged between 0.387 and 0.875, therefore no multicollinearity problems were identified among variables when conducting multiple linear regression analysis. As shown in Table 15.2, among demographic and illness characteristics, HbA1c levels [$\beta = 0.114$, $p < 0.05$] were significantly and positively associated with FoF. In terms of physical function and capability

TABLE 15.1 DISTRIBUTION OF SARCOPENIA, COGNITIVE FUNCTION, HANDGRIP STRENGTH, TIMED UP AND GO, ONE-LEG STANDING, DIABETES DISTRESS, AND FEAR OF FALLING, AND CORRELATIONS AMONG THEM ($N = 240$)

Variables	Mean (*SD*)	1	2	3	4	5	6	7
1. Sarcopenia	0.89 (1.24)	1.00	−0.148*	−0.293***	0.283***	−0.065	0.209***	0.444***
2. Cognitive function	27.85 (2.88)		1.00	0.185***	−0.388***	0.169**	0.014	−0.147*
3. Handgrip strength	26.01 (8.59)			1.00	−0.272***	0.030	−0.009	−0.182**
4. TUG	8.66 (2.57)				1.00	−0.181**	−0.016	0.322***
5. One-leg standing	19.91 (38.02)					1.00	−0.010	−0.152*
6. Diabetes distress	9.24 (7.57)						1.00	0.438***
7. Fear of falling	23.03 (7.70)							1.00

Note: *SD*, standard deviation; TUG, Timed Up and Go Test.
*$p < 0.05$, **$p < 0.01$, ***$p < 0.001$.

TABLE 15.2   MULTIPLE LINEAR REGRESSION FOR FEAR OF FALLING ($N = 240$)

Variables	B	SEB	β	Partial Correlation Coefficients
Demographics and Illness Characteristics				
Age	0.106	0.109	0.058	0.064
Sex (female)	−2.310	1.210	−0.147	−0.127
Education level (junior high and below)	−1.234	0.924	−0.078	−0.089
Insulin treatment (no)	1.104	0.984	0.069	0.075
Fall history (no)	−0.506	1.142	−0.027	−0.030
Experience of hypoglycemia (no)	0.873	1.080	0.044	0.054
HbA1c level	0.574	0.374	0.114*	0.133
Body mass index	0.018	0.108	0.009	0.011
Duration of diabetes	−8.271	0.043	0.000	0.000
Physical Function and Capability				
Sarcopenia level	1.934	0.406	0.312***	0.303
Timed Up and Go	0.591	0.198	0.198**	0.196
Handgrip strength	0.087	0.073	0.098	0.080
One-leg standing	−0.012	0.011	−0.060	−0.074
Psychosocial Factor				
Diabetes distress	0.338	0.056	0.333***	0.374
Cognitive Factor				
Cognitive function	0.081	0.158	0.030	0.034
Constant	−2.634	10.886		
R^2			0.429	
F value			11.241***	

Note: (), reference category; B, unstandardized regression coefficients; SEB, standard error of unstandardized regression coefficients; β, standardized regression coefficients.
*$p < 0.05$, **$p < 0.01$, ***$p < 0.001$.

factors, sarcopenia levels [β = 0.312, $p < 0.001$] and TUG test outcomes [β = 0.198, $p < 0.01$] were significantly and positively associated with FoF. In terms of psychosocial factor, diabetes distress [β = 0.333, $p < 0.001$] was significantly and positively associated with FoF. Regarding cognitive factors, cognitive function was not significantly associated with FoF. The multiple regression model was significant [$F(15, 224) = 11.241, p < 0.001$] and accounted for 42.9% of variance in FoF. According to the partial correlation coefficients, diabetes distress, sarcopenia levels, TUG test outcomes and HbA1c levels uniquely explained 14% (0.374^2), 9% (0.303^2), 4% (0.196^2) and 2% (0.133^2) of the variance in FoF respectively" (Inayati et al., 2022, pp. 9–10).

"Conclusions

. . . These findings highlighted that important determinants of FoF might differ according to the nature of the disease. Diabetes-specific psychosocial and illness characteristics factors should be considered to mitigate FoF among older adults with diabetes. As diabetes distress explained the largest variance in FoF in this study, healthcare providers should be especially aware of diabetes distress among older adults with diabetes and apply diabetes-tailored psychological interventions. Additionally, optimizing glycemic control should be emphasized to older adults with diabetes. Exercise-based interventions can improve sarcopenia and dynamic imbalance and have been demonstrated to reduce FoF among the general population of older adults" (Inayati et al., 2022, p. 11).

STUDY QUESTIONS

1. What is the purpose of multiple linear regression analysis?

2. In the Inayati et al. (2022) study, what was the dependent variable and what was its level of measurement? Identify the predictors (independent variables) that were significantly correlated with the dependent variable in Table 15.1.

3. What analysis technique was conducted to determine relationships among the predictor and dependent variables in Table 15.1? Was this the appropriate analysis technique? Provide a rationale for your response.

4. What is the sarcopenia level and how was it measured? What is the clinical importance of this predictor variable?

5. Which predictor variable in Table 15.1 had the highest correlation with FoF? Provide a rationale for your response.

6. Was the correlation value in Question 5 statistically significant? Provide a rationale for your response.

7. On Table 15.1, what correlation result is $r = -0.152$? Describe in words the meaning of this correlation. Was this correlation statistically significant? Provide a rationale for your response.

8. What is multicollinearity? Why is it important to test for multicollinearity before conducting multiple linear regression? Was multicollinearity a problem in this study? Provide a rationale for your response.

9. Based on the regression analysis results, was hemoglobin A1c (HbA1c) a significant predictor of FoF? Provide a rationale for your answer.

10. What percentage of the variance in FoF was explained by HbA1c? Discuss the clinical importance of this result.

Answers to Study Questions

1. Multiple linear regression analysis is conducted to predict an outcome or dependent variable using two or more predictor variables. This analysis is an extension of simple linear regression where more than one independent variable is entered into the analysis to develop a formula for predicting the dependent variable (Gray & Grove, 2021; Kim et al., 2022).

2. The dependent variable was FoF, which was measured with a 16-item, 4-point Likert scale. Likert scales produce ordinal-level data; however, if the scores are normally distributed, the data are analyzed as though at the interval level with parametric statistics. The scores from the Likert scales in this study were analyzed with parametric statistics, indicating they were normally distributed. However, Inayati et al. (2022) should have reported the normality distribution of the data in their study (see Exercise 27; Gray & Grove, 2021; Waltz et al., 2017). In Table 15.1, six predictor variables—sarcopenia level (also referred to as physical function and capability), cognitive function, handgrip strength, timed up and go (TUG), one-leg standing, and diabetes distress—were significantly correlated with the dependent variable of FoF.

3. Pearson r correlational analysis was conducted to determine the relationships of the six predictor variables with each other and with the dependent variable, FoF (see Table 15.1). Yes, Pearson r is the correct parametric analysis technique calculated to determine relationships between variables measured at the interval and ratio levels (see Exercise 12; Grove & Gray, 2023). Sarcopenia, diabetes distress, and FoF were measured with Likert scales and cognitive function was measured with MMSE, considered interval-level data (see the answer to Question 2; Gray & Grove, 2021; Waltz et al., 2017). The handgrip strength, TUG, and one-leg standing data were at the ratio level. Pearson r correlations are computed to determine the effective predictors for regression analysis, which are the variables strongly correlated with the dependent variable but only weakly correlated with each other (Gray & Grove, 2021; Kim et al., 2022).

4. Sarcopenia level is a term used to describe a person's physical function and capability. The sarcopenia level is measured with a five-item scale that assesses sluggishness, assistance in walking, rising from a chair, climbing stairs, and fall history. The items are scored from 0 to 2, with the total score ranging from 0 to 10. The higher the score, the greater the sarcopenia level, which is associated with poor physical function and capabilities. These poor physical functions increase older adults' FoF, and their potential to fall.

5. The predictor sarcopenia level has the highest correlation ($r = 0.444$) with the dependent variable FoF. This r value identifies a moderate (0.30–0.50), positive correlation between sarcopenia level and FoF (Cohen, 1988; Grove & Gray, 2023). The -1 and $+1$ are perfect correlation values, indicating the strongest relationships possible. The strength of a relationship increases as the values move toward $+1$ or -1 and away from zero. In this study, the $r = 0.444$ is the value closest to $+1$ and the farthest from 0 (Gray & Grove, 2021).

6. Yes, the $r = 0.444^{***}$ is statistically significant. Inayati et al. (2022) used asterisks (*) to identify the significant correlational values. As in the notes under Table 15.1,*** indicate that $p < 0.001$. The level of significance or alpha for this study was set at 0.05. The p value for the correlation of sarcopenia and FoF was < 0.001, which is less than alpha and is statistically significant (Grove & Gray, 2023).

7. The $r = -0.152^*$ is a weak, negative, significant relationship between one-leg standing time and FoF. Study participants who had longer one-leg standing time in seconds had lower FoF scores. This relationship was significant at $p < 0.05$, as indicated by the single asterisk (*) (see the note under Table 15.1). Because $p < 0.05$ is less than alpha = 0.05 set for this study, the result is statistically significant (Grove & Gray, 2023; Terrell, 2021).

8. Multicollinearity occurs when the predictors in the multiple regression equation are strongly correlated ($r \geq 0.85$) with each other (Kim et al., 2022). This happens in nursing studies, but it can be minimized by careful selection of predictor variables that have limited correlation with each other. If the predictor variables have multicollinearity, this reduces the percentage of variance of the dependent variable that is explained (Gray & Grove, 2021). Inayati et al. (2022, p. 9) reported: "The variance inflation factors ranged between 1.143 and 2.584 while tolerance scores ranged between 0.387 and 0.875, therefore no multicollinearity problems were identified among variables when conducting multiple linear regression analysis."

9. Yes, HbA1c was a significant predictor of FoF with $\beta = 0.114^*$ and partial correlation coefficient = 0.133. The * indicates that the value was significant at $p < 0.05$, which is less than alpha = 0.05, so it is statistically significant.

10. The percentage of variance = $R^2 \times 100\%$. The percentage of variance for HbA1c = $0.133^2 \times 100\%$ = $0.0177 \times 100\%$ = 1.77%, or rounded to the next whole percent, is 2%. The HbA1c is a limited but significant predictor of FoF. The higher the HbA1c, the greater the FoF in older adults with diabetes. Inayati et al. (2022, p. 11) recommend that "optimizing glycemic control should be emphasized to older adults with diabetes" based on the link to FoF.

Questions for Additional Study

Name: _____ Class: _____

Date: _____

Follow your instructor's directions to submit your answers to the following questions for additional study. Your instructor may ask you to write your answers below and submit them as a hard copy for evaluation. Alternatively, your instructor may ask you to submit your answers online.

1. What are the assumptions for multiple linear regression?

2. Was multiple linear regression analysis the appropriate statistical technique to calculate in the Inayati et al. (2022) study? Provide a rationale for your response.

3. On Table 15.1, what correlation result is $r = -0.016$? Was this correlation value statistically significant? What does this r value indicate for multiple linear regression?

4. What is the correlation between TUG and FoF? State in words the relationship between these variables. Was this correlational value significant? Provide a rationale for your response.

5. What independent variables were significant predictors of FoF? Provide a rationale for your response.

6. What was the strongest predictor of FoF in this regression model? What percent of the variance in FoF was uniquely explained by this variable? Provide a rationale for your response.

7. Was the regression model in the Inayati et al. (2022) study significant in predicting FoF? Provide a rationale for your response.

8. What hypothesis was stated by the researchers? Was this hypothesis accepted or rejected? Provide a rationale for your response.

9. What percentage of the variance of FoF was explained by the regression model? Provide the calculations for obtaining this value.

10. Discuss the clinical importance of the regression results in the Inayati et al. (2022) study.

Understanding the Independent Samples *t*-Test

STATISTICAL TECHNIQUE IN REVIEW

The **independent samples *t*-test** is a parametric statistical technique calculated to determine differences between the scores obtained from independent or unrelated samples or groups (Grove & Gray, 2023). Groups are independent if the assignment of one participant to a group is unrelated to the assignment of other participants to groups (see Exercise 12 for a discussion of independent groups). For example, when study participants are randomly assigned to either an intervention or control group, the groups are unrelated or independent. Because the *t*-test is considered fairly easy to calculate, researchers often use it in determining differences between two groups when variables are measured at the interval or ratio level. Jones et al. (2021) examined the statistical tests conducted to analyze data from 667 doctor of nursing practice (DNP) projects. The most frequently calculated parametric analysis techniques were the paired samples *t*-test ($n = 140$; 21%) and the independent samples *t*-test ($n = 86$; 12.9%).

The independent samples *t*-test is conducted to determine differences between the means ($\bar{X}$) of two groups in a study and adjusts that difference for the variability (computed by the standard error) among the data (Celentano & Szkla, 2018; Gray & Grove, 2021; King & Eckersley, 2019). When interpreting the results of *t*-tests, the larger the calculated *t* value in absolute value, the greater the difference between the two groups. The significance of a *t* value can be determined by comparison with the critical *t* values in the statistical table for the *t* distribution based on the degrees of freedom (*df*) for the study (see Appendix A Critical Values for Student's *t* Distribution at the back of this text). The formula for *df* for an independent *t*-test is as follows:

df = (number of participants in sample A + number of participants in sample B) − 2

Example *df* = (50 in sample A + 52 in sample B) −2 = 102−2 = 100

In a hypothetical example, researchers conducted a study to determine the effect of a structured dietary plan on adolescents' weight loss. The sample included 97 overweight adolescents who were randomly assigned to either an experimental group ($n = 48$) or a comparison group ($n = 49$). The null hypothesis was: *There is no difference in weight loss between the adolescents exposed to the structured dietary plan versus those receiving standard care.* The *df* for this example is computed as follows: $(48 + 49) - 2 = 95$. At the end of 6 months, the groups were significantly different in weight loss with $t(95) = 2.393$, $p < 0.05$. Review the critical values for the *t* distribution in Appendix A and note that $t(95) = 1.985$, $p = 0.05$. The *t* value found in this example is larger than the value in the table, so the result is significant. The $p < 0.05$ also indicates significance because it is less than the alpha $= 0.05$ set at the start of the study (Grove & Gray, 2023).

The independent samples *t*-test is best conducted once to examine differences between two groups in a study, because conducting multiple *t*-tests on study data can result in an inflated

Type I error rate. A **Type I error** occurs when the researcher rejects the null hypothesis when it is in actuality true. Researchers need to consider other statistical analysis options for their study data rather than conducting multiple *t*-tests. However, if multiple *t*-tests are conducted, researchers can perform a Bonferroni procedure to reduce the risk of a Type I error (see Exercise 18).

The Bonferroni procedure is a simple calculation in which the alpha is divided by the number of *t*-tests conducted on different aspects of the study data. For example, if a study's alpha was set at 0.05 and the researcher planned on conducting five *t*-tests on the study data, the corrected alpha would be computed as follows: $0.05 \div 5 = 0.01$. However, it should be noted that the Bonferroni procedure has long been criticized for being too stringent, resulting in overcorrection of alpha. Bender and Lange (1999, p. 601) wrote, "The Bonferroni procedure ignores dependencies among the data and is therefore much too conservative if the number of tests is large."

Assumptions for the Independent Samples *t*-Test

The *t*-test for independent samples or groups includes the following assumptions:

1. The raw scores or values in the population are normally distributed.
2. The dependent variable(s) is(are) measured at the interval or ratio levels. A dependent variable measured with a multi-item scale that has normally distributed scores can also be analyzed as though at the interval level (Waltz et al., 2017).
3. The two groups examined for differences have equal variance, which is best achieved by a random sample and random assignment to groups.
4. All scores or observations collected within each group are independent or unrelated to other study scores or observations (Gray & Grove, 2021; Kim et al., 2022).

The *t*-test is robust, meaning the results are reliable even if one of the assumptions has been violated. However, the *t*-test is not robust regarding between-samples or within-samples independence or with respect to extreme violation of normality assumptions. Groups do not need to be of equal sizes but rather of equal variance. Groups are independent if the two sets of data were not taken from the same study participants and if the scores are not related (Gray & Grove, 2021; Plichta & Kelvin, 2013). This exercise focuses on interpreting and critically appraising the *t*-tests results presented in research reports. Exercise 32 provides a step-by-step process for computing the independent samples *t*-test.

RESEARCH ARTICLE

Source

Kim, H. J., & Hwang, S. Y. (2022). Effect of website-based learning on improved monitoring and adverse drug reactions by clinical nurses. *Asian Nursing Research, 16,* 45–51. https://doi.org/10.1016/j.anr.2021.12.004

Introduction

Kim and Hwang (2022) conducted a quasi-experimental study to examine the effects of a website-based learning program on the voluntary monitoring and reporting of adverse drug reactions (ADRs) by clinical nurses. The dependent or outcome variables for this study were: (1) the knowledge on ADRs, measured with a 20-question objective test; (2) self-efficacy or level of confidence in ADR monitoring, measured with a 10-item Likert scale (1–4 points); ADR monitoring in practice, measured with a 10-item Likert scale (1–5 points); and medication performance ability related to ADR monitoring, measured with a six-item Likert-type 5-point scale (1–5 points). The results and conclusions from this study are presented in the following excerpt.

Relevant Study Results

"Methods

Study Design

This study was a quasi-experimental control group pretest-posttest design with random allocation for developing website-based learning content and verifying its effectiveness on voluntary reporting of ADRs in nurses with more than 1 year of clinical experience.

Development of Website-Based Learning Contents

The website, including the learning content, was developed according to the web-based learning design model with five steps: analysis, design, development, application, and evaluation. In the analysis stage, in July 2017, 210 clinical nurses were surveyed about their preferred educational form and content for ADR reporting. Among them, 10 individual interviews were conducted to explore the reasons for the difficulty of voluntary reporting. . . .

Setting and Participants

The number of samples in this study was calculated based on the evidence of the educational effect with a large effect size in several previous studies on ADR reporting for clinical nurses. Using G*Power program 3.1.9.2, the number of samples that fit the *t*-test with an effect size of 0.80, significance level of 0.05 for the two-tailed test, and power of 80% was at least 26 in each group. The criteria for selection of participants were nurses working at a university hospital . . . and general ward nurses with clinical experience of 1 to 25 years, excluding new nurses and chief nurses. New nurses were excluded from the participants because they had little experience with drug side effects and lacked drug-related clinical judgment skills that required critical thinking. To secure the homogeneity of clinical experience among a total of 266 participants who met the criteria, 60 participants were selected through a randomization program (Microsoft Excel), divided into 5 years and less than 5 years, and assigned to an experimental group and a control group. All 60 participants agreed to participate in the study, and there were no dropouts; 30 in the experimental group and 30 in the control group were used for the final analysis" (Kim & Hwang, 2022, pp. 46–47).

"Data Analysis

The data were analyzed using IBM SPSS Statistics Software Version 21.0 (IBM, Armonk, NY, USA). General characteristics of the participants were analyzed as real numbers, percentages, and mean and standard deviations. The prior homogeneity of the two groups was verified by the chi-square test, Fisher's exact and *t*-tests, and the Kolmogorov-Smirnov test for normality, and the Levene's test for equality of variance. To verify the effect of the intervention, the differences prior to and after the intervention were identified between the experimental group and the control group by independent *t*-test" (Kim & Hwang, 2022, pp 48–49).

"Results

Verification of the Effectiveness of the Website-Based Learning Interventions

1) Homogeneity test of participant's general characteristics and variables

    As a result of the analysis to verify the homogeneity of the general characteristics and dependent variables of the two groups, there was no statistically significant difference, and the two groups were homogeneous (Table 16.1). In this study, participants visited the website an average of 7.03 times, but mainly used learning content rather than commenting or posting, and mainly asked questions about how to use the program. This appears to be the result of the short mediation period and lack of publicity.

2) Effects of website-based learning on research-dependent variables

    The difference in ADR knowledge score of 2.93 ± 2.80 in the experimental group was significantly higher than the 1.20 ± 1.92 found in the control group ($t = -2.80$, $p = 0.007$). The score difference of self-efficacy on ADR monitoring in the experimental

TABLE 16.1   GENERAL CHARACTERISTICS OF PARTICIPANTS AND HOMOGENEITY TEST FOR DEPENDENT VARIABLES ($N = 60$)

Variables	Categories	Exp. ($n = 30$) n (%) or M±SD	Cont. ($n = 30$) n (%) or M±SD	χ^2 or t	p
Gender	Men	3(10.0)	0(0.0)	3.16	.237[b]
	Women	27(90.0)	30(100.0)		
Age (years)		31.83 ± 6.68	30.87 ± 5.57	−0.59	.559
Education	College	6(20.0)	5(163)	0.51	.774[b]
	Bachelor's	22(733)	24(80.0)		
	Master's	2(6.7)	1(3.3)		
Marital status	Married	10(33.0)	8(26.7)	0.32	.573
	Single	20(67.0)	22(73.3)		
Total clinical experience (months)		99.10 ± 82.55	88.8 ± 71.81	0.54	.911
	12~<36	7(23.3)	9(30.0)		
	36 ≤~<60	8(26.7)	6(20.0)		
	60 ≤~<120	7(23.3)	7(233)		
	≥120	8(26.7)	8(261)		
Working department	Medical ward	14(46.7)	15(50.0)	0.33	.849
	Surgical ward	12(40.0)	10(33.3)		
	Others[a]	4(13.3)	5(16.7)		
Reporting experience	Yes	16(533)	21(70.0)	136	.184
	No	14(46.7)	9(30.0)		
Education experience	Yes	18(60.0)	22(73.3)	−1.20	.273
	No	12(40.0)	8(26.7)		
Knowledge		14.57 ± 2.42	14.00 ± 2.27	−0.94	.354
Self-efficacy		35.90 ± 431	37.27 ± 5.63	1.06	.296
Monitoring practice		32.83 ± 4.54	33.50 ± 4.29	0.58	.561
Medication performance ability		2127 ± 3.15	20.60 ± 2.46	0.91	.365

Note. Cont. = control group; Exp. = experimental group; M = mean; *SD* = standard deviation.
[a] Psychiatric ward; emergency ward.
[b] Fisher exact test.
Kim, H. J., & Hwang, S. Y. (2022). Effect of website-based learning on improved monitoring and adverse drug reactions by clinical nurses. *Asian Nursing Research, 16,* 49. https://doi.org/10.1016/j.anr.2021.12.004

group was 3.50 ± 4.99 points, which was significantly higher than the −0.13 ± 5.18 points of the control group ($t = -2.77, p = 0.008$). The difference in scores of monitoring ADRs in the experimental group (5.07 ± 6.28) was higher than the 1.27 ± 6.19 found in the control group, and the difference was statistically significant ($t = -2.36, p = 0.022$). The difference in post-pre scores of medication performance ability related to ADR monitoring in the experimental group was 1.93 ± 3.29, which was higher than the 0.53 ± 3.19 evident in the control group, but the difference was not statistically significant ($t = -1.67, p = 0.100$) (Table 16.2)" (Kim & Hwang, 2022, pp. 49–50).

"Conclusion

The website content developed in this study included video lectures, case studies about ADRs, information on individual drugs, and FAQs about ADRs. In addition, various notice board functions were used to enable two-way communication such as sharing cases and providing feedback, providing drug safety information issued monthly by the local product safety center, and posting reports related to ADRs. Nurses who learned through the website significantly increased their knowledge of ADRs, self-efficacy, and monitoring practices compared with the control group. Sharing and communication through such an open website induces clinical nurses to practice monitoring for ADRs and activates voluntary reporting, leading to a safer medication culture in hospital settings" (Kim & Hwang, 2022, p. 50).

TABLE 16.2   COMPARISON OF VARIABLES BETWEEN THE TWO GROUPS (*N* = 60)

Variables	Group	Pre M±*SD*	Post M±*SD*	Difference M±*SD*	*t*	*p*
Knowledge on ADR	Exp.(*n* = 30)	14.57 ± 2.42	17.50 ± 122	2.93 ± 2.80	−2.80	.007
	Cont. (*n* = 30)	14.00 ± 2.27	1520 ± 1.85	120 ± 1.92		
Self-efficacy on ADR	Exp. (*n* = 30)	35.90 ± 4.30	39.40 ± 5.06	350 ± 4.99	−2.77	.008
	Cont. (*n* = 30)	37.27 ± 5.63	37.13 ± 6.70	−0.13 ± 5.18		
ADR monitoring practice	Exp. (*n* = 30)	32.83 ± 4.54	37.90 ± 536	5.07 ± 628	−2.36	.022
	Cont. (*n* = 30)	33.50 ± 4.30	34.77 ± 4.91	127 ± 6.19		
Medication performance ability	Exp. (*n* = 30)	21.27 ± 3.15	2320 ± 333	1.93 ± 329	−1.67	.100
	Cont. (*n* = 30)	20.60 ± 2.46	21.13 ± 239	053 ± 3.19		

ADR = adverse drug reaction; Cont. = control group; Exp. = experimental group; M = mean; *SD* = standard deviation.
Kim, H. J., & Hwang, S. Y. (2022). Effect of website-based learning on improved monitoring and adverse drug reactions by clinical nurses. *Asian Nursing Research, 16,* 49. https://doi.org/10.1016/j.anr.2021.12.004

STUDY QUESTIONS

1. What design was used in the study by Kim and Hwang (2022)? What groups were examined for differences in this study? Were these groups independent or dependent? Provide a rationale for your response with documentation.

2. What statistical test was conducted by the researchers to examine the effect of the website-based learning intervention in their study? Was this test appropriate for analyzing the data in this study? Provide a rationale for your response.

3. Kim and Hwang (2022) examined the study groups for differences prior to the implementation of the website-based learning intervention. What is the meaning of these results?

4. Were the experimental and control groups significantly different for ADR monitoring practice dependent variable preintervention? Provide a rationale for your answer.

5. What statistics were computed to describe the ADR monitoring practices pretest and posttest? What were the results from these calculations and what did these results indicate?

6. State the null hypothesis for the dependent variable knowledge on ADR in this study. What statistical test was conducted to test this hypothesis?

7. Were the groups significantly different for the dependent variable knowledge on ADR? Provide a rationale for your response. Was the null hypothesis in Question 6 accepted or rejected?

8. What can cause an increased risk for Type I errors when *t*-tests are conducted in a study? How might researchers reduce the increased risk for a Type I error in a study?

9. Were the experimental and control groups significantly different for the dependent variable self-efficacy on ADR? Provide these results and discuss the meaning of them.

10. Kim and Hwang (2022) conducted the Pearson's chi-square test to analyze the differences in marital status and working department (see Table 16.1) between the experimental and control groups. Would an independent samples *t*-test be appropriate to analyze the data for these demographic variables in this study (review algorithm in Exercise 12)? Provide a rationale for your answer.

Answers to Study Questions

1. Kim and Hwang (2022, p. 46) conducted "a quasi-experimental control group pretest-posttest design" to determine the effectiveness of a website-based learning intervention on clinical nurses' voluntary monitoring and reporting of ADRs. Study participants were randomly assigned to either the experimental group or control group, which indicates that the groups were independent or unrelated (Gray & Grove, 2021; Shadish et al., 2002).

2. Independent samples t-tests were conducted to examine the effectiveness of the website-based learning intervention on selected outcomes. The experimental group was provided the website-based content that included real cases, latest drug-related knowledge, and video lectures on ADR. The control group received a small notebook for monitoring ADRs of nurses. Yes, this analysis technique was appropriate to determine differences between the independent groups (experimental and control) created by random assignment. The knowledge variable was measured by an objective test (ratio-level data) and the other three dependent variables were measured with Likert scales (ordinal-level data). However, the data for all variables were normally distributed, so the Likert-scale data could be analyzed with t-tests (Bandalos, 2018; Waltz et al., 2017).

3. The experimental and control groups were examined for differences related to the demographic characteristics and the dependent variables at the beginning of the study. The independent samples t-tests and chi-square tests were nonsignificant for all the variables examined because the p values were all greater than the alpha set at 0.05 for this study (see Table 16.1). These nonsignificant results indicate the experimental and control groups were similar or equivalent for these variables at the beginning of the study. Therefore Kim and Hwang (2022) can conclude the significant differences found between the two groups at the end of the study were probably because of the effects of the intervention rather than sampling error or initial group differences (Gray & Grove, 2021; Kim et al., 2022; Terrell, 2021).

4. No, the experimental and control groups were not significantly different for the ADR monitoring practice variable preintervention. The $t = 0.58$, $p = 0.561$ is nonsignificant because the p value is greater than the alpha $= 0.05$ set prior to the study (Grove & Gray, 2023).

5. For the ADR monitoring practice variable, $\bar{X}$ and standard deviations (SDs) were computed for both the experimental and control groups preintervention and postintervention and also differences scores. For the experimental group, the preintervention descriptive statistics were ($\bar{X}$) $\pm$ SD $= 32.83$ $\pm$ 4.54; and those postintervention were ($\bar{X}$) $\pm$ SD $= 37.90 \pm 5.36$, with a difference score of ($\bar{X}$) $\pm$ SD $= 5.07 \pm 6.28$. For the control group, the preintervention descriptive statistics were ($\bar{X}$) $\pm$ SD $= 33.50 \pm 4.30$; and those postintervention were ($\bar{X}$) $\pm$ SD $= 34.77 \pm 4.91$, with a difference score of ($\bar{X}$) $\pm$ SD $= 1.27 \pm 6.19$. The experimental and control groups were similar for ADR monitoring practice before the intervention, but there was a greater increase in the experimental group mean (5.07 points) after the website-based intervention than the control group (1.27 points).

6. The null hypothesis is: *There is no difference in the knowledge on ADR between the clinical nurses in the experimental group receiving the website-based intervention and the control group receiving a notebook.* The independent samples t-test was conducted to examine group differences.

7. Yes, the experimental and control groups were significantly different for knowledge on ADR because $t = -2.80$, $p = 0.007$. The *p* value indicates significant results because it is less than the alpha $= 0.05$ set for this study. The study findings are significant, so the null hypothesis in Question 6 should be rejected (Gray & Grove, 2021; Terrell, 2021).

8. The computation of multiple *t*-tests on data for dependent variables can cause an increased risk for Type I errors (see Table 16.2). Computing *t*-tests on demographic characteristics (see Table 16.1) does not increase the risk of a Type I error. The Bonferroni procedure can be calculated to reduce the risk of a Type I error in studies with multiple *t*-tests; however, many researchers consider this alpha correction to be too stringent, so it should be used with caution (Celentano & Szklo, 2018).

9. The experimental and control groups were significantly different for the dependent variable of self-efficacy on ADR, because $t = -2.77$, $p = 0.008$. The *p* value is less than the alpha $= 0.05$, so the result is statistically significant. This result means that clinical nurses exposed to the website-based learning content had significantly higher self-efficacy or confidence in adapting to the ADR monitoring task than the control group (Grove & Gray, 2023; Terrell, 2021).

10. No, the independent samples *t*-test would not have been appropriate to analyze the differences in marital status and working department between the experimental and control groups. These demographic variables were measured at the nominal level because they had exhaustive and mutually exclusive categories that could not be ranked (see Exercise 1; Grove & Gray, 2023; Waltz et al., 2017). Thus the chi-square test is the appropriate statistic for analyzing these demographic variables measured at the nominal level (see Exercises 1, 12, and 19).

Name: _____ Class: _____

Date: _____

Follow your instructor's directions to submit your answers to the following questions for additional study. Your instructor may ask you to write your answers below and submit them as a hard copy for evaluation. Alternatively, your instructor may ask you to submit your answers online.

1. What does *df* mean? Kim and Hwang (2022) did not provide the *df* in their study. Why is it important to know the *df* for a *t* value? Using the *df* formula, calculate the *df* for this study.

2. What are the $\bar{X}$s and *SD*s for age for the experimental and control groups? What statistical analysis was conducted to determine the difference in means for age for the two groups at the beginning of the study? Was this an appropriate analysis technique? Provide a rationale for your answer.

3. What are the *t* and *p* values for age? What do these results mean?

4. What are the assumptions for conducting the independent samples *t*-test?

5. Were the assumptions identified in Question 4 met by Kim and Hwang (2022) in their study? Provide a rationale for your response.

6. State the null hypothesis for the ADR monitoring practice between the experimental and control groups of clinical nurses.

7. Was the null hypothesis stated in the answer to Question 6 accepted or rejected? Provide a rationale for your answer.

8. What statistics were computed to describe the medication performance ability preintervention and postintervention? What were the results from these calculations and what did these results indicate?

9. What variable had a result of $t = -1.67, p = 0.100$? Is this result significant? What does it mean?

10. Is this website-based learning intervention ready for use in practice? Provide a rationale for your response.

EXERCISE 17

Understanding the Paired Samples *t*-Test

STATISTICAL TECHNIQUE IN REVIEW

The **paired or dependent samples *t*-test** is a parametric statistical technique conducted to determine differences between two sets of repeated measures data from one group of individuals. The scores used in the analysis might be obtained from the same study participant under different conditions, such as the **one-group pretest–posttest design** (Gray & Grove, 2021). With this type of design, a single group of participants experiences the pretest, treatment or intervention, and posttest. Participants are referred to as serving as their own control during the pretest, which is then compared with the posttest scores after the intervention. Fig. 17.1 presents the pretest–posttest design (Gray & Grove, 2021; Terrell, 2021).

Paired or dependent scores also result from a one-sample repeated measures design, where one group of participants are assessed two or more times and the means ($\overline{X}$s) of these assessments are compared. Paired samples *t*-tests can also be applied to a crossover study design, in which participants receive one kind of treatment or intervention and subsequently receive a comparison treatment (Celentano & Szklo, 2018; Gliner et al., 2017). For example, one group of participants could be exposed to two different amounts, high and low, of aspartame, which is included in artificial sweeteners. The outcomes for each participant for each amount of aspartame are measured, resulting in paired scores.

The one-group design is considered a weak quasi-experimental design because it is difficult to determine the effects of a treatment without a comparison to a separate control group (Gray & Grove, 2021; Shadish et al., 2002). However, the *t*-test is the simplest statistic to conduct when comparing two means. Jones et al. (2021) examined the statistical tests conducted in 667 doctor of nursing practice (DNP) projects and found the paired samples *t*-test was the most commonly conducted statistical test ($n = 140$, 21%). Over time, DNP projects need to be conducted with stronger designs that produce data that can be analyzed with more powerful statistical techniques (Gray & Grove, 2021).

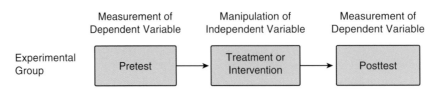

FIG. 17.1 ■ ONE-GROUP PRETEST–POSTTEST DESIGN.

Assumptions for the Paired Samples *t*-test

The assumptions for the paired samples *t* -test are as follows:

1. The distribution of scores is normal or approximately normal.
2. The dependent variable(s) is(are) measured at interval or ratio levels. A dependent variable measured with a multi-item scale that has normally distributed scores can also be analyzed as though at the interval level (Waltz et al., 2017).
3. Repeated measures data are collected from one group of study participants, resulting in paired scores.
4. The differences between the paired scores are independent (Gray & Grove, 2021; Kazdin, 2022; Shadish et al., 2002).

The degrees of freedom (*df*) for the paired samples *t*-test are calculated using the following formula: $df = N - 1$, where the N represents the sample size (Terrell, 2021). For example, if the study included a sample size of 68, the $df = 68 - 1 = 67$.

Another research design for which paired samples *t*-tests are appropriate is the case control research design (Kazdin, 2022). **Case control designs** involve a matching procedure whereby a control participant is matched to each case, in which the cases and controls are different people but matched demographically. The study participants in the two groups could be matched for age, diagnosis, or severity of illness that might affect the study outcomes. Matching the intervention and control group for selected demographic variables controls the effect of these variables and strengthens the design (Gray & Grove, 2021; Shadish et al., 2002).

RESEARCH ARTICLE

Source

Williams, T., Kennedy-Malone, L., Thompson, J., & Monge, E. C. (2022). The effect of an exergame on physical activity among older adults residing in a long-term care facility: A pilot study. *Geriatric Nursing, 44*, 48–53. https://doi.org/10.1016/j.gerinurse.2022.01.001

Introduction

Williams and colleagues (2022) conducted a quasi-experimental study to determine the effects of arranged residential video games on the health outcomes of older adults. The intervention included a Nintendo Wii video gaming system that was implemented for 6 weeks with long-term care (LTC) residents. The Wii system included several exergame options such as tennis, baseball, and bowling. The bowling option was selected because it had an option for multiple players and could be used by those who could stand, as well as those in a wheelchair. The outcome variables were exercise benefits, exercise barriers, self-efficacy or confidence in exercise ability, and physical activity levels. The dependent variables of exercise benefits and barriers were measured with the Exercise Benefits and Barriers Scale (EBBS). The EBBS was a 43-item Likert scale that included two subscales: one focused on benefits and the other on barriers. The responses for the EBBS items ranged from 4 (strongly agree) to 1 (strongly disagree). This scale was not developed for use in LTC facilities. The self-efficacy for exercise variable was measured with the Self-Efficacy for Exercise (SEE) scale. The SEE included 11 items that were scored from 0 (no confidence) to 10 (very confident) to assess the participants' confidence in their ability to exercise. The Rapid Assessment of Physical Activity (RAPA) questionnaire was used to assess the participants' level of physical activity. The RAPA included nine items with scores that ranged from 1 (rarely or never do any physical activity) to 7 ($\geq$ 20 min per day of vigorous physical activity $\geq$ 3 days a week).

Williams et al. (2022) reported limitations of sample size and lack of the sample's representation of the population. In addition, the attendance at the different sessions of the intervention was limited, with only six participants attending all 12 sessions. However, despite these limitations, the researchers encouraged directors of LTC facilities to organize exergames to improve the residents' overall purposeful physical activity. The design, sample, and key results are presented in the following study excerpt.

Relevant Study Results

"Methods

Design

A pre-posttest single group quasi-experimental cross-sectional design was chosen for this pilot study to evaluate the feasibility of the intervention implementation as well as changes in outcomes following the intervention. The intervention was conducted at four long-term care facilities in central NC [North Carolina]. The Nintendo Wii was used in a physical activity intervention. . . .

Sample

Our target population consisted of individuals capable of consenting who resided in long-term care [LTC] facilities located in two counties in central NC. . . . Within the LTC facility was a dedicated space secured by the facility liaison with a television in where the intervention took place. . . . An a priori power analysis was conducted . . . to determine an appropriate sample size. To detect medium to large effect size of 0.062 [probably a typographical error and should be 0.62] using a two-sided paired *t*-test, an alpha level of 0.05 and 80% power, this study needed at least 24 participants after accounting for 20% attrition" (Williams et al., 2022, p. 49).

"Data Analysis

Descriptive statistics (*n*, %) were conducted on participant attendance to determine feasibility of the 12-session intervention. Benefits, barriers, and self-efficacy were compared between pre- and post-intervention using paired *t*-tests and physical activity was examined using a Wilcoxon signed-rank test due to deviations from normality. Statistical analysis was conducted using IBM SPSS version 25 with alpha set to 0.05.

Results

Participant Characteristics

Of the 29 consenting participants, one had an unexpected hospitalization and subsequently passed away; three participants dropped out and did not state reasons for the withdrawal; and one contracted a contagious illness which required isolation and did not return. The final sample size for this study was $N = 24$. Participants were long-stay residents of the four facilities. . . . The majority of the participants were female ($n = 16$, 65.6%) and self-identified as Caucasian ($n = 20$, 83.3%). The ages of participants ranged from 55–93, with the average age of 79.97 ($SD = 10.35$). Most of the participants had lived in the LTC facility between 2–5 years (33.3%)" (Williams et al., 2022, p. 50).

"Perceptions of Exercise Benefits/Barriers and Self-Efficacy for Exercise

Paired *t*-test results for EBBS and SEE questionnaire mean scores are displayed in Table 17.1. The findings revealed a nonsignificant improvement in participants' perceptions of exercise benefits and barriers resulting from the intervention, though not statistically significant ($ps = 0.900$ and 0.310, respectively). The perceptions of exercise barriers scores

TABLE 17.1   PAIRED *t*-RESULTS FOR PERCEIVED EXERCISE BENEFITS/BARRIERS AND SELF-EFFICACY FOR EXERCISE

Outcome	Preintervention (mean ± *SD*)	Postintervention (mean ± *SD*)	*t*	*df*	Significance
EBBS benefits	52.1 ± 12.1	52.4 ± 12.0	−0.13	23	0.900
EBBS barriers	30.6 ± 3.4	29.6 ± 4.5	1.04	23	0.310
SEE self-efficacy	4.8 ± 2.1	5.3 ± 2.0	−1.31	23	0.200

SEE = Self-Efficacy for Exercise Scale; EBBS = Exercise Benefits and Barriers Scale.
Note: EBBS barriers are scored such that lower scores indicate fewer barriers.
Source: Williams, T., Kennedy-Malone, L., & Monge, E. C. (2022). The effect of an exergame on physical activity among older adults residing in a long-term care facility: A pilot study. *Geriatric Nursing, 44*, 51. https://doi.org/10.1016/j.gerinurse.2022.01.001

ranged from 22–37 at preintervention and 16–37 at postintervention. The perceptions of exercise benefits scores ranged from 31–81 at pretest and 29–79 at posttest. Mean self-efficacy for exercise scores as measured by the SEE questionnaire improved although not statistically significantly ($p = 0.200$). Self-efficacy for exercise scores ranged from 0.91 to 9.1 at preintervention and from 0.0 to 9.1 at postintervention.

Rapid Assessment of Physical Activity

The highest score with an affirmative response on the RAPA questionnaire was recorded for each patient at pre- and postintervention. Preliminary analyses revealed deviations from normality for the RAPA scores (Shapiro-Wilks' $p < 0.05$), therefore RAPA scores were examined using a nonparametric Wilcoxon signed rank test. The median score on the RAPA increased from 3.0, . . . albeit not significantly ($Z = -0.82$, p = 0.410)" (Williams et al., 2022, p. 51).

STUDY QUESTIONS

1. Identify and describe the design for the Williams et al. (2022) study.

2. What independent (intervention) and dependent (outcome) variables were included in this study?

3. Are independent or dependent (paired) scores examined in this study? Provide a rationale for your response.

4. What inferential statistical technique was calculated to examine differences in the participants' EBBS benefits, EBBS barriers, and self-efficacy scores before and after the 6-week physical activity intervention? Is this technique appropriate? Provide a rationale for your response.

5. What statistical techniques were calculated to describe the preintervention EBBS benefits subscale? Were these techniques appropriate? Provide a rationale for your response.

6. Compare the descriptive analysis values for the preintervention and postintervention for the EBBS benefits subscale. What do these results indicate?

7. State the null hypothesis for the EBBS benefits variable in this study.

8. What is the *t*-test value for the EBBS benefits variable preintervention and postintervention? Is this result significant? Provide a rationale for your response. Was the hypothesis in Question 7 accepted or rejected?

9. Examine the *t* values in Appendix A. What *t* value would be significant at the 0.05 level for a two-tailed *t*-test in a study with $N = 24$ participants? Discuss the meaning of these results.

10. Was there a significant difference in the participants' EBBS barriers variable between the preintervention and postintervention? Provide a rationale for your answer. Is this result clinically important?

Answers to Study Questions

1. Williams et al. (2022, p. 49) clearly reported they used "A pre-posttest single group quasi-experimental cross-sectional design." The study design is presented in Fig. 17.1 of this exercise. The study was identified as a pilot to examine the feasibility of implementing an exergame intervention with LTC residents and to examine its effects on the outcomes of benefits, barriers, self-efficacy, and physical activity level in four LTC facilities (Gray & Grove, 2021; Shadish et al., 2002).

2. The independent variable or intervention was the Nintendo Wii exergame of bowling. The dependent variables or outcomes were EBBS benefits, EBBS barriers, self-efficacy of exercise confidence, and physical activity level.

3. Dependent scores were analyzed in this study because only one group of 24 participants was included. The dependent variables for all participants were measured as the pretest followed by the 6-week exergame intervention, and then the posttest. The pretest scores served as a control to be compared with the posttest scores, resulting in paired scores (Gray & Grove, 2021; Kazdin, 2022; Terrell, 2021).

4. Paired samples t-tests were conducted to examine differences in the participants' EBBS benefits, EBBS barriers, and self-efficacy scores before and after the physical activity exergame intervention. Table 17.1 identifies the statistical technique as paired samples t-test. This statistical technique is appropriate because the study included one group and the participants' scores were dependent, obtained as a pretest prior to the intervention followed by a posttest (see answer to Question 3; Gray & Grove, 2021; Terrell, 2021). The dependent variables of EBBS benefits, EBBS barriers, and self-efficacy were measured using Likert scales, resulting in ordinal-level data. However, the scores for these variables were normally distributed and were analyzed as interval-level data using the paired t-test (Bandalos, 2018; Waltz et al., 2017).

5. A mean and standard deviation (SD) were calculated to describe the EBBS benefits variable preintervention. The $\bar{X} = 52.1$ and $SD = 12.1$. The data from the EBBS benefits subscale was ordinal (see the answer to Question 4). However, the data were normally distributed and were analyzed as interval using $\bar{X}$ and SD, which are appropriate for describing variables measured at the interval or ratio level (see Exercise 1; Bandalos, 2018; Grove & Gray, 2023; Waltz et al., 2017).

6. The EBBS benefits variable had preintervention $\bar{X} = 52.1$ and $SD = 12.1$ and postintervention $\bar{X} = 52.4$ and $SD = 12.0$. The $\bar{X}$s were essentially the same; they varied by only 0.30. These results indicate there was minimal change after the intervention. The SDs were almost the same (12.1 versus 12.0), indicating similar dispersion or spread of the EBBS benefits scores.

7. Null hypothesis: *There is no change in the EBBS benefits outcome from before and after the physical activity exergame intervention.*

8. The paired t-test result was $t(23) = -0.13$, $p = 0.900$ for the EBBS benefits variable preintervention and postintervention. This result is not statistically significant because $p = 0.900$ is greater than the alpha that was set at 0.05 for this study (Grove & Gray, 2023). When the results from a study are not statistically significant, the null hypothesis is accepted.

9. Identify the section of the table focused on two-tailed tests and the alpha = 0.05. The $df = N - 1$, which is $24 - 1 = 23$ in this study (see Table 17.1). The *t* value for alpha = 0.05, or $t(23) = 2.069$. This critical *t* value (2.069) from Appendix A supports that the *t*-test results in Table 17.1 are nonsignificant. The study *t* values are less than the critical *t* value.

10. The $t(23) = 1.04$, $p = 0.310$ for the EBBS barriers variable is a nonsignificant result. The $p = 0.310$ is greater than the alpha = 0.05 set for this study, making the result nonsignificant. The physical activity exergame intervention did not significantly change the EBBS barriers variable. The minimal change in EBBS barriers scores from preintervention to postintervention did not support the use of the exergame intervention in practice.

Name: _____ Class: _____

Date: _____

Follow your instructor's directions to submit your answers to the following questions for additional study. Your instructor may ask you to write your answers below and submit them as a hard copy for evaluation. Alternatively, your instructor may ask you to submit your answers online.

1. What are the assumptions for conducting a paired or dependent samples *t*-test in a study?

2. Which of the assumptions in Question 1 do you think were met in the Williams et al. (2022) study? Provide a rationale for your response with references.

3. Were the scores for self-efficacy, as measured by the SEE, normally distributed for the LTC residents participating in the Wii bowling exergame? Provide a rationale for your response.

4. What is the paired *t*-test value for self-efficacy for the LTC residents participating in the physical activity exergame? Is this result statistically significant? Provide a rationale for your response.

5. State the null hypothesis for self-efficacy outcome that was assessed in this study. Was this hypothesis accepted or rejected? Provide a rationale for your response.

6. Examine the *t* values in Appendix A. What *t* value would be significant at the 0.05 level for a one-tailed *t*-test in a study with 101 participants? What does this result indicate?

7. Were the scores for physical activity, as measured by the RAPA questionnaire, normally distributed for the LTC residents participating in the Wii bowling exergame? Provide a rationale for your response.

8. What analysis technique was conducted to examine preintervention and postintervention differences for physical activity level of LTC residents? Was physical activity significantly changed from preintervention to postintervention for the residents participating in the Wii bowling exergame? Provide a rationale for your response.

9. Was the sample size in this study adequate? Provide a rationale for your response with relevant sources.

10. Are the findings in the Williams et al. (2022) study ready for implementation in practice? Provide a rationale for your answer.

Understanding Analysis of Variance and Post Hoc Analyses

STATISTICAL TECHNIQUE IN REVIEW

Analysis of variance (ANOVA) is a parametric statistical technique conducted to determine whether a statistically significant difference exists among the means of three or more groups. There are different types of ANOVAs, with the most basic being the **one-way ANOVA**. This analysis is conducted when a study has one independent variable and one dependent variable. The data collected for the dependent variable should be normally distributed and achieve an interval- or ratio-level of measurement (Kim et al., 2022). This exercise focuses on the one-way ANOVA and introduces you to the repeated-measures ANOVA. The **repeated-measures ANOVA** is used to analyze data from studies where the same variable(s) is(are) repeatedly measured over time for a group or groups of study participants. The intent is to determine the change that occurs over time in the dependent variable(s) with exposure to the independent variable(s). More information about repeated-measures ANOVA and other types of ANOVA, such as multivariate ANOVA, factorial ANOVA, and analysis of covariance (ANCOVA), can be found in nursing research and statistical texts (Gray & Grove, 2021; Heavy, 2019; Kim et al., 2022; Terrell, 2021).

The outcome of ANOVA is a numerical value for the F statistic. The calculated F-ratio from ANOVA indicates the extent to which group means differ, while considering the variability within the groups.

$$F = \text{Differences between groups/Differences within groups}$$

ANOVA is similar to the independent samples t-test because both techniques are conducted to determine group differences (see Exercise 16). The null hypothesis tested is: *No differences exist between the means of the groups studied.* The null hypothesis is rejected when the analysis yields a smaller p value, such as $p = 0.022$, than the alpha $= 0.05$ set for the study. However, t-tests are conducted to determine the difference between two groups, because conducting multiple t-tests in a study with three or more groups results in an inflated Type I error. Thus ANOVA is the accurate statistic to conduct when a study includes more than two groups (Grove & Gray, 2023; Knapp, 2017).

Assuming the null hypothesis of no differences among the means of the groups studied is true, the probability of obtaining an F-ratio as large as the obtained value in each sample is determined by the calculated p value. If the p value is greater than the level of significance, or alpha, set for the study, then the study results are nonsignificant and the F-ratio will be less than the critical value for F in the statistical table (see Appendix C, Critical Values of F for alpha $= 0.05$ and alpha $= 0.01$ at the back of this text). With nonsignificant results, researchers will accept the null hypothesis of no significant differences among the groups' means. However, there is always a possibility that this decision is in error, and the probability of committing this Type I error is determined by alpha. When alpha = 0.05, there are 5 chances in 100 that the results are a Type I error or concluding something is significant when it is not. When alpha = 0.01, there is 1 chance in 100 that the results are a Type I error (Grove & Gray, 2023; Kim et al., 2022).

ANOVA Assumptions and Results

Conducting an ANOVA requires addressing the following assumptions:

1. The populations from which the samples were drawn, or the random samples, are normally distributed (i.e., the dependent variable should be normally distributed).
2. The dependent variable is measured at the interval or ratio level.
3. The measurements or observations of the dependent variable are independent.
4. The groups should be mutually exclusive.
5. The groups should have equal variance, also known as homogeneity of variance (Gray & Grove, 2021; Kim et al., 2022).

Researchers who analyze their data by conducting an ANOVA report their results in an ANOVA summary table or in the text of the research report. An example of how an ANOVA result is commonly expressed in the text of a study is as follows:

$$F(2,120) = 4.79, p = 0.01$$

where:

- F is the statistic.
- 2 is the group degrees of freedom (df) calculated by $k - 1$, where k = number of groups in the study. In this example, $k - 1 = 3 - 1 = 2$.
- 120 is the error degrees of freedom (df) that is calculated based upon the number of participants, or $N - k$. In this example, 123 participants − 3 groups = 120 error df.
- 4.79 is the F-ratio or value.
- p indicates the significance of the F-ratio in this study or $p = 0.01$.

The F value is calculated by computer with its p value to indicate its significance. As discussed earlier, the F value can also be compared with the critical values of F presented in Appendix C to determine significance. The critical F value with alpha = 0.05 for $F(2,120)$ is 3.07. In this example, the calculated F value is significant because it exceeds the critical F value in the table. In examining the critical values of F at alpha = 0.01, you note that $F(2,120) = 4.79$.

Post Hoc Analyses Following ANOVA

When a significant F value is obtained from the conduct of ANOVA, additional analyses are needed to determine the specific location of the differences in a study with more than two groups. **Post hoc analyses** were developed to determine where the differences lie, because some of the groups might be different and others might be similar. For example, a study might include three groups: an experimental group (receiving an intervention), a placebo group (receiving a pseudo or false treatment), and a comparison group (receiving standard care). The ANOVA resulted in a significant F-ratio or value, but post hoc analyses are needed to determine the exact location of the differences. With post hoc analyses, researchers might find that the experimental group is significantly different from both the placebo and comparison groups but that the placebo and comparison groups were not significantly different from each other. As discussed earlier, three t-tests could be conducted to determine differences among the groups, but that would inflate the Type I error (Grove & Gray, 2023; Kim et al., 2022). Thus post hoc analyses were developed to detect the differences after ANOVA with a significant *F* value. The frequently conducted post hoc analyses include the Newman-Keuls test, the Tukey Honestly Significant Difference (HSD) test, the Scheffé test, and the Dunnett test (Gray & Grove, 2021; Kim et al., 2022; Terrell, 2021).

With many post hoc analyses, the alpha level is reduced in proportion to the number of additional tests required to locate the statistically significant differences. As the alpha level is decreased, reaching the level of significance becomes increasingly more difficult. The Newman-Keuls test compares all possible pairs of means and is the most liberal of the post hoc tests discussed here. "Liberal" indicates that the alpha is not as severely decreased. The Tukey HSD test computes one value with which all means within the dataset are compared. It is considered more stringent than the Newman-Keuls test and requires approximately equal sample sizes in each group. The Scheffé test is one of the more conservative post hoc tests, but with the decrease in Type I error there is an increase in Type II error, which is concluding something is not significant when it is. The Dunnett test requires a control group, and the experimental groups are compared with the control group without a decrease in alpha. Exercise 35 provides the step-by-step process for calculating ANOVA and post hoc analyses.

RESEARCH ARTICLE

Source

Meehan, C. D., & Barker, N. (2021). Remediation for NCLEX-RN success in high-risk nursing students. *Teaching and Learning in Nursing, 16,* 254–257. https://doi.org/10.1016/j.teln.2021.02.003

Introduction

The pass rate on the National Council Licensure Exam for Registered Nurses (NCLEX-RN) is frequently used as one of the outcomes for determining the success of undergraduate nursing programs. Meehan and Barker (2021, p. 254) conducted a retrospective cohort study to determine whether a "remediation protocol would improve undergraduate baccalaureate predictor scores for passing the NCLEX-RN on the first attempt for high-risk students." The students completed either four semesters of remediation, two semesters of remediation, or no remediation for the classes of 2016, 2017, and 2018. This study included eight groups that are identified in Table 18.1. The eight groups included three groups of traditional students, three groups of second-degree students, and two groups of out-of-sequence students. The key results for this study are presented in the following excerpt.

Relevant Study Results

"In this study, researchers compared student scores on the Assessment Technologies Institute's (ATI) Comprehensive Predictor Exam. A comparison was made between senior students who participated in a formalized remediation program and those that did not. From the spring of 2016 through the spring of 2018, a total of 162 traditional undergraduate nursing students completed the Comprehensive Predictor Exam. Additionally, 96 second-degree nursing students completed the Comprehensive Predictor Exam from December 2016 through December 2018. Traditional students from cohort A had no implemented remediation program while cohort B had some remediation and cohort C completed two

TABLE 18.1	COMPREHENSIVE PREDICTOR SCORES FOR TRADITIONAL AND SECOND-DEGREE STUDENTS		
Groups	**Count**	**Sum**	**Average Score**
A traditional (no remediation)	50	3426.8	68.536
B traditional (two semesters remediation)	45	3093.4	68.742
C traditional (four semesters remediation)	51	3750.8	73.545
X traditional (out of sequence, 0 semesters remediation)	5	311.4	62.28
Z traditional (out of sequence, one semester remediation)	11	726	66
D Second degree (no remediation)	30	2052.3	68.41
E Second degree (two semesters remediation)	32	2354.7	73.584
F Second degree (four semesters remediation)	34	2664	78.353

years of a formalized remediation program. Similarly, second-degree students in cohort D had no implemented remediation program, cohort E had some remediation, and cohort F completed four semesters of a formalized remediation program [Table 18.1]. Additionally, 16 out-of-sequence students' data were included in the results. These students had failed one or more nursing courses. Although the Comprehensive Predictor has been determined to accurately project a student's likelihood to pass the NCLEX-RN, this study examined the effects of remediation on the Comprehensive Predictor scores in relation to remediation throughout the nursing program. . . .

A one-way between-subjects ANOVA was conducted to compare the effect of a remediation policy on nursing students enrolled in an undergraduate program in their last semester of a baccalaureate nursing program. Remediation had a significant effect on undergraduate nursing students' standardized testing at the $p < 0.05$ level for six cohorts consisting of $F(7,250) = 9.04$ and a p value of 0.0000000006 [Table 18.2]. Post hoc comparisons using the Tukey HSD test indicated that the mean score for those that received remediation was significantly different than those that did not in similar cohorts. These results would support the integration of remediation within nursing programs to improve a student's success on predictive NCLEX-RN practice exams. . . . Students who participated in the full remediation program achieved a minimal score of 73.84% and had at least a 95% likelihood of passing the NCLEX-RN on their first attempt. Students who did not participate in any remediation program did not score over 68.53%" (Meehan & Barker, 2021, p. 256).

This study indicated that the implementation of a formalized remediation program improved the predictor exam scores for students preparing for the NCLEX-RN.

TABLE 18.2	ANOVA					
Source of Variation	**SS**	**df**	**MS**	**F**	**p value**	**F crit**
Between groups	3757.095	7	536.728	9.040	0.0000000006	2.046
Within groups	14842.853	250	59.371			
Total	18599.948	257				

STUDY QUESTIONS

1. Describe the type of design used by Meehan and Barker (2021) in their study.

2. What were the independent and dependent variables included in this study?

3. How was the dependent variable measured for this study? What level of measurement was achieved for this variable? Provide a rationale for your answer.

4. Identify the number and types of groups that were examined for differences.

5. What type of analysis was conducted in this study to examine group differences? Was that an appropriate analysis technique? Provide a rationale for your answer.

6. What are the assumptions for use of ANOVA?

7. What did the researcher set the level of significance, or alpha, at for this study? What is the potential for Type I error with this level of alpha?

8. State the null hypothesis for the Meehan and Barker (2021) study.

9. What were the ANOVA results for this study? Should the null hypothesis be accepted or rejected? Provide a rationale for your answer.

10. Was group A significantly different than group C? What do these results indicate?

Answers to Study Questions

1. Meehan and Barker (2021) conducted a retrospective cohort study. Retrospective means looking back in time and involves collecting data from existing records or databases for analysis. Cohorts are groups or categories of groups that are included in a study. In this study, data were exit exam scores obtained from a convenience sample of nursing students' records in the final semester of their undergraduate program (Gray & Grove, 2021).

2. The independent variable was the remediation protocol. The dependent or outcome variable was the student scores on the ATI Comprehensive Predictor Exam.

3. The dependent variable was measured using the ATI Comprehensive Predictor Exam. This exam is a standardized test used to predict nursing students' performance on the NCLEX-RN exam. The data obtained with the ATI exam are at the ratio level with equal interval categories and an absolute zero (see Exercise 1; Grove & Gray, 2023).

4. The Meehan and Barker (2022) study included eight groups that are identified in Table 18.1. Three groups included traditional students, three groups included second-degree students, and two groups included out-of-sequence students who had failed a nursing course. The traditional and second-degree students had one of the following: no remediation, two semesters of remediation, or four semesters of remediation. The out-of-sequence students had either no remediation or one semester of remediation.

5. Meehan and Barker (2021) reported they conducted a one-way ANOVA to determine differences among the eight groups of nursing students in their study (see Table 18.1). The one-way ANOVA was appropriate because the study included one independent variable (remediation) and one dependent variable (ATI exam scores). The exam scores were independent and at the ratio level of measurement. Because this study focused on examining differences among multiple groups, the ANOVA statistical technique was the most appropriate (see Fig. 12.1; Gray & Grove, 2021).

6. The five assumptions for the ANOVA statistical technique are that there is a normal distribution of the populations from which the samples were drawn; that the dependent variable is measured at the interval or ratio level; that measurements of the dependent variable are independent; that groups should be mutually exclusive; and that groups should have equal variance or homogeneity of variance (Gray & Grove, 2021; Kim et al., 2022).

7. The level of significance, or alpha, for this study was set at 0.05. The potential for a Type I error is 5 chances in 100 (Grove & Gray, 2023).

8. The null hypothesis is: *The groups of traditional, second-degree, and out-of-sequence nursing students who received remediation had no difference in their ATI exam scores than those who did not receive remediation.*

9. According to Table 18.2 and the study narrative, $F(7,250) = 9.04$, $p = 0.0000000006$, was calculated for the ATI exam scores for the eight groups of nursing students. This F value is statistically significant because the p value is less than the alpha $= 0.05$ that was set for this study. The significant result means that there was a statistically significant difference among the eight groups of nursing students' ATI exam scores. In addition, the $F(7,250) = 9.04$ is greater than the critical value of $F = 2.046$, which indicates statistical significance (see Table 18.2). Therefore the null hypothesis was rejected (Grove & Gray, 2023).

10. Yes, groups A and C were significantly different. Meehan and Barker (2021, p. 256) reported that the "mean score for those that received remediation was significantly different than those that did not in similar cohorts." Group A (no remediation) and Group C (four semesters of remediation) were cohorts of traditional students who were reported to have significantly different ATI exam scores.

Questions for Additional Study

| Name: _____ | Class: _____ |
| Date: _____ | |

Follow your instructor's directions to submit your answers to the following questions for additional study. Your instructor may ask you to write your answers below and submit them as a hard copy for evaluation. Alternatively, your instructor may ask you to submit your answers online.

1. Examine the traditional groups of nursing students in the Meehan and Barker (2021) study. Which group had the highest average score on the ATI's Comprehensive Predictive Exam: A, B, or C? Provide a rationale for your answer.

2. Which group had the highest average score for the ATI exam? Identify the mean for this group and discuss its meaning.

3. Were the traditional out-of-sequence students in groups X and Z adequately represented in the Meehan and Barker (2021) study? Provide a rationale for your answer.

4. ANOVA was conducted by Meehan and Barker (2021) to examine group differences in their study. Would *t*-tests have also been appropriate? Provide a rationale for your answer.

5. In Table 18.2, Meehan and Barker (2021) reported the *df* for the one-way ANOVA as 7 and 250. What types of *df*s are these and how were they calculated?

6. What is the purpose for conducting post hoc analysis? What type of post hoc test was conducted in the Meehan and Barker (2021) study and was it appropriate? Provide a rationale for your answer.

7. Were adequate results reported for the calculation of the Tukey HSD test? Provide a rationale for your answer.

8. State the null hypothesis regarding the average scores for the second-degree students in groups D and F (see Table 18.1). Should the null hypothesis be accepted or rejected? Provide a rationale for your answer.

9. Hypothetically, researchers reported the following results from the one-way ANOVA in their study: $F(4,60) = 3.14$. Is this result significant? Provide a rationale for your answer.

10. Are the findings from the Meehan and Barker (2021) study ready for use in educational programs to improve nursing graduates' success on their NCLEX-RN exam? Provide a rationale for your answer.

Understanding the Pearson Chi-Square

STATISTICAL TECHNIQUE IN REVIEW

The **Pearson chi-square** (χ^2) is an inferential statistical test calculated to examine differences among groups with variables measured at the nominal level. There are different types of chi-square tests and the Pearson chi-square is commonly reported in nursing studies. The Pearson chi-square test compares the frequencies that are observed with the frequencies that were expected. The *assumptions* for the chi-square test are as follows (Daniel, 2000):

1. Only one datum entry is made for each participant in the sample. Therefore, if repeated measures from the same participant are being used for analysis, such as pretests and post-tests, chi-square is not an appropriate test.
2. The variables must be categorical (i.e., nominal), either inherently, or transformed to categorical from quantitative values.
3. For each variable, the categories are mutually exclusive and exhaustive. No cells may have an *expected* frequency of zero. In the actual data, the *observed* cell frequency may be zero. However, the Pearson chi-square test is not sensitive to small sample sizes, and other tests, such as the Fisher exact test, are more appropriate when testing very small samples (Daniel, 2000; Yates, 1934).

The chi-square values calculated are compared with the critical values in the chi-square table (see Appendix D, Critical Values of the χ^2 Distribution). If the result is greater than or equal to the value in the table, significant differences exist. If the values are statistically significant, the null hypothesis is rejected (Gray & Grove, 2021). These results indicate that the differences are probably an actual reflection of reality and not caused by random sampling error or chance.

In addition to the chi-square value, researchers often report the degrees of freedom (*df*). This statistical concept is important for calculating and determining levels of significance. The standard formula for *df* is sample size (*N*) minus 1, or $df = N - 1$; however, this formula is adjusted based on the analysis technique performed (Pett, 2016). The *df* formula for the chi-square test varies based on the number of categories examined in the analysis. The formula for *df* for the two-way chi-square test is $df = (R - 1)(C - 1)$, where *R* is the number of rows and *C* is the number of columns in a chi-square table. For example, in a 2×2 chi-square table, $df = (2 - 1)(2 - 1) = 1$. Therefore the *df* is equal to 1. Table 19.1 displays

TABLE 19.1   CONTINGENCY TABLE BASED ON THE RESULTS OF CONLON ET AL. (2021) STUDY

	COVID-19 Positive (*n* = 1,218)	COVID-19 Negative (*n* = 25,983)
Diabetes	262	2,556
No diabetes	956	23,427

a 2×2 chi-square contingency table based on the findings of a study by Conlon and colleagues (2021). In Table 19.1, the columns represent the two nominal binary categories of the novel coronavirus of 2019 (COVID-19) test results (positive/negative); and the two rows represent the two nominal binary categories of those with and without diabetes. The $df = (2 − 1) (2 − 1) = (1) (1) = 1$, and the study results were as follows: $\chi^2(1, N = 27{,}201) = 170.72$, $p < 0.001$. It is important to note that the df can also be reported without the sample size, as in $\chi^2(1) = 170.72$, $p < 0.001$. Among those with diabetes, rates of testing positive for COVID-19 were significantly higher. Alternatively, the rates of diabetes were significantly higher among those who tested positive for COVID-19 (Conlon et al., 2021).

If more than two groups are being examined, chi-square does not determine where the differences lie; it only determines that a statistically significant difference exists. A post hoc chi-square analysis will determine the location of the difference. The step-by-step process for calculating the Pearson chi-square test is presented in Exercise 37.

RESEARCH ARTICLE

Source

Conlon, A., Ashur, C., Washer, L., Eagle, K. A., & Bowman, M. A. H. (2021). Impact of the influenza vaccine on COVID-19 infection rates and severity. *American Journal of Infection Control, 49*(6), 694–700. https://doi.org/10.1016/j.ajic.2021.02.012

Introduction

Conlon and colleagues (2021) conducted a retrospective cohort study to assess the role of the influenza vaccine on COVID-19 susceptibility and severity. The primary study outcome was the comparison of positive and negative COVID-19 testing in those who received the influenza vaccine versus those who did not. Other study variables included baseline patient characteristics and the presence of comorbidities. Over 4.5 million unique patient charts within the Michigan Medicine healthcare system were extracted, and of those, 27,201 patients received laboratory testing for COVID-19. The study alpha was set to 0.05. The footnote under Table 19.2 states, "*P* values are shown from chi-square tests for categorial variables and Wilcoxon rank sum tests for continuous variables comparing probability of positive COVID-19 test."

Relevant Study Results

The following excerpt summarizes the Pearson chi-square results that indicate the differences between those with positive and negative COVID-19 test results on baseline demographic and clinical variables. "Higher rates of comorbid conditions were seen in patients testing positive for COVID-19, including chronic pulmonary disease (19.8% vs 14.6%, $P < .001$), congestive heart failure (10.3% vs 7.8%, $P = .003$), any diabetes (21.5% vs 9.8%, $P < .001$), complicated diabetes (8.5% vs 2.9%, $P < .001$), uncomplicated diabetes (13.1% vs 7.0%, $P < .001$), any hypertension (36.0% vs 22.5%, $P < .001$), complicated hypertension (14.4% vs 6.0%, $P < .001$), and uncomplicated hypertension (21.6% vs 16.5%, $P < .001$). Additionally, older patients and African Americans were more likely to test positive versus negative for COVID-19 (50.7 years vs 47.1 years, $P < .001$ and 35.5% vs 11.4%, $P < .001$, respectively). A comparison of baseline characteristics stratified by COVID-19 status is seen in [Table 19.2].

TABLE 19.2   PATIENT CHARACTERISTICS AND ASSOCIATIONS WITH COVID-19

Variable*	COVID-19 Negative (*n* = 25,983)	COVID-19 Positive (*n* = 1218)	Entire cohort (*n* = 27,201)	P value†
Influenza vaccine, n (%)	12,472 (48.0)	525 (43.1)	12,997 (47.8)	<.001
Women, n (%)	14,512 (55.9)	649 (53.3)	15,161 (55.7)	0.08
Age, mean (*SD*)	47.07 (22.21)	50.69 (18.67)	47.23 (22.07)	<.001
Age, n (%)				
<35	8143 (31.3%)	276 (22.7%)	8419 (31.0%)	<.001
35–49	4532 (17.4%)	276 (22.7%)	4808 (17.7%)	
50–64	6098 (23.5%)	349 (28.7%)	6447 (23.7%)	
≥65	6597 (25.4%)	308 (25.3%)	6905 (25.4%)	
Race, n (%)				
African American	2,972 (11.4)	432 (35.5)	3,404 (12.5)	<.001
Caucasian	20,386 (78.5)	617 (50.7)	21,003 (77.2)	
Other	1,841 (7.1)	113 (9.3)	1,954 (7.2)	
Ethnicity, n (%)				
Hispanic or Latino	824 (3.2)	27 (2.2)	851 (3.1)	0.08
Non-Hispanic or Latino	23,951 (92.2)	1111 (91.2)	25,062 (92.1)	
Chronic pulmonary disease, n (%)	3806 (14.6)	241 (19.8)	4047 (14.9)	<.001
Congestive heart failure, n (%)	2032 (7.8)	125 (10.3)	2157 (7.9)	0.003
Diabetes, n (%)	2556 (9.8)	262 (21.5)	2818 (10.4)	<.001
Complicated diabetes, n (%)	749 (2.9)	103 (8.5)	852 (3.1)	<.001
Uncomplicated diabetes, n (%)	1807 (7.0)	159 (13.1)	1966 (7.2)	<.001
Hypertension, n (%)	5847 (22.5)	438 (36.0)	6285 (23.1)	<.001
Complicated hypertension, n (%)	1549 (6.0)	175 (14.4)	1724 (6.3)	<.001
Uncomplicated hypertension, n (%)	4298 (16.5)	263 (21.6)	4561 (16.8)	<.001
BMI, SD	28.23 (9.10)	32.42 (12.28)	28.39 (9.28)	<.001
BMI, **n** (%)				
<18.5	1713 (6.6%)	17 (1.4%)	1730 (6.4%)	
18.5–24.9	4856 (18.7%)	117 (9.6%)	4973 (18.3%)	
25–29.9	5097 (19.6%)	219 (18.0%)	5316 (19.5%)	
30–39.9	5014 (19.3%)	264 (21.7%)	5278 (19.4%)	
>40	1424 (5.5%)	118 (9.7%)	1542 (5.7%)	
Elixhauser Score, SD	1.54 (2.34)	2.53 (3.19)	1.59 (2.39)	<.001
Smoking Status, n (%)				
Current smoker	1678 (6.5%)	40 (3.3%)	1718 (6.3%)	0.002
Former smoker	3635 (14.0%)	175 (14.4%)	3810 (14.0%)	
Tobacco use	91 (0.4%)	2 (0.2%)	93 (0.3%)	
Never smoker	6836 (26.3%)	348 (28.6%)	7184 (26.4%)	

*Proportions vary because of missing data on comorbid covariates chronic pulmonary disease, congestive heart failure, diabetes, complicated diabetes, uncomplicated diabetes, hypertension, complicated hypertension, and uncomplicated hypertension (*n* = 251, 0.9%), age (*n* = 622, 2.3%), race (*n* = 840, 3.1%), and ethnicity (*n* = 1,288, 4.7%), and a larger amount of missing data on BMI (*n* = 8,362, 30.7%) and smoking status (*n* = 14,396, 52.9%).
†P values are shown from Chi-square tests for categorial variables and Wilcoxon rank sum tests for continuous variables comparing probability of positive COVID-19 test.
From: Conlon, A., Ashur, C., Washer, L., Eagle, K. A., & Bowman, M. A. H. (2021). Impact of the influenza vaccine on COVID-19 infection rates and severity. *American Journal of Infection Control*, *49*(6), 694–700. https://doi.org/10.1016/j.ajic.2021.02.012

Patients receiving an influenza vaccine tended to have more comorbidities than those in the unvaccinated group, including higher rates of chronic pulmonary disease (16.4% vs 13.4%, $P < .001$), congestive heart failure (9.2% vs 6.7%, $P < .001$), diabetes (11.1% vs 9.7%, $P = .001$), and hypertension (23.9% vs 22.3%, $P = .01$). Patients receiving an influenza vaccine also tended to be older (48.4 years vs 46.1 years, $P < .001$), female (61.0% vs 50.9%, $P < .001$), and Caucasian (80.1% vs 74.6%, $P < .001$)" (Conlon et al., 2021, p. 696).

It should be noted that this article represents each *p* value with an uppercase *P* because the *American Journal of Infection Control* displays *p* as uppercase. Most journals of nursing research require formatting in accordance with the American Psychological Association (APA, 2020), which requires *p* to be lowercase.

STUDY QUESTIONS

1. What is the sample size for the Conlon et al. (2021) study? How many study participants (percentage) tested positive for COVID-19 and how many tested negative? Was this sample size adequate for the study?

2. State the null hypothesis with regard to influenza vaccine (received/not received) by COVID-19 test result (positive/negative) in the Conlon et al. (2021) study.

3. What is the p value for influenza vaccine? Was the null hypothesis accepted or rejected? Provide rationales for your answers.

4. Does a statistically significant chi-square result provide evidence of causation between the variables? Provide a rationale for your answer.

5. What is the p value for congestive heart failure? Is the p value statistically significant? Provide a rationale for your answer.

6. Is there a statistically significant difference with regard to percentage of women by COVID-19 test result (positive/negative)? Document your answer.

7. What is the *df* for smoking status? Calculate the *df* for the Pearson chi-square test comparing COVID-19 test result (positive/negative) by smoking status (current/former/tobacco use/never).

8. State the null hypothesis regarding the variable smoking status by COVID-19 test result (positive/negative).

9. Should the null hypothesis for smoking status (developed in Question 8) be accepted or rejected? Provide a rationale for your answer.

10. Would a Pearson chi-square test be appropriate for the comparison of Elixhauser Scores by COVID-19 test result (positive/negative)? Why or why not?

Answers to Study Questions

1. The sample size is $n = 27,201$ with $n = 25,983$ (95.52%) persons who tested negative for COVID-19 and $n = 1,218$ (4.48%) persons who tested positive for COVID-19 as indicated in Table 19.2. This sample size is extremely large, and the majority of the statistical results were significant, indicating adequate statistical power (see Exercise 25).

2. The null hypothesis is: *There is no difference between persons who tested negative and positive for COVID-19 on whether they received the influenza vaccine.*

3. The $p < 0.001$ for influenza vaccine. Because p is less than the study alpha of 0.05, this result is significant. The specific chi-square values are not listed in Table 19.2, which is a typical method of reporting a set of multiple chi-square tests. The null hypothesis is rejected when study results are statistically significant (Gray & Grove, 2021; Pett, 2016). It should be noted that p values never equal zero, but they may be extremely small. Per APA format, very small p values are reported as "< 0.001."

4. No, a statistically significant chi-square value does not provide evidence of causation. A statistically significant chi-square value indicates that a significant difference between groups exists, but does not provide a causal link (Grove & Gray, 2023; Shadish et al., 2002).

5. The $p = 0.003$ for congestive heart failure. Because p is less than the study alpha of 0.05, this result is significant.

6. No, there was not a statistically significant difference with regard to percentage of women by COVID-19 test result (positive/negative). Of those who tested negative for COVID-19, 55.9% were women. Of those who tested positive for COVID-19, 53.3% were women. The chi-square test was not significant because $p = 0.08$, which exceeds the study alpha of 0.05, indicating a nonsignificant result.

7. The df formula is $df = (R - 1)(C - 1)$. There are four R rows for smoking status: current, former, tobacco use, and never. There are two C columns, negative and positive COVID-19 test. Therefore $df = (4 - 1)(2 - 1) = (3)(1) = 3$.

8. The null hypothesis: *There is no difference between persons who tested negative versus those who tested positive for COVID-19 on their category of smoking status.*

9. The null hypothesis should be rejected. The $p = 0.002$ for smoking status and is therefore less than the study alpha of 0.05. The null hypothesis is rejected when study results are statistically significant (Gray & Grove, 2021; Pett, 2016).

10. No, a Pearson chi-square test is not appropriate for the comparison of Elixhauser Scores by COVID-19 test result. One of the assumptions of the Pearson chi-square test is that the data are of a nominal level of measurement. The Elixhauser Score is an ordinal variable, with higher values indicative of more medical comorbidities, and lower values indicative of fewer medical comorbidities (Elixhauser, et al., 1998). According to the footnote under Table 19.2, the Wilcoxon rank-sum test (otherwise known as the Mann-Whitney U test; see Exercises 21 and 34) was computed to compare Elixhauser Scores by COVID-19 test result.

Follow your instructor's directions to submit your answers to the following questions for additional study. Your instructor may ask you to write your answers below and submit them as a hard copy for evaluation. Alternatively, your instructor may ask you to submit your answers online.

1. According to Table 19.2 of the Conlon et al. (2021) study, name the two variables that were *not* statistically significant. Document your answer.

2. What level of measurement is appropriate for calculating the chi-square statistic? Give two examples from Table 19.2 of demographic variables measured at the level appropriate for chi-square.

3. State the null hypothesis regarding the variable of uncomplicated hypertension by COVID-19 test result (positive/negative).

4. Should the null hypothesis for uncomplicated hypertension (developed in Question 3) be accepted or rejected? Provide a rationale for your answer.

5. List the percentages of persons with uncomplicated hypertension in the two COVID-19 test groups. Show the calculations for how these percentages were derived using the values listed in Table 19.2.

6. What is the *df* for race? Calculate the *df* for the Pearson chi-square test comparing COVID-19 test result (positive/negative) by race (African American/Caucasian/other).

7. Is there a statistically significant difference with regard to presence of chronic pulmonary disease by COVID-19 test result (positive/negative)? Document your answer.

8. List the percentages of persons with chronic pulmonary disease in the two COVID-19 test groups. Show the calculations for how these percentages were derived using the values listed in Table 19.2.

9. Compare and contrast the two different statistical analyses for the variable of age presented in Table 19.2.

10. A statistically significant difference is present between persons who tested negative versus positive for COVID-19 on their category of smoking status, $p = 0.002$. Does this result provide the location of the difference? Provide a rationale for your answer.

Understanding Spearman Rank-Order Correlation Coefficient

STATISTICAL TECHNIQUE IN REVIEW

The **Spearman rank-order correlation coefficient**, or **Spearman *rho*** (also written as ρ), is a nonparametric test conducted to identify relationships or associations between two variables. The Spearman analysis technique is an adaptation of the Pearson product-moment correlation (see Exercises 13 and 29) and is calculated when the assumptions of the Pearson correlation analysis cannot be met. Thus the Spearman *rho* is computed on data that are ordinal level of measurement or variables measured at the interval or ratio levels with values that are skewed or not normally distributed (Pett, 2016; Terrell, 2021).

Each participant included in the analysis must have a score (or value) on each of two variables *x* and *y*. The values for both variables must be ranked to conduct this analysis. The values on each variable are ranked separately (Pett, 2016; Daniel, 2000). Calculation of Spearman *rho* is based on **difference scores** between a participant's ranking on the first (variable *x*) and second (variable *y*) sets of values. The formula for difference scores is $D = x - y$. Because results with negative values cancel out positive values, results are squared for use in the analysis. The formula for calculation of Spearman *rho* is:

$$\rho = 1 - \frac{6\sum D^2}{N^3 - N}$$

where:

ρ = *Rho*, the statistic for the Spearman correlation coefficient

D = Difference between the rankings of a participant's score or value on both variables *x* and *y*

N = Number of paired ranked scores (Daniel, 2000).

The Spearman rank-order correlation coefficient values range from -1 to $+1$, where a positive value indicates a positive association, and a negative value indicates a negative or inverse association. Numbers closest to $+1$ or -1 indicate the strongest associations. In comparison to the Pearson correlation coefficient (*r*), the Spearman *rho* has a statistical power of 91%, which means the Spearman *rho* has a 9% smaller probability of detecting an association if one exists. If the study sample size is greater than 50 participants, the power of the Spearman *rho* is approximately equal to the Pearson *r* in detecting a relationship in a study. The strength of *rho* values are as follows, in absolute value: <0.30 are weak relationships, 0.30 to 0.50 are moderate relationships, and >0.50 are strong relationships. A Spearman *rho* of 0 indicates no relationship between the two variables; the closer the *rho* value is to 0, the weaker the relationship (Pett, 2016; Terrell, 2021). The significance of *rho* can be determined in one of two ways: (1) by comparing the calculated value with the critical value in a Spearman *rho* table, or (2) by using statistical software to compute the Spearman *rho*, along with exact *p* values.

TABLE 20.1 ASSOCIATION BETWEEN TWO INSTRUCTORS' RANKINGS OF STUDENTS' INTRAMUSCULAR INJECTION TECHNIQUES

Student	Instructor A Ranking	Instructor B Ranking	D	D²
Amy	1	1	0	0
Jeff	3	2	1	1
John	5	4	1	1
Julie	2	3	−1	1
Mary	4	5	−1	1
Susie	6	6	0	0
Sum				**4**

The Spearman *rho* is calculated using the following hypothetical example: six students' intramuscular (IM) injection techniques were ranked by two instructors from a high score of 1 to a low score of 6. The data or rankings for this example are ordinal and presented in Table 20.1. The purpose of this example is to examine the relationship between the two instructors' rankings of the six students' IM injection techniques. The null hypothesis is: *There is no association between rankings of students' IM injection technique by instructors A and B.*

Calculations:

$$\rho = 1 - \frac{6\sum D^2}{N^3 - N} \quad \rho = 1 - \frac{6(4)}{216 - 6} = 1 - \frac{24}{210} = 1 - 0.114 = 0.886$$

In this example, a strong positive correlation or association ($\rho = 0.886$) was found between the two instructors' ranking of students on IM injection techniques. This value for *rho*, when compared with the critical value in a Spearman correlation coefficient table (Plichta & Kelvin, 2013) of 0.829 for *n* = 6 for a two-tailed test, is statistically significant because it is equal to the critical value. Because the *rho* value is statistically significant, the null hypothesis is rejected. The Spearman *rho* is usually calculated with a larger sample and using a statistical computer package, such as SPSS (IBM Corporation, 2022), that determines the *rho* value and its significance (Pett, 2016). Usually, a Spearman *rho* is calculated with data that are not rankings, and therefore the statistical software internally converts the raw data to ranks and applies the Spearman *rho* formula. Spearman *rho* values may be notated in journal articles as "*rho*," "r_s," or "ρ."

RESEARCH ARTICLE

Source

Urban, R. W., Smith, J., Wilson, S., & Cipher, D. J. (2021). Relationships among stress, resilience, and incivility in undergraduate nursing students and faculty during the COVID-19 pandemic: Policy implications for nurse leaders. *Journal of Professional Nursing, 37*(6), 1063–1070. https://doi.org/10.1016/j.profnurs.2021.08.011

Introduction

Urban and colleagues (2021) conducted a descriptive correlational study to compare associations among and differences between perceptions of incivility frequency, self-reported stress, and resilience levels in undergraduate nursing students and faculty during the COVID-19 pandemic.

An online survey was used to collect data from 710 undergraduate nursing students and faculty. The researchers measured stress and resilience using the Perceived Stress Scale-10 (*PSS-10*) and the Resilience Scale-14 (*RS-14*), respectively. Ratings of low-level and high-level incivility were collected with the Incivility in Nursing Education-Revised (*INE-R*). Higher values on each of these scales represent higher levels of the concept being measured. Examples of low-level incivility include expressions of boredom, apathy, or disinterest in the classroom. Examples of high-level incivility include using profanity, making rude remarks, or sending inappropriate emails and texts.

"Students were significantly more stressed and less resilient than faculty. Faculty reported significantly greater low- and high-level student and low-level faculty incivility behaviors than students. Understanding student and faculty perceptions of uncivil behavior frequency occurring at the intersection of high stress and moderate resilience levels is key to the creation of targeted interventions and policy development" (Urban et al., 2021, p. 1063).

Relevant Study Results

The statistical analyses in this study included descriptive statistics and the inferential statistics of Spearman correlation, chi-square (also written as χ^2) (see Exercise 19), and multiple linear regression (see Exercises 15 and 31). The level of significance, or α, was set to 0.05. "Spearman correlation coefficients were computed to assess the relationships reported by nursing faculty among the study variables (stress, resilience, and the frequency of low/high incivility behaviors in nursing students and faculty). There was a weak negative correlation between stress and resilience in faculty that approached significance (*rho* = 0.293, *p* = .08). A weak positive correlation was found between faculty stress and increased frequency of reporting high-level faculty incivility that approached significance (*rho* = 0.285, *p* = .08). Significant positive correlations existed for faculty between reporting higher frequency scores on low student incivility and reporting frequency scores for higher student incivility (*rho* = 0.876, *p* < .001) and lower faculty incivility (*rho* = 0.552, *p* < .001) but not high faculty incivility frequency scores (*rho* = 0.331, *p* < .058). Similarly, there was a significant positive correlation among nursing faculty reporting higher frequency scores on the low and high student incivility subscales (*rho* = 0.538, *p* < .006) and on the high faculty incivility subscales (*rho* = 0.388, *p* < .037)." (Urban et al., 2021, p. 1067; see Table 20.2).

TABLE 20.2   RELATIONSHIPS AMONG UNDERGRADUATE NURSING STUDENT AND FACULTY SURVEY TOTAL SCORES

		PSS–10	RS–14	SLLIB	SHLIB	FLLIB	FHLIB
Perceived Stress Scale (PSS–10)	Student	–	−0.567**	0.269**	0.119**	0.291**	0.219**
	Faculty	–	*−0.293*	*0.242*	*0.161*	*0.254*	*0.285*
Resilience Scale (RS-14)	Student		–	−0.312**	−0.163**	−0.271**	−0.202**
	Faculty		–	*−0.059*	*−0.071*	*−0.129*	*−0.058*
INE-R Student Low-Level Incivility Behaviors (SLLIB) Subscale	Student			–	0.740**	0.710**	0.592**
	Faculty			–	*0.876***	*0.552***	*0.331*
INE-R Student High-Level Incivility Behaviors (SHLIB) Subscale	Student				–	0.611**	0.616**
	Faculty				–	*0.538***	*0.388***
INE-R Faculty Low-Level Incivility Behaviors (FLLIB) Subscale	Student					–	0.836**
	Faculty					–	*0.747***
INE-R Faculty High-Level Incivility Behaviors (FHLIB) Subscale	Student						–

Note: Pooled r_s values are reported from the imputed datasets.
*Correlation is significant at the 0.05 level (2-tailed).
**Correlation is significant at the 0.01 level (2-tailed).
From: Urban, R. W., Smith, J., Wilson, S, & Cipher, D. J. (2021). Relationships among stress, resilience, and incivility in undergraduate nursing students and faculty during the COVID-19 pandemic: Policy implications for nurse leaders. *Journal of Professional Nursing*, 37(6), 1063–1070. https://doi.org/10.1016/j.profnurs.2021.08.011

STUDY QUESTIONS

1. Among the *student* respondents, what was the Spearman correlation between perceived stress (*PSS-10*) and resilience (*RS-14*)?

2. Describe the strength and direction of the correlation between student-perceived stress *(PSS-10)* and resilience *(RS-14)*. Is this correlation statistically significant? Provide a rationale for your answer.

3. What was the largest Spearman correlation value in Table 20.2? Provide an interpretation of the value.

4. What correlation is reported in Table 20.2 as Spearman $\rho = 0.219$, $p < 0.01$?

5. Describe the strength and direction of the correlation between resilience (*RS-14*) and ratings of student low-level incivility (*SLLIB*) among the *student* respondents.

6. Is there a stronger correlation between resilience (*RS-14*) and ratings of student low-level incivility (*SLLIB*) among the student respondents, or among the faculty respondents? Provide a rationale for your answer.

7. Describe the strength and direction of the association between perceived stress (*PSS-10*) and student high-level incivility (*SHLIB*) among the *faculty* respondents. Is this correlation statistically significant? Provide a rationale for your answer.

8. Examine the correlations between perceived stress (*PSS-10*) and student high-level incivility (*SHLIB*) for students versus faculty. Explain why the correlation for the student respondents was significant and the correlation for the faculty respondents was not significant.

9. How many correlations presented in Table 20.2 are statistically significant at $p < 0.01$? Provide a rationale for your answer.

10. Spearman rank-order correlation coefficients were computed to examine the associations in this study. Was this analysis appropriate? Provide a rationale for your answer. What is the preferred parametric analysis for identifying relationships between variables (review Exercise 13)?

Answers to Study Questions

1. The Spearman correlation between perceived stress (*PSS-10*) and resilience (*RS-14*) among the student respondents was $\rho = -0.567$.

2. The *rho* of -0.567** was a statistically significant inverse correlation, indicating that higher levels of stress were associated with lower levels of resilience among the student respondents. This correlation is statistically significant at $p < 0.01$, as indicated by the ** in the footnote of Table 20.2. Like most nurse researchers, Urban and colleagues (2021) set their level of significance or alpha at 0.05. Because $p < 0.01$ is smaller than alpha, the relationship is statistically significant (Pett, 2016). Note that the negative sign in $\rho = -0.567$ indicates the direction of the association, not the strength of the association (Gray & Grove, 2021; Pett, 2016).

3. The largest Spearman *rho* value in Table 20.2 is 0.876**, representing the correlation between faculty ratings of low student incivility (*SLLIB*) and faculty ratings of high student incivility (*SHLIB*). There was a strong positive association between ratings of low-level and high-level student incivility among the faculty respondents. Higher ratings of low-level incivility behaviors were associated with higher ratings of high-level incivility behaviors. Similarly, lower ratings of low-level behaviors were associated with lower ratings of high-level behaviors. This relationship was statistically significant at $p = 0.01$ as indicated by the ** displayed in the footnote to this table.

4. The correlation described in Table 20.2 with $\rho = 0.219$, $p < 0.01$ is the weak, positive association between perceived stress (*PSS-10*) and ratings of faculty high-level incivility behaviors (*FHLIB*) among the student respondents. Higher levels of perceived stress were associated with higher ratings of faculty high-level incivility, and vice versa (i.e., lower levels of perceived stress were associated with lower ratings of faculty high-level incivility).

5. There is a negative, moderate correlation between resilience (*RS-14*) and ratings of student low-level incivility (*SLLIB*) among the *student* respondents: $\rho = -0.312$ ($p < 0.01$). Among the student respondents, higher levels of resilience were associated with lower ratings of student low-level incivility, and vice versa (i.e., lower levels of resilience were associated with higher ratings of student low-level incivility).

6. The stronger correlation is between resilience (*RS-14*) and ratings of student low-level incivility (*SLLIB*) among the *student* respondents is $\rho = -0.312$ ($p < 0.01$), which is a moderate, negative, significant association. The association between resilience (*RS-14*) and ratings of student low-level incivility (*SLLIB*) among the *faculty* respondents is $\rho = -0.059$, which is a weak, negative nonsignificant association that is close to 0.0. The closer the *rho* value is to $+1$ or -1, the stronger the correlation between variables. Note that the negative sign in $\rho = -0.312$ indicates the direction of the association and not the strength of the association (Gray & Grove, 2021; Pett, 2016).

7. The correlation between perceived stress (*PSS-10*) and student high-level incivility (*SHLIB*) for the faculty respondents was not significant, with $\rho = 0.161$. This correlation was not statistically significant at $p < 0.05$ or $p < 0.01$ because there are no asterisks by the *rho* value.

8. The correlation between perceived stress (*PSS-10*) and student high-level incivility (*SHLIB*) for the student respondents was significant with $\rho = 0.119$, $p < 0.01$, whereas the correlation between perceived stress (*PSS-10*) and student high-level incivility (*SHLIB*) for the faculty respondents was not significant with $\rho = 0.161$. The student sample size was 675, while the faculty sample size was 35. Therefore a weak Spearman *rho* was statistically significant with a large N of students, but not a small N of faculty. As demonstrated in Exercise 25, the power of any inferential statistic is substantially affected by sample size. The greater the sample size, the higher the power of the statistic (Aberson, 2019; Cohen, 1988).

9. A total of 19 correlations identified in Table 20.2 are statistically significant at $p < 0.01$, as indicated by the ** beside the *rho* value and described in the footnote of Table 20.2.

10. The researchers did not explicitly state the reason(s) why Spearman rank-order correlation coefficients were computed to examine associations in this study. It is assumed that the Spearman correlations were the appropriate choice because: (1) some of the study data were considered at the ordinal level of measurement by the researchers; and/or (2) the study data were found to be nonnormally distributed and therefore inappropriate for parametric analyses. Pearson product-moment correlation is the parametric and the preferred analysis technique to identify associations between two variables when the assumptions for this test are met, which includes the study variables being measured at the interval or ratio level (see Exercise 13). The Pearson r is preferred because it is more powerful in identifying significant relationships than the Spearman *rho* (Gray & Grove, 2021; Pett, 2016).

Questions for Additional Study

20

Name: _____ Class: _____

Date: _____

Follow your instructor's directions to submit your answers to the following questions for additional study. Your instructor may ask you to write your answers below and submit them as a hard copy for evaluation. Alternatively, your instructor may ask you to submit your answers online.

1. How many correlations presented in Table 20.2 are statistically significant at $p < 0.05$? Provide a rationale for your answer.

2. What two variables from Table 20.2 have the strongest negative (i.e., inverse) correlation? Provide a rationale for your answer.

3. Provide an interpretation of the correlation value listed in Question 2.

4. What two variables from Table 20.2 have the weakest positive correlation?

5. What do the results in Question 4 mean? Provide an interpretation of the correlation value.

6. Is the correlation between resilience (*RS-14*) and ratings of faculty high-level incivility (*FHLIB*) among the student respondents significant? Provide a rationale for your answer.

7. Is there a stronger correlation between resilience (*RS-14*) and ratings of faculty high-level incivility (*FHLIB*) among the student respondents, or among the faculty respondents? Provide a rationale for your answer.

8. Describe the correlation between resilience (*RS-14*) and ratings of student low-level incivility (*SLLIB*) among the faculty respondents. What is the strength of the correlation, is it positive or negative, and is it statistically significant?

9. Using the data in Table 20.1, calculate the Spearman *rho* value on the provided data, with one change: Delete Susie's values, leaving an *n* of 5 rows. Show your calculations.

10. Compare the Spearman *rho* value from Question 9 with the *rho* value from the original data ($\rho = 0.886$). Did the value change, and why or why not? What does this mean in terms of the association between the two instructors' rankings of the students' IM injection technique?

Understanding Mann-Whitney *U* Test

STATISTICAL TECHNIQUE IN REVIEW

The **Mann-Whitney *U* test** is a nonparametric statistical technique conducted to detect differences between two independent samples. This statistical technique is the most powerful of the nonparametric tests, with 95% of the power of the *t*-test. The Mann-Whitney *U* test is often computed when the assumptions for the independent samples *t*-test cannot be satisfied, such as a dependent variable that is ordinal-level or interval/ratio whereby the distribution of values is nonnormal (Kim et al, 2022; Knapp, 2017; Terrell, 2021). Exercise 12 provides an algorithm that will assist you in determining whether the Mann-Whitney *U* test is an appropriate statistical technique. It should be noted that the Mann-Whitney *U* test is also known as the **Wilcoxon rank-sum test;** however, this test is most commonly referred to as the Mann-Whitney *U* test in nursing journals. The Mann-Whitney *U* test/Wilcoxon rank-sum test should not be confused with the **Wilcoxon signed-rank test**, which is a test for paired samples and is covered in Exercise 22.

The Mann-Whitney *U* test checks this null hypothesis: *There is no difference between two independent samples on a selected variable.* For example: *There is no difference between the education intervention group and control group regarding their self-care activities following surgery.* In this example, self-care activities data need to be measured at least at the ordinal level. When reporting the Mann-Whitney *U* test results, researchers should identify the sample size for each of the independent groups and the medians for the groups so readers will know how the sample statistics differ. For example, the education intervention group included 11 postsurgical patients (median = 16.55) and the control group included 9 postsurgical patients (median = 8.75). The medians are reported for the groups instead of means because medians are not influenced by extremely small or large values (Kim et al., 2022; Plichta & Kelvin, 2013).

To calculate the value of *U*, the data of both samples are combined, and each data value is assigned a rank. The lowest value is ranked 1, the next value is ranked 2, and so forth until all values are ranked, regardless from which sample the score was obtained. The idea is that if two distributions came from the same population, the average of the ranks of values would be equal as well.

Exercise 34 provides detailed examples that include hand calculations and SPSS computations of the Mann-Whitney *U* test. When calculating the Mann-Whitney *U* test by hand, one must compute **two** *U* values, and choose the smallest of the two *U* values when determining significance of the result (Daniel, 2000). Therefore, when reporting the Mann-Whitney *U* test results, researchers should identify the sample size of each of the independent groups, the value of the *z* statistic (converted from the smallest *U* value) and its associated *p* value, and the medians for the two groups (Terrell, 2021). The *z* statistic for the Mann-Whitney *U* test represents the extent to which the two groups differ on the dependent variable. The higher the *z* statistic, the more likely the groups significantly differ on the values of the dependent variable (Gray & Grove, 2021).

RESEARCH ARTICLE

Source

Deng, Y., Lin, Y., Yang, L., Liang, Q., Fu, B., Li, H., Zhang, H., & Liu, Y. (2021). A comparison of maternal fear of childbirth, labor pain intensity and intrapartum analgesic consumption between primiparas and multiparas: A cross-sectional study. *International Journal of Nursing Science, 8*(4), 380–387. https://doi.org/10.1016/j.ijnss.2021.09.003

Introduction

Deng and colleagues (2021) conducted a cross-sectional study to describe and compare fear of childbirth, in-labor pain intensity, and pain relief between women who were primiparas (e.g., individuals who had given birth for the first time) and multiparas (i.e., individuals who had given birth more than once). Table 21.1 displays the pain relief variables for the two groups of women, with descriptive statistics and the results of the Mann-Whitney *U* tests.

"... The clinical data of maternal and neonatal were extracted from a structured electronic medical record system. Other demographic information, such as employment and family monthly income, was collected by a questionnaire. The Numeric Rating Scale (NRS) and the Chinese version of the Childbirth Attitude Questionnaire (C-CAQ) were applied to assess maternal in-labor pain intensity and fear of childbirth. The analgesic consumption and the frequency of manual boluses as rescue analgesia were stored and collected from the analgesia pump. ...

This is a cross-sectional study conducted from February 2018 to August 2019 in a large academic specialized hospital. The annual number of births was approximately 30,000 in recent years, ranking first in Guangdong Province. Women undergoing spontaneous or induced labor were recruited by convenient sampling immediately after being admitted to the delivery and labor room at the onset of the labor process. The inclusion criteria were 20- to 45-year-old women with singleton cephalic term pregnancies (gestational age ≥37 weeks) without severe pregnancy complications, such as heart disease, uncontrolled hypertension, and gestational diabetes mellitus. Women who had a scarred uterus, underwent artificial insemination for the

TABLE 21.1   COMPARISON OF THE AMOUNT OF PAIN RELIEF BETWEEN PRIMIPARAS AND MULTIPARAS

Variables	Primiparas (*n* = 82)	Multiparas (*n* = 99)	z/χ^2	*P*
Duration of labor analgesia (h)	8.00 (4.50, 10.77)	3.25 (1.93, 6.23)	6.32[a]	<0.001
Patients requiring manual bolus, yes	75 (91.5)	94 (94.9)	0.88[b]	0.348
Total PCEA manual boluses	12.48 (6.54, 17.42)	8.20 (3.63, 13.88)	2.80[a]	0.005
PCEA successful manual boluses per hour	1.77 (0.90, 2.47)	2.68 (1.65, 3.85)	4.52[a]	<0.001
Hourly analgesic consumption (mL/h)	17.24 (11.52, 21.36)	23.00 (16.00, 28.25)	4.63[a]	<0.001
Average analgesic consumption (mL/h·kg)	0.26 (0.19, 0.35)	0.35 (0.24, 0.45)	3.92[a]	<0.001

PCEA = Patient-controlled epidural analgesia.
[a] Mann–Whitney tests; [b] chi-square tests.
Note: Data are *n* (%), Median (P_{25}, P_{75}).
From: Deng, Y., Lin, Y., Yang, L., Liang, Q., Fu, B., Li, H., Zhang, H., & Liu, Y. (2021). A comparison of maternal fear of childbirth, labor pain intensity and intrapartum analgesic consumption between primiparas and multiparas: A cross-sectional study. *International Journal of Nursing Science, 8*(4), 380–387. https://doi.org/10.1016/j.ijnss.2021.09.003

current pregnancy, had a history of a significant psychiatric disorder, could not read and write Chinese, and had any contraindication to epidural analgesia were excluded. . . . The disparities between primiparas and multiparas were compared with independent samples *t*-tests or Mann-Whitney tests for continuous variables and chi-square tests for categorical variables" (Deng et al., 2021, p. 382).

Relevant Study Results

"A total of 260 women, including 97 primiparas and 163 multiparas, were included in the final data analyses. A total of 44.2% (115/260) of the women were ≥35 years of age; of the women ≥35 years of age, more were multiparas than primiparas (57.7% vs. 21.6%, $P < 0.001$) . . .

The duration of epidural analgesia was 8.00 (4.50, 10.77) h for primiparas and 3.25 (1.93, 6.23) h for multiparas ($P < 0.001$). A similar percentage of primiparas and multiparas had manual boluses as rescue analgesia (91.5% vs. 94.9%, $P = 0.348$). Multiparas had 2.68 (1.65, 3.85) successful manual boluses per hour, and primiparas had 1.77 (0.90, 2.47) PCEA [patient-controlled epidural analgesia] successful manual boluses per hour ($P < 0.001$). To exclude the effects of weight and the duration of anesthesia, the average analgesic consumption was compared. The hourly analgesic consumption was 23.00 (16.00, 28.25) mL for multiparas and 17.24 (11.52, 21.36) mL for primiparas ($P < 0.001$). The average analgesic consumption was 0.35 (0.24, 0.45) mL/(h · kg) for multiparas and 0.26 (0.19, 0.35) mL/(h · kg) for primiparas ($P < 0.001$)" (Table 21.1; Deng et al., 2021, p. 384).

STUDY QUESTIONS

1. What is the purpose of the Mann-Whitney *U* statistical technique? Document your response.

2. Mann-Whitney *U* is the appropriate statistical test to use in which of the following situations? Provide a rationale for your answer.
   a. Correlation or relationship between two variables is being examined in a descriptive correlational study.
   b. Interval/ratio-level data with a non-normal distribution of scores for a study variable.
   c. The difference between two dependent or paired groups is being examined in a quasi-experimental study.
   d. The data collected on study variables are at the nominal level of measurement.

3. If hourly analgesic consumption by the primipara and multipara groups were normally distributed, what would be the appropriate statistic to address differences between the two groups? Provide a rationale for your answer.

4. State the null hypothesis for the Deng et al. (2021) study regarding hourly analgesic consumption by the primipara and multipara groups.

5. Was the null hypothesis in Question 4 accepted or rejected? Provide a rationale for your answer.

6. What were the median duration (in hours) of labor analgesia for each group, as displayed in Table 21.1?

7. Did the two groups significantly differ on duration (in hours) of labor analgesia? Document your answer.

8. Did the two groups significantly differ on total PCEA manual boluses? Document your answer.

9. Why was a Mann-Whitney *U* test *not* chosen to analyze the variable of patients requiring manual bolus? Provide a rationale for your response.

10. What is the clinical importance of knowing the hourly analgesic consumption by the two groups of study participants? Document your response.

Answers to Study Questions

1. The Mann-Whitney U test is a nonparametric statistical technique used to detect differences between two independent samples (review Exercises 12 and 34). If the assumptions for the independent samples t-test cannot be satisfied, such as there being a dependent variable that is ordinal-level or interval/ratio-level data with the distribution of values being non-normal, then a Mann-Whitney U test is appropriate (Kim et al, 2022; Knapp, 2017; Terrell, 2021).

2. The correct answer is: b. Interval/ratio-level data with a non-normal distribution of scores on a study variable. The Mann-Whitney U test is appropriate for analyzing interval/ratio-level data when the requirements for conducting a parametric test cannot be satisfied, such as when the collected data have a non-normal or skewed distribution. The Mann-Whitney U test is designed to determine differences between groups and does not test for relationships between variables. The Mann-Whitney U test is to be used with independent and not dependent or paired groups and is for at least ordinal-level data and not nominal-level data (Pett, 2016).

3. The independent samples t-test is the most appropriate analysis technique. If the data were normally distributed and at the interval or ratio level of measurement, a parametric statistic can be computed (de Winter & Dodou, 2010). The two groups were independent because the study participants were either primiparas or multiparas (Deng et al., 2021). The focus of the analysis is the difference between two groups, so the most appropriate analysis technique would be the independent samples t-test (see the algorithm in Exercise 12 and computational examples in Exercise 32).

4. The null hypothesis: *There is no difference between the primipara and multipara groups on hourly analgesic consumption.*

5. The null hypothesis should be rejected. The $p < 0.001$ for hourly analgesic consumption is less than the study alpha of 0.05 (Table 21.1). The null hypothesis is rejected when study results are statistically significant (Gray & Grove, 2021; Pett, 2016).

6. The median duration (in hours) of labor analgesia was 8.0 for the primipara group and 3.25 for the multipara group (Table 21.1).

7. Yes, the two groups significantly differed on duration (in hours) of labor analgesia, $p < 0.001$. The result is significant because p is less than the study alpha of 0.05.

8. Yes, the two groups significantly differed on total PCEA manual boluses, $p = 0.005$. The median number of PCEA manual boluses was 12.48 for the primipara group and 8.20 for the multipara group (see Table 21.1). The result is significant because p is less than the study alpha of 0.05.

9. A Pearson chi-square test, not a Mann-Whitney *U* test, was chosen to analyze the variable of patients requiring manual bolus. This variable is a nominal (yes/no) variable, with *yes* indicating the requirement of a manual bolus, and *no* indicating no manual bolus. Among the women in the primipara group, 75 of 82 required a manual bolus, whereas 94 of the 99 women in the multipara group required a manual bolus. As displayed in Table 21.1, the superscript letter *b* in the fourth column indicates that a chi-square test was computed.

10. The clinical importance of knowing the hourly analgesic consumption by the two groups includes planning for both the healthcare providers and the patients. If labor occurring for the first time (primiparas) requires significantly more (and longer durations of) pain management, the facilities, providers, and patients can anticipate the necessary time, costs, and resources required. The Cochrane Library in England has a large collection of systematic reviews and evidence-based guidelines and includes several resources on pain management during labor (see http://www.cochrane.org and search for "labor analgesia"). You might document with other websites, research articles, or textbooks that focus on generations of research evidence for practice (Melnyk & Fineout-Overholt, 2023).

Follow your instructor's directions to submit your answers to the following questions for additional study. Your instructor may ask you to write your answers below and submit them as a hard copy for evaluation. Alternatively, your instructor may ask you to submit your answers online.

1. State the null hypothesis for the Deng et al. (2021) study regarding the total manual patient-controlled epidural analgesia (PCEA) boluses by the primipara and multipara groups.

2. Was the null hypothesis in Question 1 accepted or rejected? Provide a rationale for your answer.

3. List the medians of average analgesic consumption (mL/h·kg) for the primipara and multipara groups.

4. What scale of measurement is the variable of hourly analgesic consumption?

5. Was there a significant difference between the primipara and multipara groups on the number of patients requiring a manual bolus?

6. What scale of measurement is the variable of PCEA successful manual boluses per hour?

7. State the null hypothesis for the Deng et al. (2021) study regarding PCEA successful manual boluses per hour by the primipara and multipara groups.

8. Was the null hypothesis in Question 7 accepted or rejected? Provide a rationale for your answer.

9. List the medians of PCEA successful manual boluses per hour for the primipara and multipara groups.

10. What is the appropriate statistic to detect differences between two independent samples, with a dependent variable that is ordinal-level and normally distributed? Document your response.

Understanding the Wilcoxon Signed-Rank Test

STATISTICAL TECHNIQUE IN REVIEW

The **Wilcoxon signed-rank test** is a nonparametric test conducted to examine differences or changes that occur between the first and second observations, such as "pretest or posttest measures for a single sample or subjects who have been matched on certain criteria" (Pett, 2016, p. 111). The term "paired samples" refers to a research design that repeatedly assesses the same group of people, an approach commonly referred to as **repeated measures**. The Wilcoxon signed-rank test is an appropriate alternative to the paired samples *t*-test when the assumptions for the *t*-test are not met. For example, the Wilcoxon signed-rank test would be computed when the data were interval or ratio level but were not normally distributed. This nonparametric test is powerful in the sense that it not only examines the direction of the change but also the degree of the change. The Wilcoxon signed-rank test requires a calculation of a difference score for each pair of scores. The greater the amount of change, the more weight the pair is given, and when no change occurs, the pair is omitted and the sample size is decreased (Daniel, 2000). This test is especially effective when the sample size is small (Pett, 2016). In summary, the Wilcoxon signed-rank test is a strong statistical technique used to examine differences for related groups when the data are ordinal level or when the data are interval/ratio level but not normally distributed (Daniel, 2000; Kim et al., 2022; Pett, 2016).

RESEARCH ARTICLE

Source

Ding, S., Lei, Q., Wu, W., Xiao, Z., Wu, Z., Chen, M., & Chen, L. (2022). Changes in lifestyle, mood, and disease management among community-dwelling older adults during the COVID-19 pandemic in China. *Aging and Health Research, 2*(1), 100059. https://doi.org/10.1016/j.ahr.2022.100059

Introduction

Ding and colleagues (2022) conducted a telephone survey to assess the effect of the novel coronavirus of 2019 (COVID-19) on the lifestyles of older adults in China. The survey was designed to assess perceived changes in lifestyle, mood, and disease management that may have occurred because of the Chinese government's social distancing, home isolation, and lockdown requirements.

The survey was administered to older adults aged 60 and above who lived in downtown Shanghai. The researchers asked respondents to retrospectively recall their prepandemic and during-pandemic levels of home inhabitation, sleep duration and quality, diet, water intake, housework, exercise, leisure activities, and mood; 156 respondents completed the survey.

"From April 13 to May 25, 2020, a telephone survey was conducted with each participant by research nurses. The survey questionnaire contained 2 parts: 1) basic characteristics and medical history, including gender, age, education, weight, height, smoking and drinking status, medical histories, and flu vaccination history. . . . .; 2) current and pre-pandemic (2019/11–2019/12) status in regard to lifestyle, chronic disease management, and mood. Information on lifestyle including: a. length of homestay; b. sleep status, including sleep quality (good, fair, poor), when to sleep, when to wake up, sleep duration at night, nap duration; c. diet, including daily intake of meat (including fish and poultry), vegetables, eggs, fruits, and water. . . .; d. exercise, including time spent on housework, walking or cycling, and other exercises per day; e. leisure activities, including time spent on playing chess, reading, and using electronic products; new hobbies; and new skills they learned during the pandemic. Chronic disease management included regular monitoring of blood pressure and glucose by older adults themselves or their caregivers; routine medication-taking; and occurrence of chronic bronchitis, asthma, or flu attack. Mood included feeling calm, nervousness, upset, fear, or irritability" (Ding et al., 2022, Study procedure and data collection section).

"Student t-test and Wilcoxon signed-rank-sum test were used for continuous variables depending on whether assumptions of normality and homogeneity of variance test were met or not. Paired χ^2 test was used for categorical variables" (Ding et al., 2022, Statistical analysis section).

Relevant Study Results

"As shown in Table 22.1, older adults spent significantly more time at home during the pandemic than before (median: 24.0, IQR [interquartile range]: 23.0–24.0 h/day vs. median: 22.0, IQR: 20.0–23.0 h/day, $P < 0.0001$). They also did significantly longer naps during the pandemic than before (median: 0.6, IQR: 0–1.0 h/day vs. median: 0.5, IQR: 0–0.6 h/day, $P < 0.0001$). No significant differences were observed for other sleep variables. During the pandemic, the proportions of older adults with adequate consumption of meat (49.4% vs. 53.1%, $P = 0.0339$), and eggs (73.7% vs. 77.6%, $P = 0.0143$) were significantly higher than before. No significant differences were observed in regard to adequate consumption of vegetables, fruits, and water before and during the pandemic. The participants during the pandemic were more likely to gain weight (median: 63.0, IQR: 55.0–70.0 kg [kilogram] vs. median: 62.0, IQR: 55.0–70.0 kg, $P = 0.0207$)" (Ding et al., 2022, Results section).

TABLE 22.1   SLEEP, DIET BEFORE AND DURING THE PANDEMIC

	Before the Pandemic (n = 156)	During the Pandemic (n = 156)	P value
Weight, kg, median (IQR)	62.0 (55.0, 70.0)	63.0 (55.0, 70.0)	0.0207
Duration at home, hour/week, median (IQR)	22.0 (20.0, 23.0)	24.0 (23.0, 24.0)	<0.0001
Sleep quality			
Good, n (%)	76 (48.7)	76 (48.7)	0.8013
Fair, n (%)	60 (38.5)	61 (39.1)	
Poor, n (%)	20 (12.8)	19 (12.2)	
Sleep duration at night, hour/day, median (IQR)	6.5 (6.0, 7.0)	6.5 (6.0, 7.0)	0.7266
Nap duration, hour/day, median (IQR)	0.5 (0, 0.6)	0.59 (0, 1.0)	<0.0001
Sufficient intake of nutrients			
Meat, n (%)	77 (49.4)	83 (53.1)	0.0339
Eggs, n (%)	115 (73.7)	121 (77.6)	0.0143
Vegetables, n (%)	13 (8.3)	14 (9.0)	0.7173
Fruits, n (%)	1 (0.6)	1 (0.6)	1.0000
Water, n (%)	42 (26.9)	43 (27.6)	0.3173

IQR = interquartile range.
From: Ding, S., Lei, Q., Wu, W., Xiao, Z., Wu, Z., Chen, M., & Chen, L. (2022). Changes in lifestyle, mood, and disease management among community-dwelling older adults during the COVID-19 pandemic in China. *Aging and Health Research, 2*(1), 100059. https://doi.org/10.1016/j.ahr.2022.100059

It should be noted that this article represents each p value with an uppercase P because the *American Journal of Infection Control* displays p as uppercase. Most journals of nursing research require formatting in accordance with the American Psychological Association (APA, 2020) which requires p to be lowercase.

The "IQR" in the Results section refers to the interquartile range. The interquartile range of a variable consists of the two values that mark the middle 50% of the variable's values. For example, one interquartile range for weight is listed as "IQR: 55.0–70.0 kg." This means that 50% of the participants' weights fell between 55.0 kilograms and 70.0 kilograms. One quarter (25%) of the participants' weights were lower than 55.0 kilograms, and 25% were higher than 70.0 kilograms.

STUDY QUESTIONS

1. What was the sample size for this study? Was the sample size adequate? Provide a rationale for your response.

2. Do the data meet criteria for "paired samples"? Provide a rationale for your answer.

3. What are the median weights in kilograms at prepandemic and during-pandemic?

4. What is the *p* value for the Wilcoxon signed-rank test for weight? Is this *p* value statistically significant? Provide a rationale for your answer.

5. What scale of measurement is the variable of nap duration in Table 22.1?

6. What are the median values for nap duration at prepandemic and during-pandemic?

7. What is the p value for the Wilcoxon signed-rank test for nap duration? Is this p value statistically significant? Provide a rationale for your answer.

8. Why do you think medians and IQR values are reported in Table 22.1 instead of means?

9. What was the research design used in this study? Was it an appropriate design to address the study purpose?

10. The researchers concluded that the "... COVID-19 pandemic affected the lifestyle, mood, and chronic disease management among community-dwelling older adults." What are some alternative explanations for these changes because of the research design of the study? Document your response.

Answers to Study Questions

1. The sample size was 156 respondents, as indicated by the study narrative and Table 22.1. The researchers did not report the results of a power analysis in this article. However, there were a number of significant findings, lending support to the conclusion that the analyses were most likely adequately powered (see Exercises 24 and 25).

2. Yes, the data meet criteria for "paired samples" because the prepandemic and during-pandemic study variables were collected from the same group of study participants during a single survey experience involving recollections of the respondents.

3. The median value for the prepandemic weight was 62.0 kg, versus 63.0 kg for weight at during-pandemic.

4. The Wilcoxon signed-rank test resulted in $p = 0.0207$ for the change in weight from prepandemic to during-pandemic, meaning weight was significantly greater during-pandemic compared with prepandemic weight. Statistical significance for this study was set at $\alpha = 0.05$. Thus the results for the change in weight is statistically significant because $p = 0.0207$ is less than $\alpha = 0.05$ (Gray & Grove, 2021). This result is statistically significant but not really clinically important, because the weight change was only 1 kg or 2.2 lb.

5. The variable of nap duration is defined as number of hours per day. Because number of hours has numerically equal intervals and an absolute zero point, it is considered a ratio (see Exercise 1).

6. The median nap durations reported for prepandemic and during-pandemic were 0.50 and 0.59 hours per day, respectively.

7. The Wilcoxon signed-rank test resulted in $p < 0.0001$ for the change in nap duration from prepandemic to during-pandemic, meaning that nap duration was significantly greater during-pandemic compared with prepandemic. Statistical significance for this study was set at $\alpha = 0.05$. Thus the results for the increase in nap duration is statistically significant because $p < 0.0001$ is less than $\alpha = 0.05$ (Gray & Grove, 2021).

8. It is likely that medians and IQR values are reported in Table 22.1 instead of means because the data did not meet the normality assumption for a paired samples t-test. When the dependent variable is not normally distributed, a nonparametric test is more appropriate (see Exercise 33). Moreover, a median can be more informative than a mean in describing a variable when the variable's frequency distribution is positively or negatively skewed (see Exercise 8). Although the mean is sensitive to or increases or decreases based on the values of the outliers, the median is relatively unaffected (see Exercises 27 and 28).

9. The researchers did not explicitly state the type of design used in the study. However, the description of the methodology indicates that the study incorporated a one-sample repeated-measures design (Gliner et al., 2017). The design could also be described as pretest– posttest.

10. When changes occur in a one-sample repeated measures design, we cannot be certain that the intervention caused the changes. Other explanations may include the passing of time, the employment of lifestyle/social/medical/pharmaceutical modifications not assessed in this survey, or statistical regression (a phenomenon that refers to artificially high baseline levels that naturally decrease to the actual population mean at postassessment, or vice versa) (Gliner et al., 2017; Gray & Grove, 2021; Shadish et al., 2002).

Name: _____ Class: _____

Date: _____

Follow your instructor's directions to submit your answers to the following questions for additional study. Your instructor may ask you to write your answers below and submit them as a hard copy for evaluation. Alternatively, your instructor may ask you to submit your answers online.

1. List each of the types of descriptive statistics reported in Table 22.1.

2. What inferential statistical test results are reported for the nominal variables in Table 22.1?

3. Why would a Wilcoxon signed-rank test be inappropriate to compare prepandemic and during-pandemic proportions of meat intake (see Table 22.1)?

4. What scale of measurement is the variable of sleep duration at night in Table 22.1?

5. What are the median values for sleep duration at night at prepandemic and during-pandemic?

6. What is the *p* value for the Wilcoxon signed-rank test for sleep duration at night? Is this *p* value statistically significant? Provide a rationale for your response.

7. What scale of measurement is the variable of duration at home in Table 22.1?

8. What are the median values for duration at home at prepandemic and during-pandemic?

9. What is the *p* value for the Wilcoxon signed-rank test for duration at home? Is this *p* value statistically significant? Provide a rationale for your answer.

10. Are the Ding et al. (2022) findings ready for use in practice? Provide a rationale for your response.

PART 2

Conducting and Interpreting Statistical Analyses

Selecting Appropriate Analysis Techniques for Studies

Multiple factors are involved in determining the suitability of a statistical procedure for a particular study. Some of these factors are related to the nature of the study, some to the nature of the researcher, and others to the nature of statistical theory. Specific factors include the following: (1) purpose of the study; (2) study hypotheses, questions, or objectives; (3) study design; (4) level of measurement of variables in a study; (5) previous experience in statistical analysis; (6) statistical knowledge level; (7) availability of statistical consultation; (8) financial resources; and (9) access and knowledge of statistical software. Use items 1 to 4 to identify statistical procedures that meet the requirements of a particular study, and then further narrow your options through the process of elimination based on items 5 through 9.

The most important factor to examine when choosing a statistical procedure is the study hypothesis or primary research question. The hypothesis that is clearly stated indicates the statistic(s) needed to test it. An example of a clearly developed hypothesis is: *There is a difference in infection occurrences between an experimental group and a control group.* This statement tells the researcher that a statistic to determine differences between two groups is appropriate to address this hypothesis. This statement also informs the researcher that the dependent variable is an occurrence, which is binary (dichotomous): infected or not infected.

One approach to selecting an appropriate statistical procedure or judging the appropriateness of an analysis technique is to use an algorithm or decision tree. A statistical algorithm directs your choices by gradually narrowing your options through the decisions you make. A statistical algorithm developed by Cipher (2021) that can be helpful in selecting statistical procedures is presented in Fig. 23.1. This is the same algorithm presented and reviewed in Exercise 12 for determining the appropriateness of the statistical tests and results presented in research reports.

One disadvantage of a statistical algorithm is that if you make an incorrect or uninformed decision (i.e., a guess), you can be led down a path in which you might select an inappropriate statistical procedure for your study. Algorithms are often constrained by space and therefore do not include all the information needed to make an appropriate selection of a statistical procedure for a study. The following examples of questions are designed to guide the selection or evaluation of statistical procedures that are reflected in Fig. 23.1. Each question confronts you with a decision, and the decision you make narrows the field of available statistical procedures.

1. Is the research question/hypothesis descriptive, associational (correlational), or difference-oriented?
2. How many variables are involved?
3. What is the measurement scale (see Exercise 1) of the independent and dependent variable(s)?
4. What is the distribution of the dependent variables (normal, non-normal)?
5. Do the data meet the assumptions for a parametric statistic (see Exercise 1)?

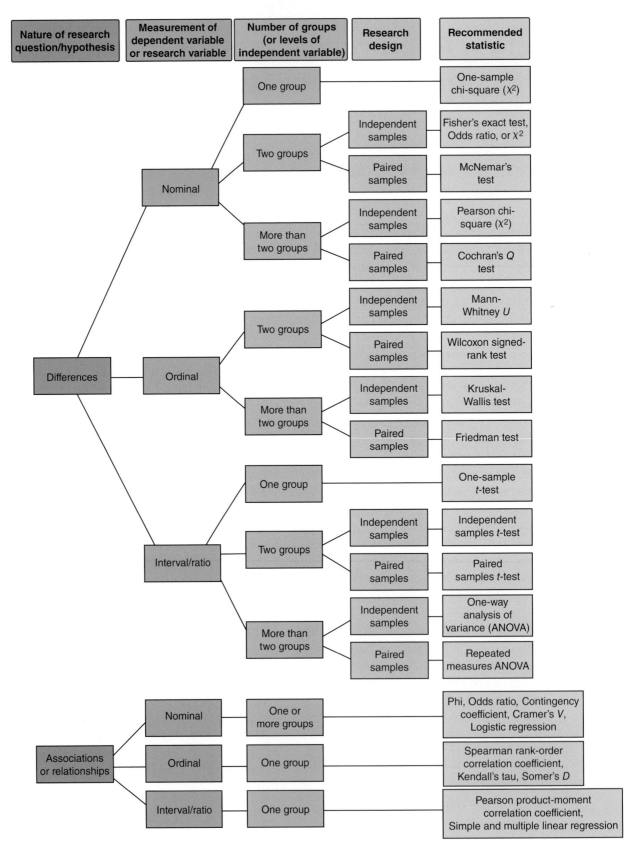

FIG. 23.1 ■ STATISTICAL SELECTION ALGORITHM.

As you can see, selecting and evaluating statistical procedures requires that you make a number of judgments regarding the nature of the data and what you want to know. Knowledge of the statistical procedures and their assumptions is necessary for selecting appropriate procedures. You must weigh the advantages and disadvantages of various statistical options. Access to a statistician can be invaluable in selecting the appropriate procedures.

STATISTICS TO ADDRESS BASIC DIFFERENCE RESEARCH QUESTIONS AND HYPOTHESES

The following statistics address research questions or hypotheses that involve differences between groups or assessments. This list is by no means exhaustive, but it represents the most common parametric and nonparametric inferential statistics involving differences. Exercises 1 and 12 discuss the concepts of parametric versus nonparametric statistics and inferential versus descriptive statistics.

t-Test for Independent Samples

One of the most common statistical tests chosen to investigate differences between two independent samples is the independent samples *t*-test, which is a parametric inferential statistic. The independent samples *t*-test only compares two groups at a time, and the dependent variable must be continuous and normally distributed (Kim et al., 2022; Zar, 2019). The independent samples *t*-test is reviewed in Exercise 16, and the process for conducting the independent samples *t*-test is in Exercise 32.

t-Test for Paired Samples

A paired samples *t*-test (also referred to as a dependent samples *t*-test) is a statistical procedure that compares two sets of data from one group of people (or naturally occurring pairs, such as siblings or spouses). This *t*-test is a parametric inferential statistical test. The dependent variable in a paired samples *t*-test must be continuous and normally distributed (Zar, 2019). The term paired samples refers to a research design that repeatedly assesses the same group of people, an approach commonly referred to as repeated measures (Kazdin, 2022). The *t*-test for paired samples is reviewed in Exercise 17, and the process for conducting the paired samples *t*-test is in Exercise 33.

One-Way Analysis of Variance

The one-way analysis of variance (ANOVA) is a parametric inferential statistical procedure that compares data between two or more groups or conditions to investigate the presence of differences between those groups on some continuous, normally distributed dependent variable (see Fig. 23.1). There are many types of ANOVAs. The one-way ANOVA involves testing one independent variable and one dependent variable (as opposed to other types of ANOVAs, such as factorial ANOVAs, that incorporate multiple independent variables). ANOVA is reviewed in Exercise 18, and the process for conducting ANOVA is presented in Exercise 35.

Repeated-Measures ANOVA

A repeated-measures ANOVA is a statistical procedure that compares multiple sets of data from one group of people. The dependent variable in a repeated-measures ANOVA must be continuous and normally distributed. The term *repeated measures* refers to a research design that repeatedly assesses the same group of people over time. Repeated measures can also refer to naturally occurring pairs, such as siblings or spouses (Gliner et al., 2017).

Mann-Whitney *U* Test

The Mann-Whitney *U* test is the nonparametric alternative to an independent samples *t*-test. Like the independent samples *t*-test, the Mann-Whitney *U* test is a statistical procedure that compares differences between two independent samples. However, the Mann-Whitney *U* is the preferred test over the independent samples *t*-test when the distribution of the dependent variable significantly deviates from normality, or the dependent variable is measured at the ordinal level and cannot be treated as an interval/ratio-scaled variable (Gray & Grove, 2021; Pett, 2016). The Mann-Whitney *U* is reviewed in Exercise 21, and Exercise 34 provides the steps for conducting this test.

Kruskal-Wallis Test

The Kruskal-Wallis test is the nonparametric alternative to the one-way ANOVA. Like the one-way ANOVA, the Kruskal-Wallis test is a statistical procedure that compares differences between two or more groups. However, the Kruskal-Wallis test is the preferred test over the ANOVA when the distribution of the dependent variable significantly deviates from normality, or the dependent variable is ordinal and cannot be treated as an interval/ratio-scaled variable (Holmes, 2018; Kim et al., 2022; Pett, 2016).

Friedman Test

The Friedman test is the nonparametric alternative to a repeated-measures ANOVA. Like the repeated-measures ANOVA, the Friedman test is a statistical procedure that compares multiple sets of data from one group of people. However, the Friedman test is the preferred test over the repeated-measures ANOVA when the dependent variable data significantly deviate from a normal distribution, or the dependent variable is ordinal and cannot be treated as an interval/ratio-scaled variable (Pett, 2016).

Wilcoxon Signed-Rank Test

The Wilcoxon signed-rank test is the nonparametric alternative to the paired samples *t*-test. Like the paired samples *t*-test, the Wilcoxon signed-rank test is a statistical procedure that compares two sets of data from one group of people. However, the Wilcoxon signed-rank test is the preferred test over the paired samples *t*-test when the dependent variable data significantly deviate from a normal distribution, or the dependent variable is ordinal and cannot be treated as an interval/ratio-scaled variable (Pett, 2016). The Wilcoxon signed-rank test is reviewed in Exercise 22.

Pearson Chi-Square Test

The Pearson chi-square test (also referred to as χ^2) is a nonparametric inferential statistical test that compares differences between groups on variables measured at the nominal level. The chi-square test compares the frequencies that are observed with the frequencies that are expected. When a study requires that researchers compare proportions (percentages) in one category versus another category, the chi-square test is a statistic that will reveal if the difference in proportion is statistically improbable. A one-way chi-square test is a statistic that compares different levels of one variable only. For example, a one-way chi-square test could be computed to identify differences in proportions of a nominal variable such as rural area versus metropolitan area. A two-way chi-square test is a statistic that tests whether proportions in levels of one nominal variable are significantly different from proportions of the second nominal variable. For example, a two-way chi-square test could be computed to identify differences between nurses working in rural areas and nurses working in urban/metropolitan areas on the proportions of patients screened for depression. The Pearson chi-square test is reviewed in Exercise 19, and Exercise 37 provides the steps for conducting this test.

STATISTICS TO ADDRESS BASIC ASSOCIATIONAL/CORRELATIONAL RESEARCH QUESTIONS AND HYPOTHESES

The following statistics address research questions or hypotheses that involve associations or correlations between variables. This list is by no means exhaustive, but it represents the most common parametric and nonparametric inferential statistics involving associations.

Pearson Product-Moment Correlation Coefficient

The Pearson product-moment correlation coefficient is a parametric inferential statistic computed between two continuous, normally distributed variables (see Fig. 23.1). The Pearson correlation is represented by the statistic r, and the value of the r is always between -1.00 and $+1.00$. A value of zero indicates absolutely no relationship between the two variables; a positive correlation indicates that higher values of x are associated with higher values of y; and a negative, or inverse, correlation indicates that higher values of x are associated with lower values of y (Grove & Gray, 2023; Kim et al., 2022). The Pearson r is reviewed in Exercise 13, and Exercise 29 provides steps for conducting this analysis.

Spearman Rank-Order Correlation Coefficient

The Spearman rank-order correlation coefficient is the nonparametric alternative to the Pearson r. Like the Pearson correlation, the Spearman rank-order correlation is a statistical procedure that examines the association between two continuous variables. However, the Spearman rank-order correlation is the preferred test over the Pearson r when one or both of the variables significantly deviate from a normal distribution, or the variables are ordinal and cannot be treated as an interval/ratio-scaled variable (Pett, 2016). The Spearman rank-order correlation is reviewed in Exercise 20.

Phi/Cramer *V*

The phi (φ) coefficient is the nonparametric alternative to the Pearson r when the two variables being correlated are both binary (dichotomous). Like the Pearson r and Spearman rank-order correlation coefficient, the phi yields a value between -1.0 and $+1.0$, where a zero represents no association between the variables. The Cramer V is the nonparametric alternative to the Pearson r when the two variables being correlated are both nominal. The Cramer V yields a value between 0 and 1, where a zero represents no association between the variables and a 1 represents a perfect association between the variables (Prett, 2016).

Odds Ratio

When both the predictor and the dependent variables are dichotomous (variables that have only two values; binary), the odds ratio is a commonly used statistic to obtain an indication of association (Gray & Grove, 2021). The odds ratio (OR) is defined as the ratio of the odds of an event occurring in one group to the odds of it occurring in another group. An OR of >1.0 indicates that the predictor is associated with higher odds of the outcome, and an OR of <1.0 indicates that predictor is associated with lower odds of the outcome (Celentano & Szklo, 2018). ORs are commonly computed in case-control studies, when the OR can identify an association between a treatment or exposure and the odds of a specific event/outcome occurring. The larger the OR, the higher the odds that the outcome will occur with treatment/exposure.

The OR can also be computed when the dependent variable is binary (dichotomous) and the predictor is continuous and would be computed by performing logistic regression analysis. Logistic regression analysis tests a predictor (or set of predictors) with a binary dependent variable. Whether the predictor is binary or continuous, an OR of 1.0 indicates that the predictor does not affect the odds of the outcome. The further the *OR* value is from 1.0 (either higher than or lower than), the greater the likelihood that a real association exists between the two variables. The steps for conducting the odds ratio are presented in Exercise 38.

Simple and Multiple Linear Regression

Linear regression is a procedure that provides an estimate of the value of a dependent variable based on the value of an independent variable or set of independent variables, also referred to as *predictors*. Knowing that estimate with some degree of accuracy, we can use regression analysis to predict the value of one variable if we know the value of the other variable. The regression equation is a mathematical expression of the influence that a predictor (or set of predictors) has on a dependent variable, based on a theoretical framework. A regression equation can be generated with a dataset containing participant's *x* and *y* values. The score on variable *y* (dependent variable, or outcome) is predicted from the same participant's known score on variable *x* (independent variable, or predictor) (Kim et al., 2022; King & Eckersley, 2019). Simple linear regression is reviewed in Exercise 14, and Exercise 30 provides the steps for conducting this analysis. Multiple linear regression is reviewed in Exercise 15, and Exercise 31 provides steps for conducting this analysis.

APPLYING INFERENTIAL STATISTICS TO POPULATION DATA

Secondary data analyses of large state and national datasets can be an economically feasible and time-efficient way for nurse researchers to address important health, epidemiologic, and clinical research questions. However, data that were collected on a national level using complex sampling procedures, such as those survey data made available to researchers by the Centers for Disease Control and Prevention or the Centers for Medicare and Medicaid Services, require specific weighting procedures before computing inferential statistics. Aponte (2010) conducted a thorough review of publicly available population datasets with nurse researchers in mind and elaborated on the advantages and disadvantages of using population survey data.

When the researcher is analyzing secondary population-based datasets, much attention must be given to the quality of the data, the extent of missing data, and the manner in which the data were sampled. Analyses of secondary population data involve much data cleaning, which can include recoding, missing data imputation, and weighting for complex sampling approaches. *Point and click* software programs such as SPSS Statistics Base (IBM SPSS Statistics for Windows, Version 22.0. Armonk, NY: IBM Corp.) can be used by the researcher for data cleaning; however, they cannot be used to adjust the data for complex sampling. There are only a handful of statistical software programs that can address the adjustments for sampling required by population survey data (Aday & Cornelius, 2006; Aponte, 2010). When such data are analyzed without adjusting for sampling, the results are at risk for Type I error and are generally considered invalid (Aday & Cornelius, 2006). In this text, the exercises focused on calculating statistical analyses (Exercises 29–38) involve data from samples and not data from populations.

STUDY QUESTIONS

1. What statistic would be appropriate for an associational research question or hypothesis involving the correlation between two normally distributed continuous variables?

2. What statistic would be appropriate for a difference research question involving the comparison of two repeated assessments from one group of participants, where the dependent variable is measured at the interval/ratio level or is continuous and the data are normally distributed?

3. A nurse educator is interested in the difference between traditional clinical instruction and simulated instruction in an undergraduate nursing pediatrics course. She randomizes students to receive 50 hours of either traditional clinical rotations in a pediatrics department or 50 hours of simulated instruction in pediatrics. At the end of the 50 hours, the students are assessed for clinical competency in pediatrics using a standardized instrument that yields a continuous score, where higher values represent higher levels of competency. Her research question is: *Is there a difference between the traditional clinical group and the simulation group on clinical competency?* What is the appropriate statistic to address the research question if the scores are normally distributed?

4. What is the appropriate statistic to address the research question in Question 3 if the scores are *NOT* normally distributed?

5. What statistic would be appropriate for a difference research question involving the comparison of two groups on a dichotomous dependent variable? Provide a rationale for your answer.

6. A researcher surveyed a sample of college students with two measures. The first measure was an assessment of loneliness, and the second measure was an assessment of stress. The two variables are normally distributed continuous variables. Her research question is: *Does loneliness predict stress levels among college students?* What is the appropriate statistic to address the research question?

7. A diabetes educator wants to track diabetic patients' progress throughout an educational program for glycemic control. She collects each of her patients' hemoglobin A1c (HbA1c) levels at baseline, again halfway through the educational program, and once again at the end of the program (a total of three HbA1c values). Her research question is: *Did the patients' glycemic control (as measured by HbA1c values) change over the course of the program, from baseline to the end of program?* What is the appropriate statistic to address the research question if the HbA1c values are normally distributed?

8. What is the appropriate statistic to address the research question in Question 7 if the scores are *NOT* normally distributed?

9. In the scenario presented in Question 7, the researcher also collected data on the participants, such as gender, duration of disease, age, and depression levels. Her research question is: *Do gender, duration of disease, age, and depression levels predict baseline HbA1c levels?* What is the appropriate statistic to address the research question if the baseline HbA1c levels are normally distributed?

10. What statistic would be appropriate for a difference research question involving the comparison of three independent groups on a normally distributed continuous dependent variable?

Answers to Study Questions

1. A Pearson *r* is an appropriate statistic to test an association between two normally distributed continuous variables or variables measured at the interval or ratio level.

2. A paired samples *t*-test is an appropriate statistic to compare two repeated assessments from one group of participants, where the dependent variable is continuous or measured at the interval/ratio level and the data are normally distributed.

3. An independent samples *t*-test is an appropriate statistic to compare two groups on a normally distributed continuous dependent variable (such as clinical competency scores).

4. The Mann-Whitney *U* is an appropriate statistic to compare two independent groups on a non-normally distributed continuous dependent variable.

5. A Pearson chi-square test is an appropriate statistic to compare two groups on a dichotomous dependent variable.

6. Simple linear regression is the appropriate statistical procedure that tests the extent to which a single variable predicts a normally distributed dependent variable.

7. A repeated-measures ANOVA is an appropriate statistic to compare three or more repeated assessments of the HbA1c from one group of diabetic patients where the dependent variable is normally distributed.

8. A Friedman test is an appropriate statistic to compare three or more repeated assessments from one group of participants where the dependent variable is not normally distributed.

9. Multiple linear regression is the appropriate statistical procedure that tests the extent to which a set of variables predicts a normally distributed dependent variable.

10. A one-way ANOVA is an appropriate statistic to compare three independent groups on a normally distributed continuous dependent variable.

Questions for Additional Study

Name: _____ Class: _____

Date: _____

Follow your instructor's directions to submit your answers to the following questions for additional study. Your instructor may ask you to write your answers below and submit them as a hard copy for evaluation. Alternatively, your instructor may ask you to submit your answers online.

1. A researcher surveyed a sample of college students with two measures. The first measure was an assessment of loneliness, and the second measure was an assessment of stress. Her research question is: *Is there an association between loneliness and stress among college students?* She finds that the distributions of her two continuous variables are non-normally distributed. What is the appropriate statistic to address the research question?

2. A nurse practitioner (NP) tested his clinic patients (all of whom had a diagnosis of diabetes mellitus) for their levels of health literacy. He compared two groups of patients: those with a comorbid diagnosis of depression and those without a diagnosis of depression. His research question is: *Is there a difference between those with and without comorbid depression on health literacy scores among persons with diabetes?* What is the appropriate statistic to address the research question, if the scores are continuous and normally distributed?

3. What statistic would be appropriate for an associational research question involving the correlation between two nominal binary variables?

4. A researcher is interested in the extent to which years of practice among NPs predicts level of support for expanded prescription privileges, measured on a 10-point Likert scale. She finds that both of the variables, years of practice and level of support, are normally distributed. Her research question is: *Does years of practice among NPs predict level of support for expanded prescription privileges?* What is the appropriate statistic to address the research question?

5. A nursing professor tests her students' level of clinical competency regarding resuscitation at the beginning of the semester and administers the same test at the end of the semester. She compares the two sets of interval scores on a 100-point clinical competency exam. Her research question is: *Is there a difference in competency pertaining to resuscitation from the beginning to the end of the semester?* What is the appropriate statistic to address the research question if the scores are normally distributed?

6. What is the appropriate statistic to address the research question in Question 5 if the scores are *NOT* normally distributed?

7. What is the appropriate statistic to identify the association between two dichotomous variables, where the researcher is interested in identifying the odds of an outcome occurring?

8. A researcher wants to compare cortisol levels among a group of patients taking dehydroepiandros-terone (DHEA) and a control group. Her research question is: *Is there a difference between the two groups on cortisol levels?* She finds that her two continuous dependent variables are non-normally distributed. What is the appropriate statistic to address the research question?

9. What is the appropriate statistic to address the research question in Question 8 if the scores were normally distributed?

10. A nurse educator is interested in the role of different kinds of clinical instruction in undergraduate nursing students taking a pediatrics clinical course. She randomizes students to one of three groups: group 1: 100% simulation hours; group 2: 50% simulation hours and 50% traditional clinical hours; and group 3: 100% traditional clinical hours. At the end of the course, the students are assessed for clinical competency using a standardized instrument that yields a continuous score. Her research question is: *Is there a difference between the three groups on clinical competency in pediatrics?* What is the appropriate statistic to address the research question if the scores are normally distributed?

Describing the Elements of Power Analysis: Power, Effect Size, Alpha, and Sample Size

The deciding factor in determining an adequate sample size for descriptive, correlational, quasi-experimental, and experimental studies is power. **Power** is the probability that a statistical test will detect an effect when it actually exists. Therefore, power is the inverse of Type II error and is calculated as $1 - \beta$. Type II error is the probability of retaining the null hypothesis when it is in fact false. When the researcher sets Type II error at the conventional value of 0.20 prior to conducting a study, this means that the power of the planned statistic has been set to 0.80. In other words, the statistic will have an 80% chance of detecting an effect if an effect actually exists.

Power analysis can address the number of participants required for a study or, conversely, the extent of the power of a statistical test. A power analysis performed prior to the study beginning to determine the required number of participants needed to identify an effect is termed an **a priori power analysis**. A power analysis performed after the study ends to determine the power of the statistical result is termed a **post hoc power analysis**. Optimally, the power analysis is performed prior to the study so that the researcher can plan to include an adequate number of participants. Otherwise, the researcher risks conducting a study with an inadequate number of participants and putting the study at risk for Type II error (Aberson, 2019; Taylor & Spurlock, 2018). The four factors involved in a power analysis are as follows:

1. Level of significance (α, or alpha level), usually 0.05.
2. Probability of obtaining a significant result (power desired, or $1 - \beta$), usually 0.80.
3. The hypothesized or actual effect (association among variables or difference between your groups).
4. Sample size.

Knowing any of the three factors listed above allows researchers to compute the fourth (Cohen, 1988; Hayat, 2013). Significance (α) level and sample size are fairly straightforward. **Effect size** is "the degree to which the phenomenon is present in the population, or the degree to which the null hypothesis is false" (Cohen, 1988, pp. 9-10). For example, suppose you were measuring changes in anxiety levels, measured first when the patient is at home and then just before surgery. The effect size would be large if you expected a great change in anxiety. If you expected only a small change in the level of anxiety, the effect size would be small.

Small effect sizes require larger samples to detect these small differences. If the power is too low, it may not be worthwhile conducting the study unless a sample large enough to detect an effect can be obtained. Deciding to conduct a study in these circumstances is costly in terms of time and money, minimally adds to the body of nursing knowledge, and can actually lead to false conclusions (Taylor & Spurlock, 2018). Power analysis can be conducted via hand calculations, computer software, or online calculators and should be performed to determine the sample size necessary for a particular study (Aberson, 2019). For example, a power analysis can be calculated by using the free power analysis software G*Power (Faul et al., 2009) or statistical software such as NCSS, SAS, and SPSS. Moreover, there are many free sample size calculators online that are easy to use and understand.

The notion of whether researchers should conduct a post hoc power analysis after a study fails to reject the null hypothesis has been greatly debated (Hayat, 2013). This is because there is a strong association between the p value of the finding and the post hoc power; the lower the p value, the higher the power, and vice versa. Therefore any finding that fails to yield statistical significance will inevitably be associated with low power (Levine & Ensom, 2001). Because of this phenomenon, reporting a post hoc power analysis may be considered redundant. On the other hand, if power was high, the post hoc power analysis may strengthen the meaning of the findings. Many researchers advocate the reporting of effect sizes and confidence intervals in the results of research articles in addition to or instead of post hoc power analyses (Hayat, 2013; Levine & Ensom, 2001).

One appropriate context for a post hoc power analysis might be an exploratory pilot study, when a researcher analyzes the study data and reports the obtained effect size on which to base a future study (Hayat, 2013). For any study that results in low statistical power, the researcher needs to address this issue in the discussion of limitations and implications of the study findings. Modifications in the research methodology that resulted from the use of power analysis also need to be reported. Therefore, the researcher must evaluate the elements of the methodology that affect the required sample size, which include the following:

1. Statistical power corresponds to one type of statistical test at a time. If the researcher is planning to compute different categories of statistical tests, in order to adequately power the study one must perform a power analysis for each planned statistical procedure (Hayat, 2013). For example, if the researcher is planning an analysis of variance (ANOVA) to address the first research question, and a chi-square test (χ^2) to address the second research question, the study will not be adequately powered unless both statistical tests are addressed with power analyses. In this example, the researcher would need to perform two power analyses, one for each research objective or hypothesis.
2. The more stringent the α (e.g., 0.001 vs. 0.05), the greater the necessary sample size due to the reduced probability of a Type I error. With $\alpha = 0.001$, the probability of Type I error is 1 chance in 1000; with $\alpha = 0.05$, there are 5 chances for error in 100 analyses conducted.
3. Two-tailed statistical tests require larger sample sizes than one-tailed tests because two-tailed tests require a larger critical statistical value to yield significance than a one-tailed test (Kim et al., 2022; Zar, 2010).
4. The smaller the effect size, the larger the necessary sample size because the effect size indicates how strong the relationship is between variables and the strength of the differences between groups (Taylor & Spurlock, 2018).
5. The larger the power required, the larger the necessary sample size. For example, a power set at 0.90 requires a larger sample size than the standard power set at 0.80.
6. The smaller the sample size, the smaller the power of the study (Cohen, 1988).

EFFECT SIZE

Cohen (1988) defined effect size as "the degree to which the phenomenon is present in the population." There are many different types of effect size measures, and each corresponds to the type of statistic computed. A decision tree developed by Cipher (2023) that can be helpful in selecting statistical procedures is presented in Fig. 23.1 of Exercise 23 in this text. The researcher needs to have identified the statistic(s) required to address the research question or hypothesis prior to conducting the power analysis. For example, if we were planning to compute an independent samples t-test, then the effect size in the power analysis would be a

Effect Size	Cohen's d	Cohen's d_z	Cohen's f	r	R_2	OR	d
Small	0.20	0.20	0.10	0.10	0.02	1.5	0.05
Moderate	0.50	0.50	0.25	0.30	0.13	2.5	0.15
Large	0.80	0.80	0.40	0.50	0.26	4.3	0.25

TABLE 24.1   MAGNITUDE RANGES OF SEVEN COMMON EFFECT SIZES

Cohen's d = difference between two groups in standard deviation units
Cohen's d_z = difference between two paired assessments when the correlation between the pairs is r = 0.50
Cohen's f = difference between more than two groups
r = Pearson r
R^2 = variance explained in linear regression model
OR = odds ratio
d = difference between proportions when one of the two groups' rates = 50%

Cohen's d (Cohen, 1988). If we were planning to compute one-way ANOVA, then the effect size in the power analysis would be a Cohen's f. A Pearson correlation coefficient (r) serves as its own effect size, as does the odds ratio (OR). Table 24.1 is a compilation of seven of the most common effect sizes used in power analyses. This table was created by extracting the information presented in the seminal text on power analysis by Cohen (1988) and provides three magnitudes of effects: small, moderate, and large.

Cohen's d

The most common effect size measure for a two-sample design (that is, a two-group comparison) is Cohen's d. Cohen's d is calculated as follows:

$$d = \frac{\bar{X}_1 - \bar{X}_2}{SD}$$

where $\bar{X}_1$ and $\bar{X}_2$ are the means for Groups 1 and 2, respectively, and the SD would be the standard deviation of either group, considering that both groups are assumed to have approximately equal SDs.

The resulting d value represents the difference between the means of Groups 1 and 2, in SD units. Thus a value of 1.0 means that the two groups differed exactly 1 SD unit from one another. One can still compute the Cohen's d even if the design has more than two groups, but the Cohen's d is calculated one pair at a time. However, the more appropriate effect size for comparing three or more groups, such as a one-way ANOVA, is the f.

Cohen's d_z

Cohen's d_z is almost identical to Cohen's d above, except the d_z applies to paired samples instead of independent samples. Like Cohen's d, Cohen's d_z also represents the difference between two means in SD units. However, Cohen's d_z is computed with two means of paired values. These paired values are most often from one group of people, but they can also be composed of paired data from naturally occurring pairs, such as siblings or spouses.

When the correlation (r) between the paired values is approximately r = 0.50, then the ranges of the magnitude of effect in terms of small, moderate, and large are the same as that of Cohen's d, where small = 0.20, moderate = 0.50, and large = 0.80 or greater. However, when the correlation between the paired values is smaller, then the resulting magnitude of effect is smaller. Likewise, when the correlation between the paired values is larger, the resulting magnitude of effect is larger. For example, if there is a 0.50 mean difference between two paired samples, with a high r of the paired values at r = 0.80, the d_z = 0.79 (a large effect). On the other hand, if there is a 0.50 mean difference between two paired samples, with a low r of the paired values at r = 0.20, the d_z = 0.40 (a small to moderate effect). Therefore the magnitude of the association between the pairs has a direct impact on the magnitude of the d_z value (Cohen, 1988).

Cohen's *f*

Like Cohen's *d,* Cohen's *f* also expresses effect size in standard deviation units but does so for two or more groups. When planning a one-way ANOVA, Cohen's *f* can be computed to determine the differences between the groups. Like the ANOVA, the Cohen's *f* will identify the magnitude of the differences among all of the groups, but it will not explain differences between specific groups. For two groups, $f = 1/2d$. Conversely, $d = 2f$ (Cohen, 1988).

Pearson *r*

The Pearson product-moment correlation coefficient was the first of the correlation measures developed and is computed on two continuous, approximately normally distributed variables (see Exercises 13 and 29). This coefficient (statistic) is represented by the letter *r*, and the value of the *r* is always between -1.00 and $+1.00$. A value of zero indicates absolutely no relationship between the two variables; a positive correlation indicates that higher values of *x* are associated with higher values of *y*; and a negative, or inverse, correlation indicates that higher values of *x* are associated with lower values of *y* and vice versa. The *r* value is indicative of the slope of the line (called a regression line) that can be drawn through a standard scatterplot of the two variables (see Exercise 11). The strengths of different relationships are identified in Table 24.1.

R^2

The R^2, also referred to as the **coefficient of determination,** is the effect size for linear regression. The R^2 represents the percentage of variance explained in *y* by the predictor (see Exercises 14 and 30). Simple linear regression provides a means to estimate the value of a dependent variable based on the value of an independent variable. Multiple regression analysis is an extension of simple linear regression in which more than one independent variable is entered into the analysis to predict a dependent variable (see Exercises 15 and 31).

Odds Ratio

When both the predictor and the dependent variable are dichotomous, the odds ratio (*OR*) is a commonly used statistic to obtain an indication of association (see Exercise 38). The odds ratio is defined as the ratio of the odds of an event occurring in one group to the odds of it occurring in another group (Celentano & Szklo, 2018). Put simply, the *OR* is a way of comparing whether the odds of a certain event is the same for two groups. The *OR* can also be computed when the dependent variable is dichotomous and the predictor is continuous, and would be computed by performing logistic regression analysis. Logistic regression analysis tests a predictor (or set of predictors) with a dichotomous dependent variable. The output yields an adjusted *OR,* meaning that each predictor's *OR* represents the relationship between that predictor and *y*, after adjusting for the presence of the other predictors in the model (Tabachnick & Fidell, 2019).

d

For a two-sample comparative design where the dependent variable is dichotomous, the d is the effect size used in the power analysis. The letter "d" represents the difference in percentages in Group 1 versus Group 2. One example might be to compare employment rates in an intervention and control groups. We have evidence that our control group will have a 50% employment rate, and the intervention will be 15% higher, at 65%. Thus, our anticipated d would be 65% $-$ 50% = 15%. In Exercise 25, we will present a power analysis using each of the effect sizes described in this exercise.

STUDY QUESTIONS

1. Define statistical power.

2. List the four components of a power analysis.

3. Define power and beta and discuss the importance of power and beta in a study.

4. What is the difference between Cohen's d and Cohen's d_z?

5. Using the values in Table 24.1, what would be considered a small Pearson r? How would this value affect sample size for a study?

6. Prior to conducting a power analysis, a researcher reviewed the literature and discovered that a study similar to hers reported an *OR* value of 2.75. According to Table 24.1, how would you characterize the magnitude of that effect?

7. Prior to conducting a power analysis, a researcher reviewed the literature and discovered a similar study reported an R^2 value of 0.30, or 30%. According to Table 24.1, how would you characterize the magnitude of that effect?

8. Prior to performing the power analysis, a researcher debates whether to set the study α at 0.05 or 0.01. Which α level will require more study participants? Provide a rationale for your answer.

9. Prior to performing the power analysis, a researcher debates whether to set the study beta (β) at 0.15 or 0.20. Which beta level will require more study participants? Provide a rationale for your answer.

10. What is the difference between Cohen's *d* and d?

Answers to Study Questions

1. Power is the probability that a statistical test will detect an effect (that is, a difference between groups or a relationship between variables) when it actually exists.

2. The four components of a power analysis are alpha, power, effect size, and sample size (Aberson, 2019).

3. Beta (β) is the probability of making a Type II error, and power is the inverse of beta, or $1 - \beta$. Because of the inverse association between beta and power, lower values of beta allow for a larger likelihood of finding an effect when one is present (power).

4. Cohen's d is the effect size for a two-sample design for a continuous, normally distributed dependent variable, whereas Cohen's d_z is the effect size for a one-sample design for a continuous, normally distributed dependent variable. Both Cohen's d and Cohen's d_z represent the difference between two means in SD units. However, Cohen's d is computed with two independent means, and Cohen's d_z is computed with two means of paired values.

5. A small Pearson r would be any value equal to or less than 0.10, and would result in a lower required sample size because a small effect size requires a higher critical statistical value to yield significance (Cohen, 1988; Taylor & Spurlock, 2018).

6. An OR value of 2.75 would be considered a moderate effect size.

7. An R^2 value of 30% would be considered a large effect size.

8. Setting the alpha at 0.01 will require more study participants. A smaller alpha requires a larger sample size because the statistical test will require a larger critical statistical value to yield significance (Gray & Grove, 2021).

9. Setting the beta at 0.15 will require more study participants because there is less potential for error than with beta set at 0.20. With beta set at 0.15, the power is stronger (85%) than with beta set at 0.20 (80%) (Cohen, 1988).

10. Cohen's d is the effect size for a two-sample design for a continuous, normally distributed dependent variable, whereas d is the effect size for a two-sample design for a dichotomous dependent variable (Aberson, 2019; Cohen, 1988).

Questions for Additional Study

Name: _____ Class: _____

Date: _____

Follow your instructor's directions to submit your answers to the following questions for additional study. Your instructor may ask you to write your answers below and submit them as a hard copy for evaluation. Alternatively, your instructor may ask you to submit your answers online.

1. When is the optimal time to perform a power analysis—before the beginning of the study or after the study ends? Provide a rationale for your answer.

2. Define effect size.

3. A researcher is planning to compute a Pearson r. What effect size measure should be used in the power analysis? Provide a rationale for your answer.

4. A researcher is planning to compute a one-way ANOVA. What effect size measure should be used in the power analysis? Provide a rationale for your answer.

5. A researcher is planning to compute an independent samples t-test. What effect size measure should be used in the power analysis?

6. A researcher is planning to perform a paired samples t-test. What effect size measure should be used in the power analysis?

7. A study reported an OR of 1.58, which was not significant. The authors note that their *a priori* power analysis was based on a large effect size. Are they able to confidently accept the null hypothesis? Why or why not?

8. Before conducting a power analysis, you reviewed the literature and discovered that two similar studies reported Cohen d values of 0.30 and 0.50. Which effect will require more study participants? Provide a rationale for your answer.

9. Before conducting a power analysis, a researcher reviews the literature and discovered a similar study comparing differences between groups. The authors reported a d value of 31%. How would you characterize the magnitude of that effect?

10. A researcher plans a study whereby she will compute three statistical tests: a Pearson r, a one-way analysis of variance (ANOVA), and an odds ratio. She performs a power analysis based on an anticipated Pearson r and enrolls the required number of participants based on the results of that power analysis, declares that the study has adequate statistical power, and begins the study. Is the researcher correct? Provide a rationale for your answer.

Conducting Power Analysis

Exercise 24 described the components of a power analysis: α, power (1 − β), hypothesized effect, and sample size (*N*). Seven common effect sizes were presented: *r*, R^2, Cohen's *d*, Cohen's d_z, Cohen's *f*, d, and *OR* (Table 25.1). For an *a priori* power analysis, the researcher has already stated the research problem and the corresponding research question or hypothesis. Because the size of the effect in a power analysis is directly linked to the required sample size, it is crucial that the hypothesized effect be accurate. Sometimes, prior reports of a similar study or studies exist in the literature to determine the magnitude of the hypothesized effect chosen for the power analysis. Other times, a paucity of published studies hinders the researcher's ability to find effect size information. Effect size information includes any values in the study that allow the reader to directly or indirectly calculate an effect size. For example, reporting means and *SD*s would allow the reader to calculate a Cohen's *d*. A table of percentages for different groups would allow the reader to compute a d value (difference between rates).

It is very important to conduct an extensive search of the literature to yield the most accurate effect size information possible (Taylor & Spurlock, 2018). Sometimes, effect sizes found in the literature differ in magnitude. For example, a researcher may be investigating effects for an association between two variables of interest, and finds studies reporting Pearson *r* values of varying sizes. The process of deciding which effect size to use in one's own power analysis can be very difficult. The researcher must take into account the sample sizes of each study, the quality of the methodology, the quality of the measurement, and the similarity of the population to which the researcher plans to investigate. A study with a larger sample size using a sample with characteristics similar to the researcher's own target population is likely to yield the highest generalizability.

If the literature review does not produce any helpful effect size information, then the researcher may consider contacting other investigators in the field to obtain guidance (Hulley et al., 2013). A small pilot study could be conducted to obtain effect size information, although the typically smaller sample sizes used in pilot studies yield less stable or reliable effect size estimates because sample size affects power. If these options are not available, then the planned study should be considered a pilot study, because it has been established that it is the first of its kind to address the research question. Pilot studies, by and large, are by definition underpowered studies. Therefore, although a pilot study can provide useful information about the presence of an effect, the researcher should take caution in relying solely on this information when conducting a power analysis (Hayat, 2013). Ultimately, effects from prior published empirical studies are the preferred method to obtaining effect sizes for a *priori* power analyses.

G*Power 3.1 is a free power analysis software available for download (Faul et al., 2009). The download is available at http://www.gpower.hhu.de/en.html. Exercise 25 presents seven power analyses using G*Power 3.1, one for each of the effect sizes presented in Exercise 24. Each of the seven power analyses present hypothetical effect sizes in the small, moderate, or large ranges, in order to provide the reader with the opportunity to perform power analyses using G*Power.

TABLE 25.1	MAGNITUDE RANGES OF SEVEN COMMON EFFECT SIZES						
Effect Size	**Cohen's d**	**Cohen's d_z**	**Cohen's f**	**r**	**R^2**	**OR**	**d**
Small	0.20	0.20	0.10	0.10	0.02	1.5	0.05
Moderate	0.50	0.50	0.25	0.30	0.13	2.5	0.15
Large	0.80	0.80	0.40	0.50	0.26	4.3	0.25

Cohen's d = difference between two groups in standard deviation units
Cohen's d_z = difference between two paired assessments when the correlation between the pairs is $r = 0.50$
Cohen's f = difference between more than two groups
r = Pearson r
R^2 = variance explained in linear regression model
OR = Odds ratio
d = difference between proportions when one of the two groups' rates = 50%

POWER ANALYSIS 1: COHEN'S *d*

Cohen's d is an effect that represents the magnitude of the difference between two groups expressed in standard deviation units. The following instructions outline the steps required to perform a hypothetical power analysis with a *moderate* anticipated effect size of Cohen's $d = 0.50$ (see Table 25.1), $\alpha = 0.05$, and power = 0.80.

Step 1: Open G*Power 3.1.
Step 2: Select "t-tests" from the pull-down menu labeled "Test family."
Step 3: Select "Means: Differences between two independent means (two groups)" from the pull-down menu labeled "Statistical test."
Step 4: Make sure that the type of power analysis listed is "A priori: Compute required sample size—given α, power, and effect size." This is the default setting.
Step 5: In the "Input parameters" section, select a two-tailed test.
Step 6: Enter the hypothesized effect next to "Effect size d." For our example, it will be 0.50.
Step 7: Enter the α next to "α err prob." For our example, it will be 0.05.
Step 8: Enter the desired power next to "Power (1 − β err prob)." For our example, it will be 0.80.
Step 9: Leave "Allocation ratio N2/N1" at 1 unless there is a specific reason to anticipate unequal sample sizes.
Step 10: Click Calculate. The window should look like the screen shot in Fig. 25.1.

As can be observed in Fig. 25.1, 128 total participants are required (64 in each group) to test a study hypothesis using an independent samples t-test, based on a *moderate* Cohen's d of 0.50, $\alpha = 0.05$, and power = 0.80.

POWER ANALYSIS 2: COHEN'S *d*_Z

Cohen's d_z is an effect that represents the magnitude of the difference between two sets of paired data expressed in standard deviation units. The following instructions outline the steps required to perform a hypothetical power analysis with a *small* anticipated effect size of Cohen's $d_z = 0.20$ (see Table 25.1), $\alpha = 0.05$, and power = 0.80.

Step 1: Open G*Power 3.1.
Step 2: Select "t-tests" from the pull-down menu labeled "Test family."
Step 3: Select "Means: Differences between two dependent means (matched pairs)" from the pull-down menu labeled "Statistical test."

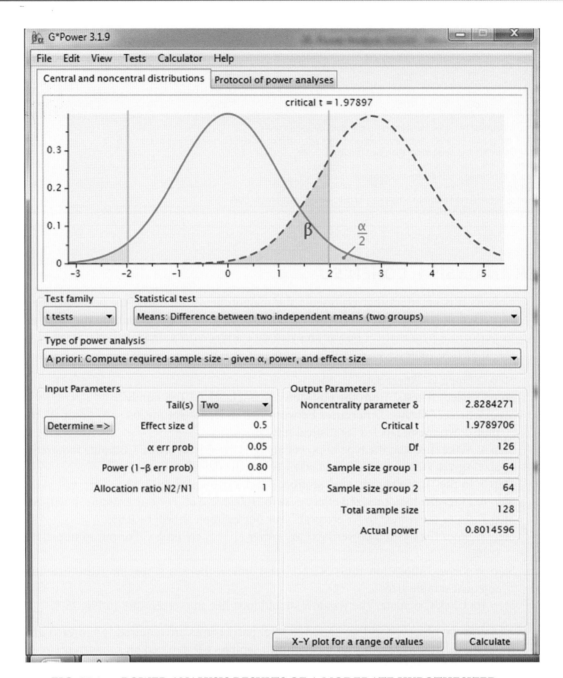

FIG. 25.1 ■ **POWER ANALYSIS RESULTS OF A MODERATE HYPOTHESIZED COHEN'S *d*, α = 0.05, AND POWER = 0.80.**

Step 4: Make sure that the type of power analysis listed is "A priori: Compute required sample size—given α, power, and effect size." This is the default setting.

Step 5: In the "Input parameters" section, select a two-tailed test.

Step 6: Enter the hypothesized effect next to "Effect size d_z." For our example, it will be 0.20.

Step 7: Enter the α next to "α err prob." For our example, it will be 0.05.

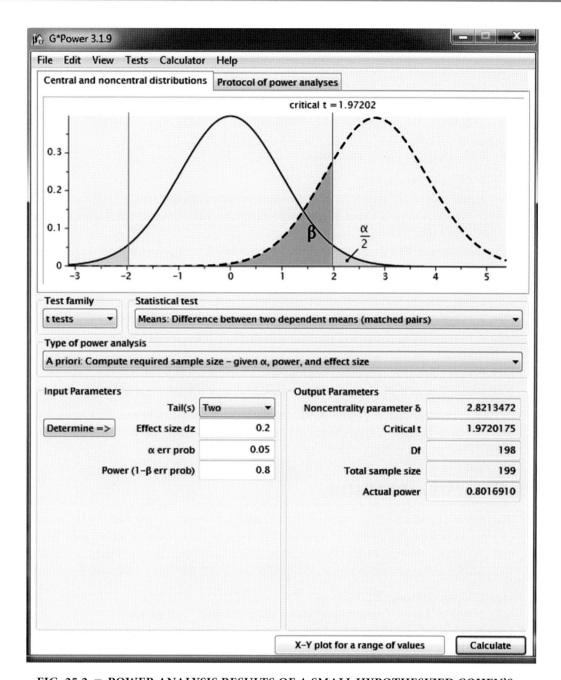

FIG. 25.2 ■ **POWER ANALYSIS RESULTS OF A SMALL HYPOTHESIZED COHEN'S**
d_Z, α = 0.05, AND POWER = 0.80.

Step 8: Enter the desired power next to "Power (1 – β err prob)." For our example, it will be
0.80.

Step 9: Click Calculate. The window should look like the screen shot in Fig. 25.2.

As can be observed in Fig. 25.2, 199 total participants are required to test a study
hypothesis using a paired samples *t*-test, based on a *small* Cohen's d_z of 0.20, α = 0.05, and
power = 0.80.

POWER ANALYSIS 3: COHEN'S *f*

When planning a one-way analysis of variance (ANOVA), Cohen's *f* can be computed to determine the differences between the groups. Like the ANOVA, Cohen's *f* will identify the magnitude of the differences among the groups, but it will not explain differences between specific groups. The following instructions outline the steps required to perform a hypothetical power analysis for a three-group design with a *small* anticipated effect size of $f = 0.10$ (see Table 25.1), $\alpha = 0.05$, and power = 0.80.

Step 1: Open G*Power 3.1.
Step 2: Select "F-tests" from the pull-down menu labeled "Test family."
Step 3: Select "ANOVA: Fixed effects, omnibus, one-way" from the pull-down menu labeled "Statistical test."
Step 4: Make sure that the type of power analysis listed is "A priori: Compute required sample size—given α, power, and effect size." This is the default setting.
Step 5: In the "Input parameters" section, select a two-tailed test.
Step 6: Enter the hypothesized effect next to "Effect size *f*." For our example, it will be 0.10.
Step 7: Enter the α next to "α err prob." For our example, it will be 0.05.
Step 8: Enter the desired power next to "Power (1 − β err prob)." For our example, it will be 0.80.
Step 9: Enter 3 next to "Number of groups."
Step 10: Click Calculate. The window should look like the screen shot in Fig. 25.3.

As can be observed in Fig. 25.3, 969 total participants are required (323 in each group) to test a study hypothesis using a three-group one-way ANOVA based on a Cohen's *f* of 0.10, α = 0.05, and power = 0.80.

POWER ANALYSIS 4: PEARSON *r*

The Pearson product-moment correlation is always between −1.00 and +1.00, where a value of zero indicates absolutely no relationship between the two variables (see Exercises 13 and 29). The following instructions outline the steps required to perform a power analysis with a *large* anticipated effect size of $r = 0.50$ (see Table 25.1), $\alpha = 0.05$, and power = 0.80.

Step 1: Open G*Power 3.1.
Step 2: Select "Exact" from the pull-down menu labeled "Test family."
Step 3: Select "Correlation: Bivariate normal model" from the pull-down menu labeled "Statistical test."
Step 4: Make sure that the type of power analysis listed is "A priori: Compute required sample size—given α, power, and effect size." This is the default setting.
Step 5: In the "Input parameters" section, choose a two-tailed test.
Step 6: Enter the hypothesized effect next to "Correlation ρ H1." For our example, it will be 0.50.
Step 7: Enter the α next to "α err prob." For our example, it will be 0.05.
Step 8: Enter the desired power next to "Power (1 − β err prob)." For our example, it will be 0.80.

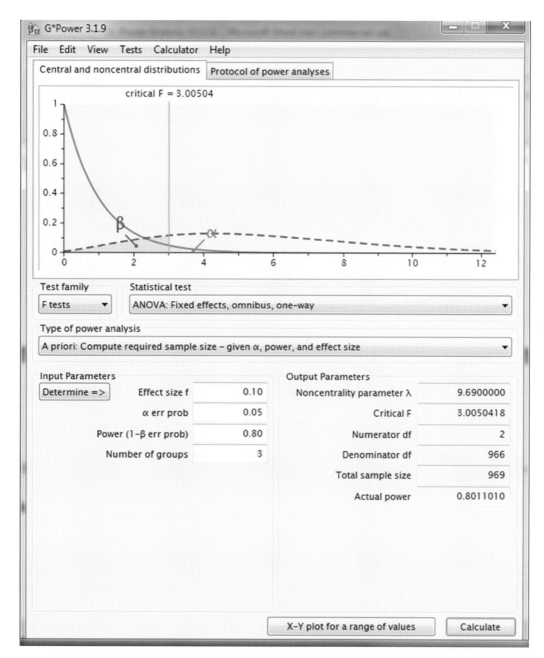

FIG. 25.3 ■ **POWER ANALYSIS RESULTS OF A SMALL HYPOTHESIZED COHEN'S *f*, α = 0.05, AND POWER = 0.80, WITH THREE GROUPS.**

Step 9: Enter 0 next to "Correlation ρ H0." This means that the null hypothesis states that there is no correlation between the two variables ($r = 0.0$).

Step 10: Click Calculate. The window should look like the screen shot in Fig. 25.4.

As can be observed in Fig. 25.4, 29 total participants are required to test a study hypothesis using a Pearson correlation coefficient, based on a Pearson *r* of 0.50, α = 0.05, and power = 0.80.

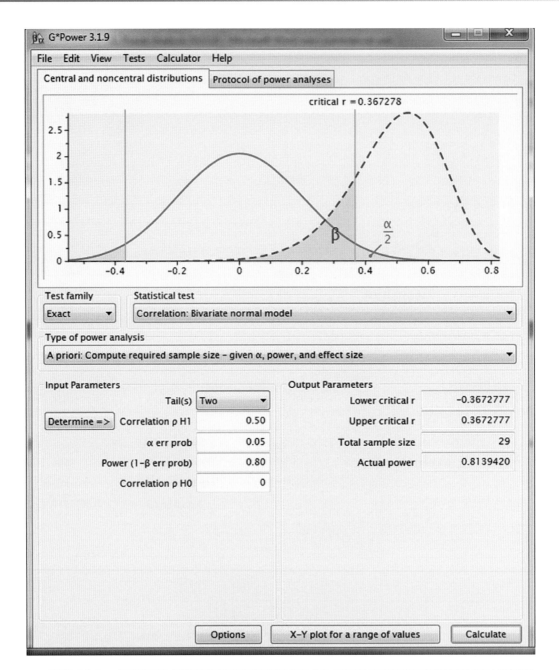

FIG. 25.4 ■ POWER ANALYSIS RESULTS OF A LARGE HYPOTHESIZED PEARSON *r*, α = 0.05, AND POWER = 0.80.

POWER ANALYSIS 5: R^2

The R^2 is the effect size for linear regression. The R^2 represents the percentage of variance explained in *y* by the predictor (see Exercises 15 and 30). The following instructions outline the steps required to perform a hypothetical power analysis with a *moderate* anticipated effect size of $R^2 = 0.15$ (see Table 25.1), α = 0.05, and power = 0.80, with a three-predictor model.

Step 1: Open G*Power 3.1.

Step 2: Select "F-Tests" from the pull-down menu labeled "Test family."

Step 3: Select "Linear multiple regression: Fixed model, R^2 deviation from zero" from the pull-down menu labeled "Statistical test."

Step 4: Make sure that the type of power analysis listed is "A priori: Compute required sample size—given α, power, and effect size." This is the default setting.

Step 5: Underneath the phrase "Input parameters," click "Determine." A window will slide out to the right of your screen. This is so you can convert your hypothesized R^2 value to an f^2 value, which is what G*Power uses to perform a power analysis for multiple regression.

Step 6: Enter the hypothesized effect next to "Squared multiple correlation ρ^2." For our example, it will be 0.15.

Step 7: Click "Calculate and transfer to main window."

Step 8: Enter the α next to "α err prob." For our example, it will be 0.05.

Step 9: Enter the desired power next to "Power (1 − β err prob)." For our example, it will be 0.80.

Step 10: Enter 3 next to "Number of predictors."

Step 11: Click Calculate. The window should look like the screen shot in Fig. 25.5.

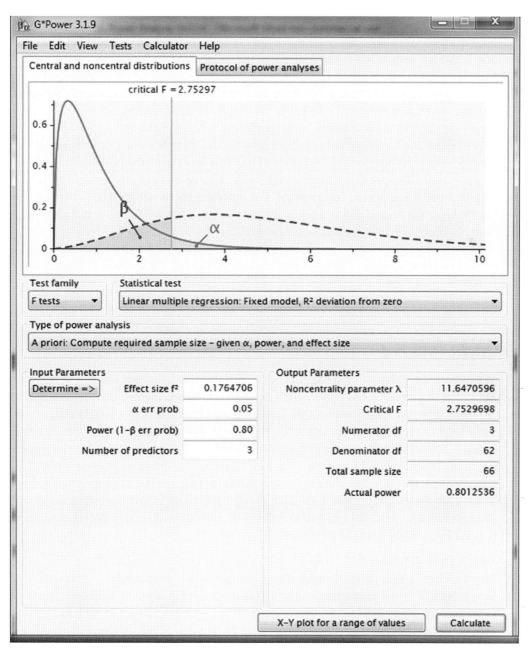

FIG. 25.5 ▪ POWER ANALYSIS RESULTS OF A MODERATE HYPOTHESIZED R^2, α = 0.05, AND POWER = 0.80.

As can be observed in Fig. 25.5, 66 total participants are required to test a study hypothesis using a three-predictor multiple regression model, based on an R^2 of 0.15, $\alpha = 0.05$, and power $= 0.80$.

POWER ANALYSIS 6: ODDS RATIO

An *OR* is computed when the dependent variable is dichotomous and the predictor is either continuous or dichotomous. With multiple predictors, *OR*s are computed by performing logistic regression analysis. Logistic regression analysis tests a predictor (or set of predictors) with a dichotomous dependent variable (Tabachnick & Fidell, 2019). Because an *OR* in a power analysis is often being planned within the context of logistic regression, the following example uses the logistic regression feature of G*Power. The following instructions outline the steps required to perform a hypothetical power analysis with a *small* anticipated effect size of $OR = 1.5$ (see Table 25.1), $\alpha = 0.05$, and power $= 0.80$.

Step 1: Open G*Power 3.1.
Step 2: Select "z-tests" from the pull-down menu labeled "Test family."
Step 3: Select "Logistic regression" from the pull-down menu labeled "Statistical test."
Step 4: Make sure that the type of power analysis listed is "A priori: Compute required sample size—given α, power, and effect size." This is the default setting.
Step 5: In the "Input parameters" section, choose a two-tailed test.
Step 6: Enter the hypothesized effect next to "Odds ratio." For our example, it will be 1.5.
Step 7: Enter 0.30 next to "Pr(Y=1|X=1) H0." This represents the probability that y is 1 when x is 1, and 30% would represent a small to moderate association between x and y.
Step 8: Enter the α next to "α err prob." For our example, it will be 0.05.
Step 9: Enter the desired power next to "Power (1 − β err prob)." For our example, it will be 0.80.
Step 10: Leave the default value of 0 next to "R^2 other predictors."
Step 11: Select "Binomial" from the pull-down menu next to "X distribution."
Step 12: Click Calculate. The window should look like the screen shot in Fig. 25.6.

As can be observed in Fig. 25.6, 853 total participants are required to test a study hypothesis using an unadjusted odds ratio, based on an *OR* of 1.5, $\alpha = 0.05$, and power $= 0.80$.

POWER ANALYSIS 7: d

When both the predictor and the dependent variable are dichotomous, you may use either the *OR* or the d as the effect size in a power analysis. However, the d is the preferred effect size in a power analysis for a two-sample comparative design where the dependent variable is dichotomous. Recall that the letter "d" represents the difference in percentages in Group 1 versus Group 2. A power analysis based on the effect size d can involve any two pairs of proportions. However, in this exercise, for ease of understanding one proportion will always be 0.50, or 50%. This is because the ranges of effect size magnitudes in Table 25.1 for d only apply when one group's proportion is 50% (Cohen, 1988). The following instructions outline the steps required to perform a hypothetical power analysis with a *large* anticipated effect size of d $= 0.25$, $\alpha = 0.05$, and power $= 0.80$.

Step 1: Open G*Power 3.1.
Step 2: Select "Exact" from the pull-down menu labeled "Test family."
Step 3: Select "Proportions: Inequality, two independent groups (Fisher's exact test)" from the pull-down menu labeled "Statistical test."
Step 4: Make sure that the type of power analysis listed is "A priori: Compute required sample size—given α, power, and effect size." This is the default setting.

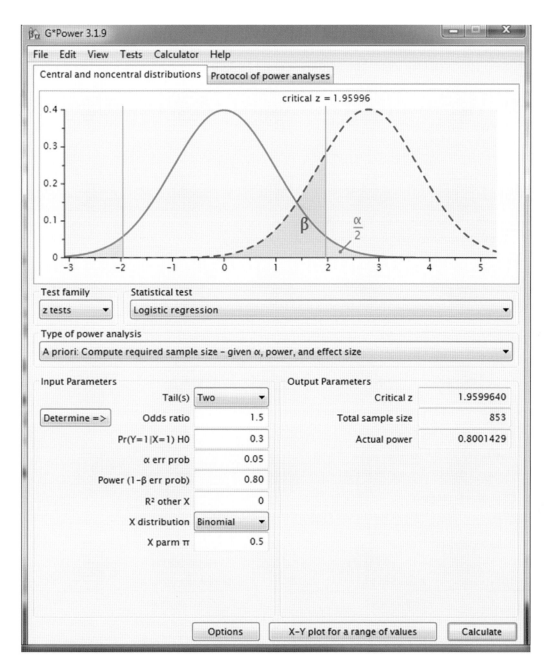

FIG. 25.6 ■ **POWER ANALYSIS RESULTS OF A SMALL HYPOTHESIZED *OR*, α = 0.05, AND POWER = 0.80.**

Step 5: In the "Input parameters" section, choose a two-tailed test.

Step 6: Enter the hypothesized proportions next to "Proportion p1 and Proportion p2." For our example, it will be 0.50 and 0.25 to represent a 25% difference. It does not matter which proportion, p1 or p2, is 0.25 and 0.50. Thus, 0.25 and 0.50 can be entered in p1 and p2, or vice versa.

Step 7: Enter the α next to "α err prob." For our example, it will be 0.05.

Step 8: Enter the desired power next to "Power (1 − β err prob)." For our example, it will be 0.80.

Step 9: Leave "Allocation ratio N2/N1" at 1 unless there is a specific reason to anticipate unequal sample sizes.

Step 10: Click Calculate. The window should look like the screen shot in Fig. 25.7.

As can be observed in Fig. 25.7, 128 total participants are required (64 in each group) to test a study hypothesis using a Fisher's exact test, based on a large d of 0.25, $\alpha = 0.05$, and power = 0.80.

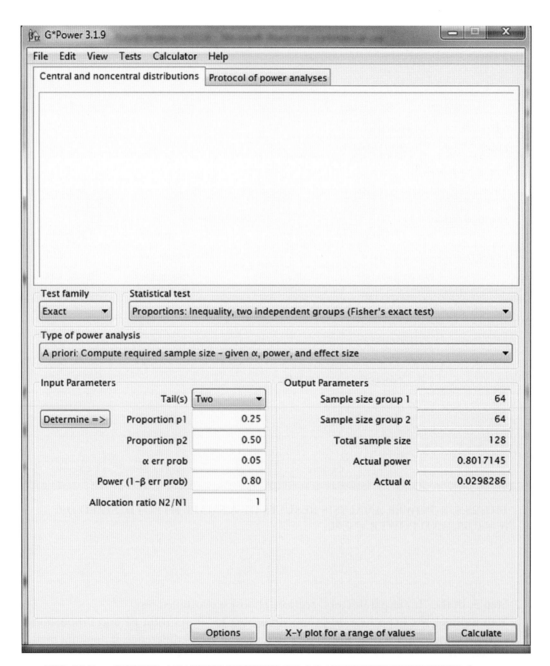

FIG. 25.7 ■ **POWER ANALYSIS RESULTS OF A LARGE HYPOTHESIZED d, $\alpha = 0.05$, AND POWER = 0.80.**

STUDY QUESTIONS

1. Perform a power analysis based on a moderate hypothesized Cohen's d_z, $\alpha = 0.05$ and power = 0.80, two-tailed test, using G*Power. What is the required N?

2. Perform a power analysis based on a large hypothesized R^2 with four predictors in the model, $\alpha = 0.05$, and power = 0.80 using G*Power. What is the required N?

3. Perform a power analysis based on a large hypothesized three-group Cohen's f, $\alpha = 0.05$, and power = 0.80 using G*Power. What is the required N?

4. Redo your power analysis from Question 3 using a moderate hypothesized Cohen's f. How many more participants are required? Provide a rationale for the difference in the sample size.

5. Perform a power analysis based on a moderate hypothesized d where Group 1 = 50% and Group 2 = 65%, $\alpha = 0.05$, and power = 0.80, two-tailed test, using G*Power. What is the required N?

6. Redo your power analysis from Question 5, using an α of 0.01. How many more participants are required? Provide a rationale for your difference in sample size.

7. Prior to conducting a power analysis, a researcher reviewed the literature and discovered that a study similar to hers reported a Cohen's *d* of 0.22. According to Table 25.1, how would you characterize the magnitude of that effect?

8. Perform a power analysis based on a moderate Pearson *r*, α = 0.05, and power = 0.80, two-tailed test, using G*Power. What is the required *N*?

9. Redo your power analysis from Question 8, using a power of 85% instead of 80%. How many more participants are required? Provide a rationale for the change in sample size.

10. Prior to conducting a power analysis, a researcher reviewed the literature and discovered a similar study reported a Pearson *r* of 0.34. According to Table 25.1, how would you characterize the magnitude of that effect?

Answers to Study Questions

1. The required *N* would be 34.

Input Parameters			Output Parameters	
	Tail(s)	Two	Noncentrality parameter δ	2.9154759
Determine =>	Effect size dz	0.50	Critical t	2.0345153
	α err prob	0.05	Df	33
	Power (1−β err prob)	0.80	Total sample size	34
			Actual power	0.8077775

2. The required *N* would be 40.

Input Parameters			Output Parameters	
Determine =>	Effect size f²	0.3513514	Noncentrality parameter λ	14.0540560
	α err prob	0.05	Critical F	2.6414652
	Power (1−β err prob)	0.8	Numerator df	4
	Number of predictors	4	Denominator df	35
			Total sample size	40
			Actual power	0.8127117

3. The required *N* would be 66.

Input Parameters			Output Parameters	
Determine =>	Effect size f	0.4	Noncentrality parameter λ	10.5600000
	α err prob	0.05	Critical F	3.1428085
	Power (1−β err prob)	0.8	Numerator df	2
	Number of groups	3	Denominator df	63
			Total sample size	66
			Actual power	0.8180744

4. The required *N* would be 159, which would be 93 more participants than would be needed in Question 3. This example demonstrates that the smaller the anticipated effect size, the larger the sample size required to conduct the study (Gray & Grove, 2021).

Input Parameters			Output Parameters	
Determine =>	Effect size f	0.25	Noncentrality parameter λ	9.9375000
	α err prob	0.05	Critical F	3.0540042
	Power (1−β err prob)	0.8	Numerator df	2
	Number of groups	3	Denominator df	156
			Total sample size	159
			Actual power	0.8048873

5. The required *N* would be 366.

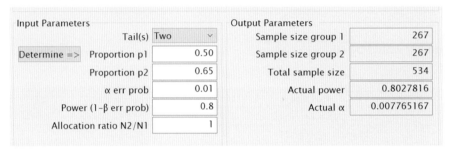

6. The required *N* would be 534, which would be 168 more participants than would be needed in Question 5. This example demonstrates that the smaller the alpha, the larger the sample size required to conduct the study (Kim et al., 2022).

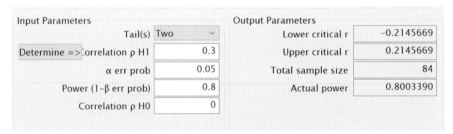

7. A Cohen's *d* of 0.22 would be considered a small effect according to Table 25.1.

8. The required *N* would be 84.

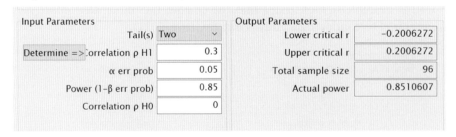

9. The required *N* would be 96, which would be 12 more participants than would be needed in Question 8. This example demonstrates that the larger the desired statistical power, the larger the sample size required to conduct the study (Terrell, 2021).

10. A Pearson *r* of 0.34 would be considered a moderate effect, because it is so close to 0.30 (a moderate effect according to Table 25.1).

Name: _____ Class: _____

Date: _____

Follow your instructor's directions to submit your answers to the following questions for additional study. Your instructor may ask you to write your answers below and submit them as a hard copy for evaluation. Alternatively, your instructor may ask you to submit your answers online.

1. What is one approach a researcher can take when there is a lack of information in the literature concerning effect sizes that can be used as a basis for her power analysis?

2. Perform a power analysis based on a large hypothesized Cohen's *d*, $\alpha = 0.05$, and power $= 0.80$, two-tailed test, with two groups of equal size using G*Power. What is the required *N*?

3. Redo your power analysis from Question 2 using a power of 85% instead of 80%. How many more participants are required? Provide a rationale for the difference in sample size.

4. Perform a power analysis based on a small hypothesized Cohen's f with a four-group design, $\alpha = 0.05$, and power $= 0.80$ using G*Power. What is the required N?

5. Redo your power analysis from Question 4 using an α of 0.01. How many more participants are required? Provide a rationale for the difference in sample size.

6. Perform a power analysis based on a large hypothesized R^2 with two predictors in the model, $\alpha = 0.05$, and power $= 0.80$ using G*Power. What is the required N?

7. Redo your power analysis from Question 6 using six predictors instead of two. How many more participants are required? Provide a rationale for the difference in sample size.

8. Perform a power analysis based on a moderate hypothesized d where Group 1 $= 32\%$ and Group 2 $= 50\%$, $\alpha = 0.05$, and power $= 0.80$, two-tailed test, using G*Power. What is the required N?

9. Redo your power analysis from Question 8 using a one-tailed test. How many fewer participants are required? Provide a rationale for the difference in sample size.

10. Perform a power analysis based on a moderate Pearson r, $\alpha = 0.01$, and power $= 0.85$, two-tailed test, using G*Power. What is the required N?

Handling Missing Data

Handling missing values within a dataset is important for all statistical analyses. Missing data can occur when participants are lost to follow-up; where there is a failure of instrumentation, mistakes, and/or omissions by the researcher; refusal of response; and many other possible reasons. Assessment of the missing data problem begins with knowing the extent, pattern, and reasons for the missing data (Little & Rubin, 1987). Improper handling of missing values will distort the statistical analyses because, until proven otherwise, the researcher must assume that missing cases differ in important ways from the cases where values are present. Although the extent of missing data (the degree or scope of missing values in a dataset) is important, the current consensus among experts is that the pattern of the missingness is much more of an issue than the extent of the missingness (Cheema, 2014). A clear pattern of missing data is an indicator that the remaining dataset is biased in some way (Little & Rubin, 1987; Tabachnick & Fidell, 2019).

PATTERNS OF THE MISSING DATA

The pattern of missing data refers to whether the data are missing because of random chance or because of a particular reason. The ability to identify whether the data are missing randomly will inform the researcher on how to remedy the missing data problem.

Random Patterns of Missing Data

A random pattern of missing data occurs when the data are randomly missing throughout the dataset, with no apparent explanation or pattern. The chance of a missing value occurring would be likened to a flip of a coin. Missing data that are scattered randomly throughout the dataset pose the least threat to internal and external validity of the analyses (Gray & Grove, 2021; Little & Rubin, 1987; Tabachnick & Fidell, 2019).

Data are considered to be missing at random (either completely or partially) if the missing data are unrelated to the study variables. The assumption that the data are *missing completely at random* (MCAR) can be tested with the Little test, a type of chi-square statistic that tests a quantitative dataset against the assumption of MCAR (Little, 1988). If the Little test is nonsignificant at alpha > 0.05, then the researcher can proceed with missing data imputation (summarized later in this exercise) with the least probable effect on internal and external validity of the analyses (Little, 1988; Little & Rubin, 1987).

NonRandom Patterns of Missing Data

Nonrandom missing data occur when values are missing with an obvious pattern in the dataset. Nonrandom patterns can exist along a continuum from a partial, fragmented pattern to a pervasive, predictable pattern of missingness. The assessment of this continuum should

TABLE 26.1	EXAMPLE OF A NONRANDOM PATTERN OF MISSING DATA	
ID	Gender	Hopefulness at Discontinuation, Nonrandom Pattern
1	F	4
2	F	
3	F	1
4	F	
5	F	
6	F	5
7	F	2
8	F	
9	F	
10	F	3
11	M	3
12	M	3
13	M	4
14	M	3
15	M	1
16	M	4
17	M	3
18	M	2
19	M	3
20	M	4

F, female; M, male.

TABLE 26.2	EXAMPLE OF A RANDOM PATTERN OF MISSING DATA	
ID	Gender	Hopefulness with Randomly Missing Data
1	F	4
2	F	2
3	F	
4	F	3
5	F	
6	F	5
7	F	2
8	F	5
9	F	2
10	F	3
11	M	3
12	M	3
13	M	
14	M	3
15	M	1
16	M	
17	M	3
18	M	2
19	M	
20	M	4

F, female; M, male.

be conducted with statistical software. These nonrandom patterns, when not addressed in the analyses, can distort the internal and external validity of the findings (Kim et al., 2022; Tabachnick & Fidell, 2019). Table 26.1 displays an example of a nonrandom pattern of missing data. Using an example from a study by Cipher and Urban (2022), survey data were collected from recently discontinued nursing students. Among the study variables were gender and ratings of hopefulness. Among these hypothetical data, note that the hopefulness variable consists of missing values for the females, but not the males. In contrast, Table 26.2 displays an example of a random pattern of missing data. The hopefulness variable in Table 26.2 consists of values that are missing evenly across both genders. When a nonrandom pattern of missing data is observed, it is highly recommended that the researcher consults with a statistician before performing the planned statistical analyses (Gray & Grove, 2021).

IMPUTATION METHODS

The term **imputation** in research refers to the process of estimating missing data values and inserting those estimations into a dataset where the missing values are located (Little & Rubin, 1987). There are several approaches to imputing missing data, and each has advantages and disadvantages. This exercise will not provide a comprehensive review, but for those who are interested in the theoretical underpinnings of each approach, including mathematical explanations, the seminal text on missing data imputation is Little and Rubin (1987).

Missing data are generally imputed for quantitative variables (ordinal/interval/ratio), not categorical (nominal) variables. The approach implemented to address missing data depends on (1) the extent (degree or scope) of the missing data and (2) the randomness of the missing data. Generally, when less than 5% of the data in a dataset are missing, the missing data procedures described as follows yield similar results (Tabachnick & Fidell, 2019). There are many different methods of handling missing data, each of which can have substantially different effects on estimation (Cheema, 2014). For this reason, it is important to consult with a statistician to obtain assistance with missing data estimations.

Listwise and Pairwise Deletion

Listwise deletion of missing values refers to deleting an entire case (one participant's data) when one or more data point(s) for that case is(are) missing. The subsequent analysis is performed only on complete sets of data. Pairwise deletion of missing values refers to the partial use of a participant's data. The statistical procedure would include the participant's data only for the variables that are nonmissing. Deletion methods of handling missing data can be problematic when statistical power is at risk, because deleting cases can make a small sample even smaller (Little & Rubin, 1987). Recall from Exercises 24 and 25 that a small sample size is a detriment to statistical power.

Mean and Median Replacement

A frequently applied imputation approach is estimating the missing values using the means or medians of a particular variable. For example, if a participant is missing a value for a variable representing a pain visual analog score, the mean pain score can be calculated from the nonmissing values and inserted into the participant's missing cell. Likewise, a median approach can be implemented whereby the median pain score can be calculated from the nonmissing values and inserted into the participant's missing cell. The main disadvantage to imputing missing data with means or medians is that the variance of the imputed variable is artificially lowered and consequently, this will affect the results of subsequent inferential statistics (Tabachnick & Fidell, 2019).

One method to increase the accuracy of imputation with means or medians is to estimate missing data within subgroups wherever possible. For example, if a researcher plans to analyze the data in Table 26.2 by comparing males versus females on hopefulness ratings, it is advisable to impute missing data within each gender subgroup. Table 26.3 displays the missing data imputed regardless of gender, followed by imputation by the gender subgroups using the mean replacement method. Note that the first mean replacement method imputes the value of 3 into all missing cells, whereas the second mean replacement method imputes different values based on whether the participant is a female or male. The mean hopefulness rating for the females is 3.25, and the mean hopefulness rating for the males is 2.71. Therefore we can observe that any subsequent inferential statistics computed on the newly imputed data (such as an independent samples *t*-test) would differ depending on which mean replacement method were used.

Regression

Multiple regression may be used for data imputation by using nonmissing data to predict the values of missing data. The regression method has similar disadvantages as the mean replacement method, in that all of the cases with the same values on the independent variables will be imputed with the same value on the missing variable. As with the mean replacement method, imputation with multiple regression results in the variance of the imputed variable being artificially lower, and consequently, this will affect the results of subsequent inferential statistics. Moreover, the regression method can be a disadvantage if the variables being used as the predictors in the imputation have a low or no association with the variable(s) with the missing data (Tabachnick & Fidell, 2019).

TABLE 26.3	EXAMPLE OF A MEAN REPLACEMENT METHOD FOR MISSING DATA			
ID	Gender	Hopefulness with Randomly Missing Data	Mean Replacement, Whole Sample	Mean Replacement by Gender Group
1	F	4	4	4
2	F	2	2	2
3	F		3	3.25
4	F	3	3	3
5	F		3	3.25
6	F	5	5	5
7	F	2	2	2
8	F	5	5	5
9	F	2	2	2
10	F	3	3	3
11	M	3	3	3
12	M	3	3	3
13	M		3	2.71
14	M	3	3	3
15	M	1	1	1
16	M		3	2.71
17	M	3	3	3
18	M	2	2	2
19	M		3	2.71
20	M	4	4	4

F, female; M, male.

Expectation Maximization

The expectation maximization (EM) method is a two-step iterative process that begins with correlations among the variables in the dataset. The EM method subsequently uses a type of regression called maximum likelihood estimation to iteratively fill in missing values and adjusts the imputed values to ensure that realistic estimates of variance are obtained (Little & Rubin, 1987; Tabachnick & Fidell, 2019). Thus the EM method is an improvement over the mean replacement and regression methods by ensuring that variances are not artificially lowered during the imputation process (Cheema, 2014).

Multiple Imputation

Multiple imputation (MI) is a method of generating multiple simulated values for each missing value, then iteratively analyzing datasets with each simulated value substituted in turn. The purpose of MI is to generate estimates that better reflect true variability and uncertainty in the data than those of other imputation methods (Cheema, 2014). The MI method involves the creation of more than one newly imputed dataset (typically, five datasets are created by the researcher). Statistical software is used to subsequently compute the planned inferential statistic(s) on each of the new datasets and combines the results, yielding a composite as the final estimate. Like the EM method, the MI method ensures that realistic estimates of variance are obtained (Little & Rubin, 1987; Tabachnick & Fidell, 2019).

In general, the consensus among statisticians is that among all available missing data imputation methods, the two best approaches are EM and MI (Cheema, 2014). Both approaches ensure that realistic estimates of variance are obtained (Little & Rubin, 1987;

Tabachnick & Fidell, 2019). The EM method creates one newly imputed dataset, while the MI method creates multiple datasets. Therefore the MI method is a more complicated process, because multiple analyses are conducted that may yield different results, and it is the responsibility of the researcher to collate and report the composite findings.

SPSS COMPUTATION

A cross-sectional survey study investigated the attitudes and future plans among registered nurse–to–bachelor of science in nursing (RN-to-BSN) students who had recently discontinued their program (Cipher & Urban, 2022). Age at program enrollment, recent grade point average (GPA), and feelings of stress and hopefulness were among the study variables examined. The study variables of stress at discontinuation and of hopefulness at discontinuation were single items that were assessed on a 5-point Likert scale. Higher values of the stress variable are indicative of higher self-reported stress levels, and higher values of the hopefulness variable are indicative of higher self-reported levels of hopefulness. A simulated subset of the study data is presented in Table 26.4.

TABLE 26.4   AGE, GPA, AND FEELINGS OF STRESS AND HOPEFULNESS AMONG FORMER RN-TO-BSN STUDENTS

ID	Age at Enrollment	GPA at Discontinuation	Stress at Discontinuation	Hopefulness at Discontinuation
1	27	4.00	3	
2	25	4.00	2	2
3	29	1.49	5	1
4	29			3
5	28	4.00	1	3
6	30	3.00	5	5
7	32	2.34	5	2
8	37			5
9	28	3.90	4	2
10	40	2.67	5	
11	33	3.00	2	3
12	34	4.00	4	3
13	38	3.14	4	4
14	41			3
15	43	3.75	4	1
16	48	3.79	3	
17	39	1.80	5	3
18	49	4.00	3	
19	62	2.14	2	3
20	68	4.00	3	4

GPA, grade point average.

This is how our dataset looks in SPSS.

	ID	Age	GPA	Stress	Hopeful	va
1	1	27	4.00	3	.	
2	2	25	4.00	2	2	
3	3	29	1.49	5	1	
4	4	29	.	.	3	
5	5	28	4.00	1	3	
6	6	30	3.00	5	5	
7	7	32	2.34	5	2	
8	8	37	.	.	5	
9	9	28	3.90	4	2	
10	10	40	2.67	5	.	
11	11	33	3.00	2	3	
12	12	34	4.00	4	3	
13	13	38	3.14	4	4	
14	14	41	.	.	3	
15	15	43	3.75	4	1	

Step 1: From the "Analyze" menu, choose "Missing Value Analysis." Move the four study variables over to the right. Check "EM."

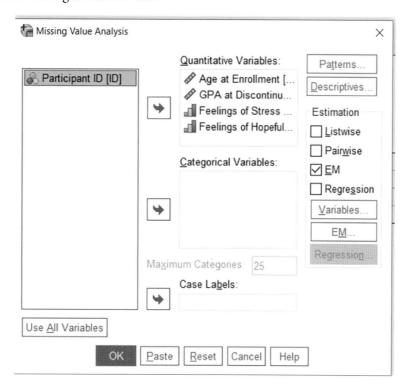

Step 2: Click "Patterns." Check "Tabulated cases, grouped by missing values." Click "Continue."

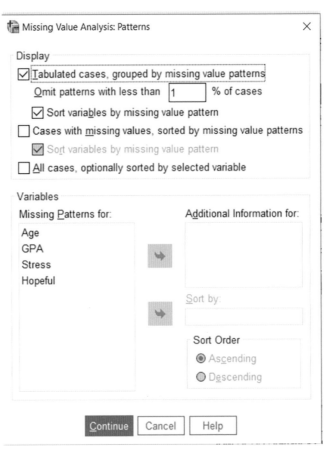

Step 3: Click "Descriptives." Check "Univariate Statistics" and "t tests with groups formed by indicator variables." Click "Continue" and then "OK."

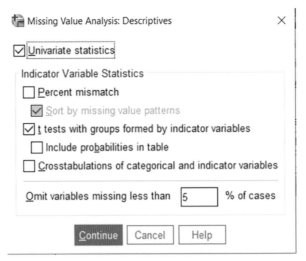

INTERPRETATION OF SPSS OUTPUT

The following tables are generated from SPSS. The first table contains descriptive statistics of the four study variables, along with information about the extent to which each variable contains missing data. Note that in the row labeled "Age," the last column notes that there is one extreme value, and this value is high, not low. When looking at the actual dataset, that outlier is the value of 68. The variable of age is also the only variable in the dataset to have no missing values. The extent of missing data can be calculated by adding the values in the column in the table labeled "Count" and dividing by the total possible values: $(0 + 3 + 3 + 4) \div 80 = 0.125 \times 100\% = 12.5\%$. Thus 12.5% of the data in this dataset are missing.

MVA

Univariate Statistics

	N	Mean	Std. Deviation	Missing Count	Missing Percent	No. of Extremes[a] Low	No. of Extremes[a] High
Age	20	38.00	11.539	0	.0	0	1
GPA	17	3.2365	.86864	3	15.0	0	0
Stress	17	3.53	1.281	3	15.0	0	0
Hopeful	16	2.94	1.181	4	20.0	0	0

a. Number of cases outside the range (Q1 - 1.5*IQR, Q3 + 1.5*IQR).

The next two tables contain means and standard deviations for each study variable. The first row, labeled "All Values," displays the means and standard deviations as computed in the dataset, excluding the missing values. The second row, labeled "EM," displays the means and standard deviations if the EM method were used to impute all of the missing values (IBM Corporation, 2022).

Summary of Estimated Means

	Age	GPA	Stress	Hopeful
All Values	38.00	3.2365	3.53	2.94
EM	38.00	3.2531	3.53	2.98

Summary of Estimated Standard Deviations

	Age	GPA	Stress	Hopeful
All Values	11.539	.86864	1.281	1.181
EM	11.539	.86898	1.279	1.179

The next table, titled "Separate Variance t Tests," displays independent samples *t*-test results with missingness as the independent variable (missing versus present) and the study variable as the dependent variable. Note the first column for "Age" and the results for "Hopefulness." The mean age for participants that had nonmissing (present) values for hopefulness is 37.25, while the mean age for participants that had missing values for hopefulness is 41.00. If the *t*-test were significant, it would indicate a pattern of missing data whereby older participants were less likely to provide hopefulness ratings than younger participants. However, the t value is -0.60, which is not significant, indicating no pattern of missingness between age and hopefulness ratings.

Separate Variance t Tests[a]

		Age	GPA	Stress	Hopeful
GPA	t	.6	.	.	-1.2
	df	5.6	.	.	3.0
	# Present	17	17	17	13
	# Missing	3	0	0	3
	Mean(Present)	38.41	3.2365	3.53	2.77
	Mean(Missing)	35.67	.	.	3.67
Stress	t	.6	.	.	-1.2
	df	5.6	.	.	3.0
	# Present	17	17	17	13
	# Missing	3	0	0	3
	Mean(Present)	38.41	3.2365	3.53	2.77
	Mean(Missing)	35.67	.	.	3.67
Hopeful	t	-.6	-1.2	.1	.
	df	5.3	7.3	7.0	.
	# Present	16	13	13	16
	# Missing	4	4	4	0
	Mean(Present)	37.25	3.1202	3.54	2.94
	Mean(Missing)	41.00	3.6143	3.50	.

For each quantitative variable, pairs of groups are formed by indicator variables (present, missing).

a. Indicator variables with less than 5% missing are not displayed.

The table titled "Tabulated Patterns" displays an "X" where there is a possibility of missing data patterns. The column for "Age" is blank, indicating that the variable of age contains no missing data. The second and third columns for "GPA" and "Stress," respectively, displays an "X" together on the same row, indicating that there are three instances where three participants were missing pairs of GPA and stress values. There were 13 participants who had complete sets of data, with no missing values for any variable.

Tabulated Patterns

	Missing Patterns[a]				
Number of Cases	Age	GPA	Stress	Hopeful	Complete if …[b]
13					13
4				X	17
3		X	X		16

a. Variables are sorted on missing patterns.

b. Number of complete cases if variables missing in that pattern (marked with X) are not used.

The table titled "EM Means" contains the same information provided in the earlier tables by displaying the means of the study variables if the EM method were used to impute all of the missing values. The new piece of information is found in the footnote below the table: Little's MCAR test. Little's test is reported as a type of chi-square test, with an exact p value of 0.652. This statistic tests the assumption that the data are missing completely at random (Little, 1988). If the result is not significant, then the researcher can assume that the data are missing completely at random and the researcher can proceed with missing data imputation with the least probable effect on internal and external validity of the analyses (Gray & Grove, 2021; Shadish et al., 2002). If the result is significant, then the researcher can assume that there is evidence of nonrandom patterns of missing data (Little, 1988). In this example, Little's test is not significant, suggesting that the data are missing completely at random, and that any possible patterns of missing data that exist in the dataset are too small and not meaningful enough to be detected by Little's statistic (Little, 1988).

EM Estimated Statistics

EM Means[a]

Age	GPA	Stress	Hopeful
38.00	3.2531	3.53	2.98

a. Little's MCAR test: Chi-Square = 3.313, DF = 5, Sig. = .652

STUDY QUESTIONS

1. Provide one possible cause or reason for missing data in a dataset.

2. What is meant by the *extent* of missing data? Define and give an example.

3. What is meant by the *pattern* of missing data? Define and give an example.

4. Which is the most important component of assessing missing data: the extent of the missingness or the pattern of the missingness? Provide a rationale for your response and include documentation.

5. What does a significant Little's test indicate?

6. Name one disadvantage of using the mean replacement method for missing data imputation.

7. In the example data, calculate the extent of missing data for the variable of stress. Show your work.

8. In the example data, calculate the extent of missing data for the variable of hopefulness. Show your work.

9. In the example data, does there appear to be a pattern of missing data for GPA? Provide a rationale for your response.

10. In the SPSS output tabled titled "Separate Variance t Tests," the mean stress rating for participants that had nonmissing (i.e., present) values for the variable of hopefulness is 3.54. What is the mean stress rating for participants that had missing values for hopefulness? Is there a disparity between the two means?

Answers to Study Questions

1. No follow-up of study participants is a common cause of missing data. Other reasons include failure of instrumentation, mistakes and/or omissions by the researcher, and refusal of response (Tabachnick & Fidell, 2019).

2. The *extent* of missing data refers to the amount of data missing in a dataset. For example, in a hypothetical dataset with 10 participants and two study variables (for a total of 20 potential values), if one value is missing from the first variable, and two values missing from the second variable, the extent of missing data is calculated as: $(1 + 2) \div 20 = 0.15 \times 100\% = 15.0\%$.

3. The *pattern* of missing data refers to whether the data are missing because of random chance or because of a particular reason. One example of data that have a nonrandom pattern would be the presence of missing income for study participants who are retired, but no missing income data for those who are currently employed. This pattern would suggest that the retired participants were less likely to divulge their income than the employed participants. One reason might be that the participants might have no income related to a job, so they left this item blank.

4. The pattern of the missing data is the most important component of assessing missing data. A clear pattern of missing data is an indicator that the remaining dataset is biased in some way (Little & Rubin, 1987; Tabachnick & Fidell, 2019). The ability to identify whether the data are missing randomly will inform the researcher on how to remedy the missing data problem.

5. A significant Little's test indicates that there is evidence of nonrandom patterns of missing data (Little, 1988). This finding implies a more complicated approach to the imputation process because a nonrandom pattern of missing data is an indicator that the remaining dataset is biased in some way (Little & Rubin, 1987; Tabachnick & Fidell, 2019).

6. The main disadvantage of imputing missing data with means or medians is that the variance of the imputed variable is lowered and, consequently, this will affect the results of subsequent inferential statistics (Tabachnick & Fidell, 2019).

7. The extent of missing data for the variable of stress is calculated as: $(3 \div 20) \times 100\% = 0.15 \times 100\% = 15.0\%$.

8. The extent of missing data for the variable of hopefulness is calculated as: $(4 \div 20) \times 100\% = 0.20 \times 100\% = 20.0\%$.

9. Yes, there appears to be a pattern of missing data for GPA. Upon visual inspection of the raw data, it appears that with every missing value for GPA, there is also a missing value for stress. Moreover, in the SPSS output tabled titled "Tabulated Patterns," the columns for GPA and stress display an "X" together on the same rows, indicating that there are three instances where three participants were missing pairs of GPA and stress values. There are zero instances where there is a missing value for GPA but not for stress, and vice versa.

10. The mean stress rating for participants that had missing values for the variable of hopefulness is 3.50. No, there is no notable disparity between the stress ratings for participants with present and missing hopefulness data because the difference between 3.50 and 3.54 is clinically insignificant (Gray & Grove, 2021).

DATA FOR ADDITIONAL COMPUTATIONAL PRACTICE

The following questions for additional study refer to the same example from Cipher and Urban (2022). The data are presented in Table 26.4.

Name: _____ Class: _____

Date: _____

Answer the following questions with hand calculations using the data presented in Table 26.4 or the SPSS dataset called "Exercise 26 Example" available on the Evolve website. Follow your instructor's directions to submit your answers to the following questions for additional study. Your instructor may ask you to write your answers below and submit them as a hard copy for evaluation. Alternatively, your instructor may ask you to submit your answers online.

1. In the example data, calculate the extent of missing data for grade point average (GPA). Show your work.

2. In the SPSS output table titled "Tabulated Data," the column titled "Complete if ..." lists 13 "complete cases." Explain the meaning of this number.

3. In a hypothetical dataset, a Little's MCAR test is computed. The results are $\chi^2(2) = 8.83$, $p = 0.02$. How would you interpret this result?

4. In a hypothetical dataset, a Little's MCAR test is computed. The results are $\chi^2(4) = 1.92$, $p = 0.36$. How would you interpret this result?

5. Explain one reason why the expectation maximization (EM) method is an improvement over the mean replacement and regression methods for missing data imputation.

6. In a hypothetical example, a dataset contains 100 participants and two study variables, for a total of 200 potential values. If one value is missing from the first variable, and zero values missing from the second variable, calculate the extent of missing data. Show your work.

7. In the example in Question 6, what are the implications of the extent of the missing data on the imputation procedure? In other words, will the imputation procedure significantly affect the final results? Provide a rationale for your response.

8. The following hypothetical table is generated with SPSS with two variables: pain score and health score. What is the extent of missing data for pain score? Show your calculations, or alternatively, indicate where the answer is found in the table.

Univariate Statistics

	N	Mean	Std. Deviation	Missing Count	Missing Percent	No. of Extremes[a] Low	No. of Extremes[a] High
Pain Score	16	7.73	1.64	4	20.0	0	0
Health Score	19	5.47	2.12	1	5.0	1	0

a. Number of cases outside the range (Q1 - 1.5*IQR, Q3 + 1.5*IQR).

9. In the same hypothetical table from Question 8, there is one outlier noted. Which variable contains the outlier? Note whether the outlier is an unusually small value or large value. Provide a rationale for your response.

10. Does the table from Question 8 provide information on the pattern of missing data? Provide a rationale for your response.

Determining the Normality of a Distribution

Most parametric statistics require that the variables being studied are normally distributed. The normal curve has a symmetric or equal distribution of scores around the mean with a small number of outliers in the two tails. The first step to determining normality is to create a frequency distribution of the variable(s) being studied. A frequency distribution can be displayed in a table or figure. A line graph figure can be created whereby the x axis consists of the possible values of that variable, and the y axis is the tally of each value. The frequency distributions presented in this exercise focus on values of continuous variables. With a continuous variable, higher numbers represent more of that variable and the lower numbers represent less of that variable, or vice versa. Common examples of continuous variables are age, income, blood pressure, weight, height, pain levels, and health status (see Exercise 1; Grove & Gray, 2023; Waltz et al., 2017).

The frequency distribution of a variable can be presented in a **frequency table,** which is a way of organizing the data by listing every possible value in the first column of numbers, and the frequency (tally) of each value as the second column of numbers. For example, consider the following hypothetical age data for patients from a primary care clinic. The ages of 20 patients were: 45, 26, 59, 51, 42, 28, 26, 32, 31, 55, 43, 47, 67, 39, 52, 48, 36, 42, 61, and 57.

First, we must sort the patients' ages from lowest to highest values:

26
26
28
31
32
36
39
42
42
43
45
47
48
51
52
55
57
59
61
67

Next, each age value is tallied to create the frequency. This is an example of an ungrouped frequency distribution. In an **ungrouped frequency distribution**, researchers list all categories of the variable on which they have data and tally each datum on the listing (Grove & Gray, 2023). In this example, all the different ages of the 20 patients are listed and then tallied for each age.

Age	Frequency
26	2
28	1
31	1
32	1
36	1
39	1
42	2
43	1
45	1
47	1
48	1
51	1
52	1
55	1
57	1
59	1
61	1
67	1

Because most of the ages in this dataset have frequencies of "1," it is better to group the ages into ranges of values. These ranges must be mutually exclusive (i.e., a patient's age can only be classified into one of the ranges). In addition, the ranges must be exhaustive, meaning that each patient's age will fit into at least one of the categories (Exercise 1). For example, we may choose to have ranges of 10, so that the age ranges are 20 to 29, 30 to 39, 40 to 49, 50 to 59, and 60 to 69. We may choose to have ranges of 5, so that the age ranges are 20 to 24, 25 to 29, 30 to 34, etc. The grouping should be devised to provide the greatest possible meaning to the purpose of the study. If the data are to be compared with data in other studies, groupings should be similar to those of other studies in this field of research. Classifying data into groups results in the development of a **grouped frequency distribution**. Table 27.1 presents a grouped frequency distribution of patient ages classified by ranges of 10 years. Note that the range starts at "20" because there are no patient ages lower than 20, nor are there ages higher than 69.

Table 27.1 also includes percentages of patients with an age in each range; the cumulative percentages for the sample should add up to 100%. This table provides an example of a percentage distribution that indicates the percentage of the sample with scores falling into a specific group. Percentage distributions are particularly useful in comparing this study's data with results from other studies.

TABLE 27.1   GROUPED FREQUENCY DISTRIBUTION OF PATIENT AGES WITH PERCENTAGES

Adult Age Range	Frequency (f)	Percentage (%)	Cumulative Percentage
20–29	3	15%	15%
30–39	4	20%	35%
40–49	6	30%	65%
50–59	5	25%	90%
60–69	2	10%	100%
Total	20	100%	

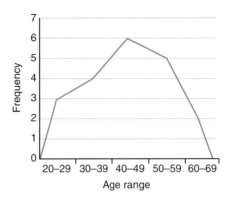

FIG. 27.1 ▪ **FREQUENCY DISTRIBUTION OF PATIENT AGE RANGES.**

As discussed earlier, frequency distributions can be presented in figures. The common figures used to present frequencies include graphs, charts, histograms, and frequency polygons (Gray & Grove, 2021). Fig. 27.1 is a line graph of the frequency distribution for age ranges, where the x axis represents the different age ranges and the y axis represents the frequencies (tallies) of patients with ages in each of the ranges.

THE NORMAL CURVE

The theoretical normal curve is an expression of statistical theory. It is a theoretical frequency distribution of all *possible* scores (Fig. 27.2). However, no real distribution exactly fits the normal curve. This theoretical normal curve is symmetric, unimodal, and has continuous values. The mean, median, and mode are equal in a normal curve (see Fig. 27.2). The distribution is completely defined by the mean and standard deviation (s), which are calculated and discussed in Exercises 8, 9 and 28.

SKEWNESS

Any frequency distribution that is not symmetric is referred to as **skewed** or **asymmetric** (Holmes, 2018). Skewness may be exhibited in the curve in a variety of ways. A distribution may be **positively skewed**, which means that the largest portion of data is below the mean. For example, data on length of enrollment in hospice are positively skewed because most of the people die within the first 3 weeks of enrollment, whereas increasingly smaller numbers of people survive as time increases. A distribution can also be **negatively skewed**, which

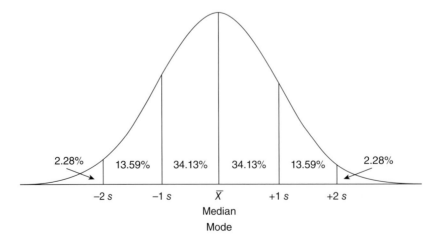

FIG. 27.2 ▪ **THE NORMAL CURVE.**

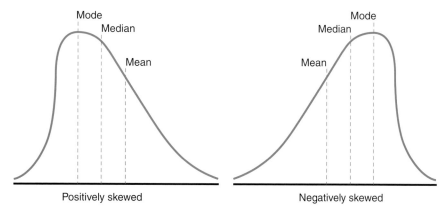

FIG. 27.3 ■ EXAMPLES OF POSITIVELY AND NEGATIVELY SKEWED DISTRIBUTIONS.

means that the largest portion of data is above the mean (Terrell, 2021). For example, data on the occurrence of chronic illness in an older age group are negatively skewed, because more chronic illnesses occur in seniors. Fig. 27.3 includes both a positively skewed distribution and a negatively skewed distribution (Gray & Grove, 2021).

In a skewed distribution, the mean, median, and mode are not equal. Skewness interferes with the validity of many statistical analyses; therefore statistical procedures have been developed to measure the skewness of the distribution of the sample being studied. Few samples will be perfectly symmetric; however, as the deviation from symmetry increases, the seriousness of the effect on statistical analysis increases. In a positively skewed distribution, the mean is greater than the median, which is greater than the mode. In a negatively skewed distribution, the mean is less than the median, which is less than the mode (see Fig. 27.3; Terrell, 2021). The effects of skewness on the types of statistical analyses conducted in a study are discussed later in this exercise.

KURTOSIS

Another term used to describe the shape of the distribution curve is kurtosis. **Kurtosis** explains the degree of peakedness of the frequency distribution, which is related to the spread or variance of scores. An extremely peaked distribution is referred to as **leptokurtic**, an intermediate degree of kurtosis as **mesokurtic**, and a relatively flat distribution as **platykurtic** (see Fig. 27.4; Terrell, 2021). Extreme kurtosis can affect the validity of statistical analysis because the scores have little variation. Many computer programs analyze kurtosis before conducting statistical analyses. A kurtosis of zero indicates that the curve is mesokurtic, kurtosis values above zero indicate that the curve is leptokurtic, and values below zero that are negative indicate a platykurtic curve (Gray & Grove, 2021; Holmes, 2018).

TESTS OF NORMALITY

Skewness and kurtosis should be assessed prior to statistical analysis, and the importance of such non-normality needs to be determined by both the researcher and the statistician. Skewness and kurtosis statistic values of $\geq +1$ or ≥ -1 are fairly severe and could affect the outcomes from parametric analysis techniques (Kim et al., 2022). Because the severity of the deviation from symmetry compromises the validity of the parametric tests, nonparametric analysis techniques should be computed instead (Field, 2013). Nonparametric statistics have no assumption that the distribution of scores be normally distributed (Daniel, 2000; Pett, 2016).

There are statistics that obtain an indication of *both* the skewness and kurtosis of a given frequency distribution. The Shapiro-Wilk W test is a formal test of normality that assesses whether a variable's distribution is skewed and/or kurtotic (Kim et al., 2022; Tabachnick &

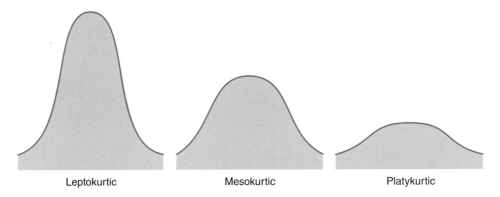

Leptokurtic   Mesokurtic   Platykurtic

FIG. 27.4 ■ **EXAMPLES OF KURTOTIC DISTRIBUTIONS.**

Fidell, 2018). Thus this test has the ability to calculate both skewness and kurtosis by comparing the shape of the variable's frequency distribution to that of a perfect normal curve. For large samples ($n > 2000$) the Kolmogorov-Smirnov D test is an alternative test of normality for large samples (Field, 2013; Marsaglia et al., 2003).

SPSS COMPUTATION

A cross-sectional survey study investigated the attitudes and future plans among former registered nurse–to–bachelor of science in nursing (RN-to-BSN) students who had recently discontinued their program (Cipher & Urban, 2022). Age at program enrollment, recent grade point average (GPA), and feelings of stress and hopefulness were among the study variables examined. The study variables of stress at discontinuation and of hopefulness at discontinuation were assessed on a 5-point Likert scale. Higher values of the variable of stress are indicative of higher self-reported stress levels, and higher values of the variable of hopefulness are indicative of higher self-reported levels of hopefulness. A simulated subset of the study data is presented in Table 27.2. Below is how our dataset looks in SPSS.

File	Edit	View	Data	Transform	Analyze	Graphs	Utilities	Extensions	Window	Help

	ID	Age	GPA	Stress	Hopeful	var
1	1	27	4.00	3	4	
2	2	25	4.00	2	2	
3	3	29	1.49	5	1	
4	4	29	3.10	4	3	
5	5	28	4.00	1	3	
6	6	30	3.00	5	5	
7	7	32	2.34	5	2	
8	8	37	3.85	3	5	
9	9	28	3.90	4	2	
10	10	40	2.67	5	3	
11	11	33	3.00	2	3	
12	12	34	4.00	4	3	
13	13	38	3.14	4	4	
14	14	41	2.90	5	3	
15	15	43	3.75	4	1	
16	16	48	3.79	3	4	

TABLE 27.2   AGE, GPA, AND FEELINGS OF STRESS AND HOPEFULNESS AMONG FORMER RN-TO-BSN STUDENTS

ID	Age at Enrollment	GPA at Discontinuation	Stress at Discontinuation	Hopefulness at Discontinuation
1	27	4.00	3	4
2	25	4.00	2	2
3	29	1.49	5	1
4	29	3.10	4	3
5	28	4.00	1	3
6	30	3.00	5	5
7	32	2.34	5	2
8	37	3.85	3	5
9	28	3.90	4	2
10	40	2.67	5	3
11	33	3.00	2	3
12	34	4.00	4	3
13	38	3.14	4	4
14	41	2.90	5	3
15	43	3.75	4	1
16	48	3.79	3	4
17	39	1.80	5	3
18	49	4.00	3	2
19	62	2.14	2	3
20	68	4.00	3	4

GPA, grade point average.

Step 1: From the "Analyze" menu, choose "Descriptive Statistics" and "Frequencies." Move the four study variables over to the right.

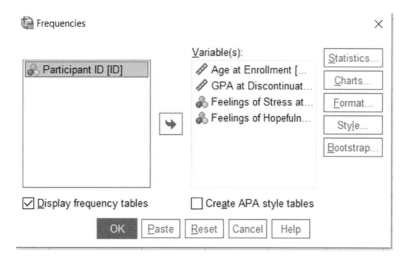

Step 2: Click "Statistics." Check "Skewness" and "Kurtosis." Click "Continue."

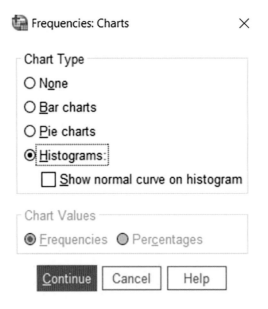

Step 3: Click "Charts." Check "Histograms." Click "Continue" and then "OK."

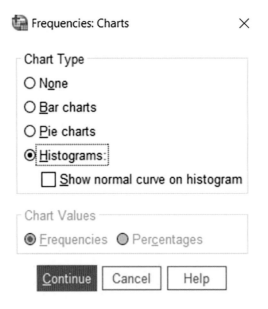

INTERPRETATION OF SPSS OUTPUT

The following tables are generated from SPSS. The first table contains the skewness and kurtosis statistics for the four variables.

Frequencies

Statistics

		Age at Enrollment	GPA at Discontinuation	Feelings of Stress at Discontinuation	Feelings of Hopefulness at Discontinuation
N	Valid	20	20	20	20
	Missing	0	0	0	0
Skewness		1.348	-.798	-.444	.000
Std. Error of Skewness		.512	.512	.512	.512
Kurtosis		1.552	-.488	-.735	-.279
Std. Error of Kurtosis		.992	.992	.992	.992

The next four tables contain the frequencies, or tallies, of the variable values. The last four tables contain the frequency distributions of the four variables.

Frequency Table

Age at Enrollment

		Frequency	Percent	Valid Percent	Cumulative Percent
Valid	25	1	5.0	5.0	5.0
	27	1	5.0	5.0	10.0
	28	2	10.0	10.0	20.0
	29	2	10.0	10.0	30.0
	30	1	5.0	5.0	35.0
	32	1	5.0	5.0	40.0
	33	1	5.0	5.0	45.0
	34	1	5.0	5.0	50.0
	37	1	5.0	5.0	55.0
	38	1	5.0	5.0	60.0
	39	1	5.0	5.0	65.0
	40	1	5.0	5.0	70.0
	41	1	5.0	5.0	75.0
	43	1	5.0	5.0	80.0
	48	1	5.0	5.0	85.0
	49	1	5.0	5.0	90.0
	62	1	5.0	5.0	95.0
	68	1	5.0	5.0	100.0
	Total	20	100.0	100.0	

GPA at Discontinuation

		Frequency	Percent	Valid Percent	Cumulative Percent
Valid	1.49	1	5.0	5.0	5.0
	1.80	1	5.0	5.0	10.0
	2.14	1	5.0	5.0	15.0
	2.34	1	5.0	5.0	20.0
	2.67	1	5.0	5.0	25.0
	2.90	1	5.0	5.0	30.0
	3.00	2	10.0	10.0	40.0
	3.10	1	5.0	5.0	45.0
	3.14	1	5.0	5.0	50.0
	3.75	1	5.0	5.0	55.0
	3.79	1	5.0	5.0	60.0
	3.85	1	5.0	5.0	65.0
	3.90	1	5.0	5.0	70.0
	4.00	6	30.0	30.0	100.0
	Total	20	100.0	100.0	

Feelings of Stress at Discontinuation

		Frequency	Percent	Valid Percent	Cumulative Percent
Valid	1	1	5.0	5.0	5.0
	2	3	15.0	15.0	20.0
	3	5	25.0	25.0	45.0
	4	5	25.0	25.0	70.0
	5	6	30.0	30.0	100.0
	Total	20	100.0	100.0	

Feelings of Hopefulness at Discontinuation

		Frequency	Percent	Valid Percent	Cumulative Percent
Valid	1	2	10.0	10.0	10.0
	2	4	20.0	20.0	30.0
	3	8	40.0	40.0	70.0
	4	4	20.0	20.0	90.0
	5	2	10.0	10.0	100.0
	Total	20	100.0	100.0	

Histogram

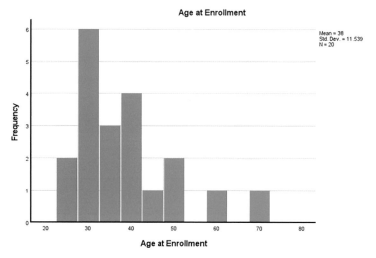

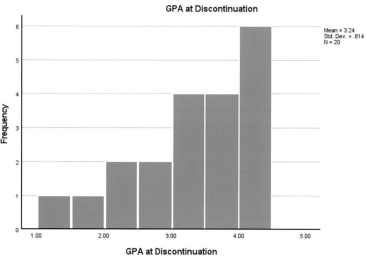

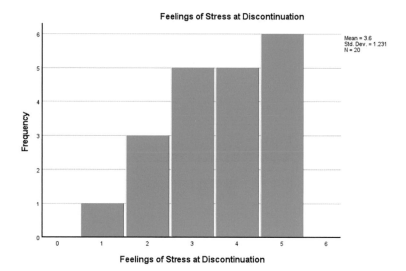

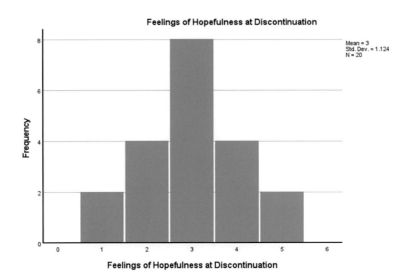

In terms of skewness, the frequency distribution for the variable of age at enrollment appears to be positively skewed, the variables of GPA and stress are negatively skewed, and the variable of hopefulness is normally distributed. The absolute values of the skewness statistics for the variable of age at enrollment is greater than 1.0. The kurtosis statistic for the variable of age at enrollment is also greater than 1.0. No other skewness or kurtosis statistics were greater than 1.0. Note that the skewness statistic for the variable of hopefulness is 0.00, indicating no skewness.

In order to obtain a comparison of the study variables' deviation from normality (and thereby assessing skewness and kurtosis simultaneously), we must compute a Shapiro-Wilk test of normality.

Step 1: From the "Analyze" menu, choose "Descriptive Statistics" and "Explore." Move the four study variables over to the box labeled "Dependent List."

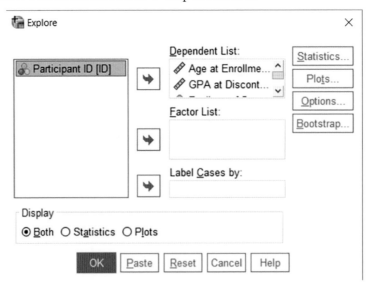

Step 2: Click "Plots." Check "Normality plots with tests." Click "Continue" and "OK."

For this example, SPSS produces many tables and figures. In the interest of saving space, we will focus on the table of interest, titled "Tests of Normality." This table contains the Shapiro-Wilk tests of normality for the four study variables. The last column contains the p values of the Shapiro-Wilk statistics. Of the four p values, three are significant at $p < 0.05$. Hopefulness is the only variable that did not significantly deviate from normality ($p = 0.126$).

Explore

Tests of Normality

	Kolmogorov-Smirnov[a]			Shapiro-Wilk		
	Statistic	df	Sig.	Statistic	df	Sig.
Age at Enrollment	.147	20	.200[*]	.869	20	.011
GPA at Discontinuation	.233	20	.006	.855	20	.006
Feelings of Stress at Discontinuation	.177	20	.099	.893	20	.030
Feelings of Hopefulness at Discontinuation	.200	20	.035	.925	20	.126

*. This is a lower bound of the true significance.

a. Lilliefors Significance Correction

In summary, the skewness statistics, Shapiro-Wilk values, and visual inspections of the variables of age at enrollment, of GPA, and of stress indicated significant deviations from normality. Hopefulness did not yield skewness, kurtosis, or Shapiro-Wilk values that indicated deviations from normality. Sometimes, Shapiro-Wilk values may conflict with skewness and kurtosis statistics because the Shapiro-Wilk test examines the entire shape of the distribution, while skewness and kurtosis statistics examine only skewness and kurtosis, respectively. When a Shapiro-Wilk value is significant *and* visual inspection of the frequency distribution indicates non-normality, the researcher must consider a nonparametric statistical alternative (Field, 2013; Pett, 2016). See Exercise 23 for a review of nonparametric statistics that would be appropriate when the normality assumption for a parametric statistic is not met.

STUDY QUESTIONS

1. Define skewness.

2. Define kurtosis.

3. Given this set of numbers, plot the frequency distribution:
    1, 2, 9, 9, 11, 11, 11, 12, 12, 12, 12, 13, 13, 13, 14, 14.

4. How would you characterize the skewness of the distribution in Question 3: positively skewed, negatively skewed, or approximately normal? Provide a rationale for your answer.

5. Given this set of numbers, plot the frequency distribution:
    1, 2, 2, 2, 3, 3, 3, 3, 3, 4, 4, 4, 5, 5, 10, 11.

6. How would you characterize the skewness of the distribution in Question 5: positively skewed, negatively skewed, or approximately normal? Provide a rationale for your answer.

7. Given this set of numbers, plot the frequency distribution:
   4, 4, 4, 5, 5, 5, 5, 5, 5, 5, 5, 5, 6, 6, 6, 6.

8. How would you characterize the kurtosis of the distribution in Question 7: leptokurtic, mesokurtic, or platykurtic? Provide a rationale for your answer.

9. When looking at the frequency distribution for the variable of stress in the example data, where is the mean in relation to the median?

10. What is the mode for the variable of hopefulness?

Answers to Study Questions

1. Skewness is defined as a frequency distribution that is not symmetric (Gray & Grove, 2021; Terrell, 2021).

2. Kurtosis is defined as the degree of peakedness of the frequency distribution (Terrell, 2021).

3. The frequency distribution approximates the following plot:

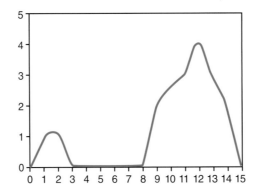

4. The skewness of the distribution in Question 3 is negatively skewed, as evidenced by the tail of the distribution appearing below the mean (Gray & Grove, 2021; Holmes, 2018).

5. The frequency distribution approximates the following plot:

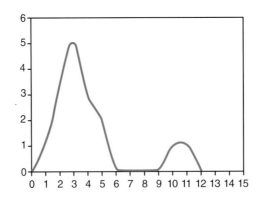

6. The skewness of the distribution in Question 5 is positively skewed, as evidenced by the tail of the distribution appearing above the mean.

7. The frequency distribution approximates the following plot:

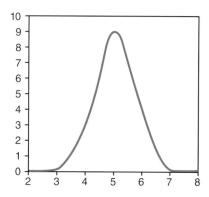

8. The kurtosis of the distribution in Question 7 is leptokurtic, as evidenced by the peakedness of the distribution and the limited variance of the values (Terrell, 2021).

9. The mean for the variable of stress is less than (below) the median because of its negatively skewed distribution: 3.60 versus 4.00, respectively.

10. The mode for the variable of hopefulness is 3.00, which is the most frequently occurring value (Grove & Gray, 2023).

DATA FOR ADDITIONAL COMPUTATIONAL PRACTICE

Using the same example from Cipher and Urban (2022), the following data include only the last 15 observations (the first five were deleted). The data are presented in Table 27.3.

TABLE 27.3   AGE, GPA, AND FEELINGS OF STRESS AND HOPEFULNESS AMONG FORMER RN-TO-BSN STUDENTS

ID	Age at Enrollment	GPA at Discontinuation	Stress at Discontinuation	Hopefulness at Discontinuation
6	30	3.00	5	5
7	32	2.34	5	2
8	37	3.85	3	5
9	28	3.90	4	2
10	40	2.67	5	3
11	33	3.00	2	3
12	34	4.00	4	3
13	38	3.14	4	4
14	41	2.90	5	3
15	43	3.75	4	1
16	48	3.79	3	4
17	39	1.80	5	3
18	49	4.00	3	2
19	62	2.14	2	3
20	68	4.00	3	4

GPA, grade point average.

Questions for Additional Study

Name: _____ Class: _____

Date: _____

Answer the following questions with hand calculations using the data presented in Table 27.3 or the SPSS dataset called "Exercise 27 Example 2.sav" available on the Evolve website. Follow your instructor's directions to submit your answers to the following questions for additional study. Your instructor may ask you to write your answers below and submit them as a hard copy for evaluation. Alternatively, your instructor may ask you to submit your answers online.

1. Plot the frequency distribution for the variable of hopefulness by hand or by using SPSS.

2. How would you characterize the skewness of the distribution in Question 1—positively skewed, negatively skewed, or approximately normal? Provide a rationale for your answer.

3. Compare the original skewness statistic and Shapiro-Wilk statistic with those of the smaller dataset ($n = 15$) for the variable of grade point average (GPA). How did the statistics change, and how would you explain these differences?

4. Plot the frequency distribution for the variable of stress by hand or by using SPSS.

5. How would you characterize the skewness of the distribution in Question 4—positively skewed, negatively skewed, or approximately normal? Provide a rationale for your answer.

6. What is the skewness statistic for the variable of age at enrollment? How would you characterize the magnitude of the skewness statistic for the variable of age at enrollment?

7. What is the kurtosis statistic for the variable of hopefulness? How would you characterize the magnitude of kurtosis for the variable of hopefulness? Provide a rationale for your answer.

8. Using SPSS, compute the Shapiro-Wilk statistic for the variable of stress. What would you conclude from the results?

9. In the SPSS output table titled "Tests of Normality," the Shapiro-Wilk statistic is reported along with the Kolmogorov-Smirnov statistic. Why is the Kolmogorov-Smirnov statistic inappropriate to report for these example data?

10. How would you explain the skewness statistic for a particular frequency distribution being low and the Shapiro-Wilk statistic still being significant at $p < 0.05$?

Calculating Descriptive Statistics

There are two major classes of statistics: descriptive statistics and inferential statistics. Descriptive statistics are computed to reveal characteristics of the sample dataset and to describe study variables. Inferential statistics are computed to gain information about effects and associations in the population being studied. For some types of studies, descriptive statistics will be the only approach to analysis of the data. For other studies, descriptive statistics are the first step in the data analysis process, to be followed by inferential statistics. For all studies that involve numerical data, descriptive statistics are crucial in understanding the fundamental properties of the variables being studied. Exercise 28 focuses only on descriptive statistics and will illustrate the most common descriptive statistics computed in nursing research and provide examples using actual study data from empirical publications.

MEASURES OF CENTRAL TENDENCY

A **measure of central tendency** is a statistic that represents the center or middle of a frequency distribution. The three measures of central tendency commonly used in nursing research are the **mode, median** (*MD*), and **mean** ($\overline{X}$). The mean is the arithmetic average of all of a variable's values in a study. The median is the exact middle value (or the average of the middle two values if there is an even number of observations). The mode is the most commonly occurring value or values (see Exercise 8).

The following data were collected during a cross-sectional survey study that investigated the attitudes and future plans among former registered nurse–to–bachelor of science in nursing (RN-to-BSN) students who had recently discontinued their program (Cipher & Urban, 2022). Table 28.1 contains a simulated subset of data collected from 10 former nursing students who discontinued their programs, and the variable represents the extent to which the student reported feeling relieved at the time of discontinuation, with higher values representing more self-reported relief.

Because the number of study participants represented is 10, the correct statistical notation to reflect that number is:

$$n = 10$$

Note that the *n* is lowercase because we are referring to a sample of discontinued nursing students. If the data being presented represented the entire population of discontinued nursing students, the correct notation is the uppercase *N*. Because most nursing research is conducted using samples, not populations, all formulas in the subsequent exercises will incorporate the sample notation, *n*.

TABLE 28.1   RATINGS OF RELIEF AMONG NURSING STUDENTS WHO DISCONTINUED THEIR PROGRAMS ($n = 10$)
Self-Reported Ratings of Relief at Discontinuation
1
2
2
2
2
3
3
3
4
5

n, sample size.

Mode

The mode is the numerical value or score that occurs with the greatest frequency; it does not necessarily indicate the center of the dataset. The data in Table 28.1 contain one mode: 2.0. This value occurred four times in the dataset. When two modes exist, the dataset is referred to as **bimodal**; a dataset that contains more than two modes would be **multimodal** (Gray & Grove, 2021).

Median

The median or *MD* is the value at the exact center of the ungrouped frequency distribution. It is the 50th percentile. To obtain the *MD,* sort the values from lowest to highest. If the number of values is an uneven number, the *MD* is the exact middle number in the dataset. If the number of values is an even number, the *MD* is the average of the two middle values. Thus the *MD* may not be an actual value in the dataset. For example, the data in Table 28.1 consist of 10 observations, and therefore the *MD* is calculated as the average of the two middle values (Gray & Grove, 2021).

$$MD = \frac{(2.0 + 3.0)}{2} = 2.50$$

Mean

The most commonly reported measure of central tendency is the mean. The mean is the sum of the values divided by the number of values being summed. Thus like the median, the mean may not be a member of the dataset. The formula for calculating the mean is as follows:

$$\bar{X} = \frac{\Sigma X}{n}$$

where

$\bar{X}$ = mean
Σ = sigma, the statistical symbol for summation
X = a single value in the sample
n = total number of values in the sample

The mean of the self-reported ratings for the variable of relief is calculated as follows:

$$\bar{X} = \frac{(1+2+2+2+2+3+3+3+4+5)}{10} = 2.70$$

The mean is an appropriate measure of central tendency for approximately normally distributed populations with variables measured at the interval or ratio level. It is also appropriate for ordinal-level data such as the Likert scale variable of relief, where higher numbers represent more of the construct being measured and lower numbers represent less of the construct. Common examples of ordinal data include pain levels, patient satisfaction, depression, and health status (Waltz et al., 2017).

The mean is sensitive to extreme values such as outliers. An **outlier** is a value in a sample dataset that is unusually low or unusually high in the context of the rest of the sample data (Kim et al., 2022). An example of an outlier in the data presented in Table 28.1 might be a value such as 10. The existing values range from 1 to 5, meaning that no participant rated their relief level beyond a value of 5. If a study participant accidentally rated their level of relief as a 10, the mean would be much larger: 3.36 instead of 2.70. The outlier would also change the frequency distribution. Without the outlier, the frequency distribution is slightly positively skewed, with a skewness statistic of 0.73, as shown in Fig. 28.1. Including the outlier changes the shape of the distribution to appear substantially positively skewed, with a skewness statistic of 2.24.

Outliers can also be identified by using the approach called the *three-sigma rule*, which involves taking the suspected outlier and determining its distance from the mean (Lehmann, 2013). First, the suspected outlier is subtracted from the mean. If that result (in absolute value) is greater than $3 \times SD$, then the suspected value is identified as an outlier. Using the example from Fig. 28.1, the mean of the data with the suspected outlier of 10 is 3.60, and the **standard deviation** or SD is 2.10. When the suspected outlier is subtracted from the mean, the result in absolute value is: $10 - 3.60 = 6.40$. This difference is compared with $3 \times SD$: $3 \times 2.10 = 6.30$. Because the suspected outlier of 10 lies outside of three standard deviations above the mean, the value is identified as an outlier.

Although the use of summary statistics has been the traditional approach to describing data or describing the characteristics of the sample before inferential statistical analysis, its ability to clarify the nature of data is limited. For example, using measures of central tendency, particularly the mean, to describe the nature of the data obscures the effect of extreme values or deviations in the data. Thus significant features in the data may be concealed or misrepresented. Often, anomalous, unexpected, or problematic data and discrepant patterns are evident, but are not regarded as meaningful. Measures of dispersion, such as the range, difference scores, variance, and standard deviation, provide important insights into the nature of the data (King & Eckersley, 2019; Terrell, 2021).

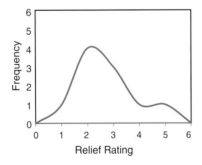 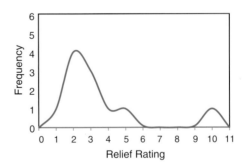

FIG. 28.1 ■ **FREQUENCY DISTRIBUTION OF SELF-REPORTED RATINGS OF RELIEF, WITHOUT AND WITH AN OUTLIER.**

MEASURES OF DISPERSION

Measures of dispersion, or variability, are measures of individual differences of the members of the population and sample. They indicate how values in a sample are dispersed around the mean. These measures provide information about the data that is not available from measures of central tendency. They indicate how different the values are—the extent to which individual values deviate from one another. If the individual values are similar, measures of variability are small, and the sample is relatively **homogeneous** in terms of those values. **Heterogeneity** (i.e., wide variation in values) is important in some statistical procedures, such as correlation. Heterogeneity is determined by measures of variability. The measures of variability most commonly conducted include range, difference scores, variance, and *SD* (see Exercise 9; Gray & Grove, 2021; Kim et al., 2022).

Range

The simplest measure of dispersion is the **range**. In published studies, range is presented in two ways: (1) the range is the set of lowest and highest values, or (2) the range is calculated by subtracting the lowest value from the highest value. The range for the values in Table 28.1 is 1.0 to 5.0, or it can be calculated as follows: $5.0 - 1.0 = 4.0$. In this form, the range is a difference score that uses only the two extreme values for the comparison. Therefore a very large range can indicate the presence of an outlier.

Difference Scores

Difference scores are obtained by subtracting the mean from each value. Sometimes a difference score is referred to as a **deviation score** because it indicates the extent to which a score (or value) deviates from the mean. Of course, most variables in nursing research are not "scores," yet the term **difference score** is used to represent a value's deviation from the mean. The difference score is positive when the value is above the mean, and it is negative when the value is below the mean (see Table 28.2). Difference scores are the basis for many statistical analyses and can be found within many statistical equations. The formula for difference scores is:

$$X - \bar{X}$$

Σ of absolute values: 9.0

TABLE 28.2	**DIFFERENCE SCORES OF SELF-REPORTED RELIEF RATINGS**		
X	$-\bar{X}$	$X - \bar{X}$	$\lvert X - \bar{X} \rvert$
1	2.70	−1.70	1.70
2	2.70	−.70	.70
2	2.70	−.70	.70
2	2.70	−.70	.70
2	2.70	−.70	.70
3	2.70	.30	.30
3	2.70	.30	.30
3	2.70	.30	.30
4	2.70	1.30	1.30
5	2.70	2.30	2.30

The **mean deviation** is the average difference score, using the absolute values. The formula for the mean deviation is:

$$\bar{X}_{deviation} = \frac{\Sigma|X-\bar{X}|}{n}$$

In this example, the mean deviation is 0.90. This value was calculated by taking the sum of the absolute value of each difference score (1.70, 0.70, 0.70, 0.70, 0.70, 0.30, 0.30, 0.30, 1.30, 2.30) and dividing by 10. The result indicates that, on average, participants' ratings of the variable of relief deviated from the mean by 0.90 units.

Variance

Variance is another measure commonly used in statistical analysis. The equation for a sample variance (s^2) is below.

$$s^2 = \frac{\Sigma(X-\bar{X})^2}{n-1}$$

Note that the lowercase letter s^2 is used to represent a sample variance. The lowercase Greek sigma (σ^2) is used to represent a population variance, in which the denominator is N instead of $n - 1$. Because most nursing research is conducted using samples, not populations, formulas in the subsequent exercises that contain a variance or standard deviation will incorporate the sample notation, using $n - 1$ as the denominator. Moreover, many statistical software packages compute the variance and standard deviation using the sample formulas, not the population formulas, unless otherwise programmed.

The variance is always a positive value and has no upper limit. In general, the larger the variance, the larger the dispersion of sample values. The variance is most often computed to derive the standard deviation because, unlike the variance, the standard deviation reflects important properties about the frequency distribution of the variable it represents. Table 28.3 displays how we would compute a variance by hand, using the discontinued nursing student variable of relief.

$$s^2 = \frac{12.10}{9}$$

$$s^2 = 1.3444, \text{ rounded to } 1.34$$

TABLE 28.3   VARIANCE COMPUTATION OF SELF-REPORTED RELIEF RATINGS

X	$-\bar{X}$	$X-\bar{X}$	$(X-\bar{X})^2$
1	2.70	−1.70	2.89
2	2.70	−.70	.49
2	2.70	−.70	.49
2	2.70	−.70	.49
2	2.70	−.70	.49
3	2.70	.30	.09
3	2.70	.30	.09
3	2.70	.30	.09
4	2.70	1.30	1.69
5	2.70	2.30	5.29
		Σ	**12.10**

X, a single value in the sample; $\bar{X}$, mean.

Standard Deviation

Standard deviation is a measure of dispersion that is the square root of the variance. The standard deviation is represented by the notation *s* or *SD*. The equation for obtaining a standard deviation is

$$SD = \sqrt{\frac{\Sigma\left(X - \bar{X}\right)^2}{n-1}}$$

Table 28.3 displays the computations for the variance. To compute the *SD*, simply take the square root of the variance. We know that the variance of the variable of relief is $s^2 = 1.3444$, rounded to 1.34. Therefore the *s* of relief is $SD = 1.1595$, rounded to 1.16. The *SD* is an important statistic, both for understanding dispersion within a distribution and for interpreting the relationship of a particular value to the distribution (Gray & Grove, 2021).

SAMPLING ERROR

A standard error describes the extent of sampling error. For example, a standard error of the mean is calculated to determine the magnitude of the variability associated with the mean. A small standard error is an indication that the sample mean is close to the population mean, while a large standard error yields less certainty that the sample mean approximates the population mean. The formula for the standard error of the mean ($s_{\bar{x}}$) is:

$$s_{\bar{x}} = \frac{s}{\sqrt{n}}$$

Using the discontinued nursing student data, we know that the standard deviation of the relief variable is *s* or $SD = 1.16$. Therefore the standard error of the mean for relief is computed as follows:

$$s_{\bar{x}} = \frac{1.16}{\sqrt{10}}$$

$$s_{\bar{x}} = 0.367, \text{ rounded to } 0.37$$

The standard error of the mean for relief is 0.367.

Confidence Intervals

To determine how closely the sample mean approximates the population mean, the standard error of the mean is used to build a confidence interval (CI). For that matter, a CI can be created for many statistics, such as a mean, proportion, and odds ratio. To build a CI around a statistic, you must have the standard error value and the *t* value to adjust the standard error. The **degrees of freedom (*df*)** to use to compute a CI is $df = n - 1$.

To compute the CI for a mean, the lower and upper limits of that interval are created by multiplying the s_x by the *t* statistic, where $df = n - 1$. For a 95% CI, the *t* value should be selected at $\alpha = 0.05$. For a 99% CI, the *t* value should be selected at $\alpha = 0.01$.

Using the discontinued nursing student data, we know that the standard error of the mean for the variable of relief is $s_{\bar{x}} = 0.37$. The mean for relief is 2.70. Therefore the 95% CI for the mean of relief is computed as follows:

$$\bar{X} \pm s_{\bar{x}} t$$

$$2.70 \pm (0.37)(2.262)$$

$$2.70 \pm 0.84$$

As referenced in Appendix A, the *t* value required for the 95% CI with *df* = 9 is 2.262 for a two-tailed test. The computation here results in a lower limit of 1.86 and an upper limit of 3.54. This means that our CI of 1.86 to 3.54 estimates the population mean of the relief rating with 95% confidence (Kline, 2004). Technically and mathematically, it means that if we computed the mean relief ratings on an infinite number of discontinued nursing students, exactly 95% of the intervals would contain the true population mean, and 5% would not contain the population mean (Gliner et al., 2017). If we were to compute a 99% CI, we would require the *t* value of 3.25 that is referenced at α = 0.01. Therefore the 99% CI for the mean relief rating is computed as follows:

$$2.70 \pm (0.37)(3.25)$$

$$2.70 \pm 1.20$$

As referenced in Appendix A, the *t* value required for the 99% CI with *df* = 9 is 3.250 for a two-tailed test. This computation results in a lower limit of 1.50 and an upper limit of 3.90. This means that our CI of 1.50 to 3.90 estimates the population mean variable of relief rating with 99% confidence.

Degrees of Freedom

The concept of *df* was used in reference to computing a CI. For any statistical computation, *df* means the number of independent pieces of information that are free to vary to estimate another piece of information (Zar, 2010). In the case of the CI, the degrees of freedom are *n* − 1. This means that there are *n* − 1 independent observations in the sample that are free to vary (to be any value) to estimate the lower and upper limits of the CI.

SPSS COMPUTATIONS

A cross-sectional survey study was conducted to investigate the attitudes and future plans among former RN-to-BSN students who had recently discontinued their program (Cipher & Urban, 2022). Gender, age at program enrollment, recent grade point average (GPA), ratings of hopefulness and relief, and potential reasons for discontinuation (e.g., family responsibilities and financial issues) were among the study variables examined. The study variables of hopefulness at discontinuation and relief at discontinuation were assessed on a 5-point Likert scale. Higher values of hopefulness and relief are indicative of higher self-reported levels of hopefulness and relief, respectively. The variables of family (i.e., family responsibilities) and finance (i.e., financial issues) are binary variables that represent potential reasons for discontinuation, assessed as yes/no. A simulated subset of the study data is presented in Table 28.4.

TABLE 28.4   SELECTED VARIABLES OF SURVEY STUDY

Participant ID	Gender	Age	GPA	Hopefulness	Relief	Family	Finance
1	Female	27	4.00	4	3	Yes	Yes
2	Female	25	4.00	2	2	No	Yes
3	Male	30	3.00	5	5	No	No
4	Female	32	2.34	2	3	Yes	Yes
5	Female	33	3.00	3	4	No	Yes
6	Female	38	3.14	4	2	No	No
7	Female	43	3.75	1	2	No	No
8	Male	48	3.79	4	3	Yes	No
9	Female	39	1.80	3	1	Yes	Yes
10	Female	68	4.00	4	2	No	No

This is how our dataset looks in SPSS.

File	Edit	View	Data	Transform	Analyze	Graphs	Utilities	Extensions	Window	Help

	ID	Female	Age	GPA	Hopeful	Relieved	Family	Finance	v
1	1	Female	27	4.00	4	3	Yes	Yes	
2	2	Female	25	4.00	2	2	No	Yes	
3	3	Male	30	3.00	5	5	No	No	
4	4	Female	32	2.34	2	3	Yes	Yes	
5	5	Female	33	3.00	3	4	No	Yes	
6	6	Female	38	3.14	4	2	No	No	
7	7	Female	43	3.75	1	2	No	No	
8	8	Male	48	3.79	4	3	Yes	No	
9	9	Female	39	1.80	3	1	Yes	Yes	
10	10	Female	68	4.00	4	2	No	No	
11									
12									
13									

Step 1: For a nominal variable, the appropriate descriptive statistics are frequencies and percentages. There are three nominal variables in this dataset: gender, family, and finance. From the "Analyze" menu, choose "Descriptive Statistics" and "Frequencies." Move gender over to the right. Click "OK."

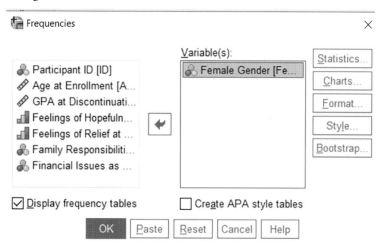

Step 2: For ordinal and interval/ratio variables, the appropriate descriptive statistics are means and standard deviations. There are four ordinal and interval/ratio variables in this dataset: age, GPA, hopefulness, and relief. From the "Analyze" menu, choose "Descriptive Statistics" and "Explore." Move GPA and relief over to the right. Click "OK."

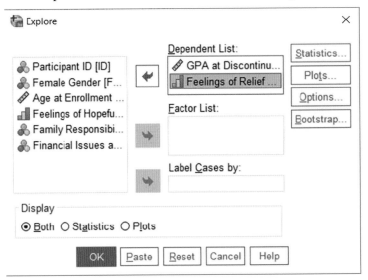

INTERPRETATION OF SPSS OUTPUT

The following tables are generated from SPSS. The first set of tables (from the first set of SPSS commands in Step 1) contains the frequencies of gender. Most participants (80%) were female.

Frequencies

Frequency Table

Female Gender

		Frequency	Percent	Valid Percent	Cumulative Percent
Valid	Male	2	20.0	20.0	20.0
	Female	8	80.0	80.0	100.0
	Total	10	100.0	100.0	

The second set of output (from the second set of SPSS commands in Step 2) contains the descriptive statistics for the variables of GPA and relief, including the mean, SD (standard deviation), SE, 95% CI for the mean, median, variance, minimum value, maximum value, range, and skewness and kurtosis statistics.

Explore

Descriptives

			Statistic	Std. Error
GPA at Discontinuation	Mean		3.2823	.24234
	95% Confidence Interval for Mean	Lower Bound	2.7341	
		Upper Bound	3.8305	
	5% Trimmed Mean		3.3248	
	Median		3.4465	
	Variance		.587	
	Std. Deviation		.76636	
	Minimum		1.80	
	Maximum		4.00	
	Range		2.20	
	Interquartile Range		1.17	
	Skewness		-.864	.687
	Kurtosis		-.201	1.334
Feelings of Relief at Discontinuation	Mean		2.70	.367
	95% Confidence Interval for Mean	Lower Bound	1.87	
		Upper Bound	3.53	
	5% Trimmed Mean		2.67	
	Median		2.50	
	Variance		1.344	
	Std. Deviation		1.160	
	Minimum		1	
	Maximum		5	
	Range		4	
	Interquartile Range		1	
	Skewness		.727	.687
	Kurtosis		.512	1.334

STUDY QUESTIONS

1. Define mean.

2. What does this symbol, s^2, represent?

3. Define outlier.

4. Are there any outliers among the values of the variable relief? Provide a rationale for your answer.

5. List the 95% CI (lower and upper limits) for the mean of GPA. How would you interpret these values?

6. What percentage of participants listed family responsibilities as a reason for program discontinuation?

7. Can you compute the variance for the variable of GPA by using the information presented in the SPSS output in the example? If so, calculate the variance.

8. Plot the frequency distribution of the variable of age.

9. Where is the mean in relation to the median in the frequency distribution of the variable of age? What does this mean indicate regarding the distribution of values?

10. When would a median be more informative than a mean in describing a variable?

Answers to Study Questions

1. The mean is defined as the arithmetic average of a set of numbers.

2. s^2 represents the sample variance of a given variable.

3. An outlier is a value in a sample dataset that is unusually low or unusually high in the context of the rest of the sample data (Gray & Grove, 2021; Kim et al., 2022).

4. There are no outliers among the ratings of the variable relief at discontinuation. The frequency distribution is approximately normal. Using the three-sigma rule, there are no values for ratings of relief that exceed three standard deviations from the mean in absolute value (Lehmann, 2013).

5. The 95% CI is 2.73 to 3.83, meaning that our CI of [2.73, 3.83] estimates the population GPA with 95% confidence.

6. Forty percent of participants (4 of 10) listed family responsibilities as a reason for program discontinuation.

7. Yes, the variance for GPA can be computed by squaring the SD presented in the SPSS table. The SD is listed as 0.77; therefore, the variance is $0.77^2 = 0.5929$, rounded to 0.59.

8. The frequency distribution approximates the following plot:

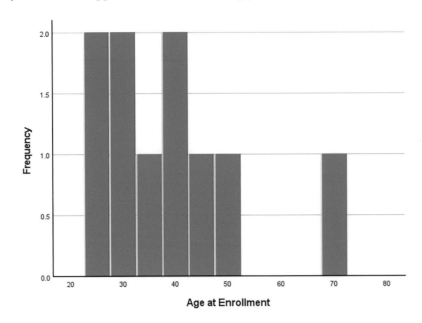

9. The mean is 38.30 and the median is 35.50. Therefore the median is lower in relation to the mean in the frequency distribution of age, indicating that the distribution is positively skewed.

10. A median can be more informative than a mean in describing a variable when the variable's frequency distribution is positively or negatively skewed. While the mean is sensitive to or increases or decreases based on the values of the outliers, the median is relatively unaffected (Kim et al., 2022).

Questions for Additional Study

Name: _____ Class: _____

Date: _____

Answer the following questions with hand calculations using the data presented in Table 28.4 or the SPSS dataset called "Exercise 28 Example.sav" available on the Evolve website. Follow your instructor's directions to submit your answers to the following questions for additional study. Your instructor may ask you to write your answers below and submit them as a hard copy for evaluation. Alternatively, your instructor may ask you to submit your answers online.

1. What is the mean age of the sample data?

2. What percentage of participants listed financial issues as a reason for program discontinuation?

3. What is the standard deviation for the variable of hopefulness?

4. Are there outliers among the values of hopefulness ? Provide a rationale for your answer.

5. What is the range of values for GPA?

6. Among only those participants who listed financial issues as a reason for program discontinuation, calculate the mean relief rating.

7. What percentage of participants did *not* report family responsibilities as a reason for program discontinuation?

8. Among only the female participants, what percentage of participants listed family responsibilities as a reason for program discontinuation?

9. List the 95% confidence interval (CI; lower and upper limits) for the mean age of participants. How would you interpret these values?

10. Among only the male participants, calculate the mean GPA.

Calculating the Pearson Product-Moment Correlation Coefficient

Correlational analyses identify associations between two variables. There are many different kinds of statistics that yield a measure of correlation. All of these statistics address a research question or hypothesis that involves an association or relationship. Examples of research questions that are answered with correlation statistics are: *Is there an association between weight loss and depression?* and *Is there a relationship between patient satisfaction and health status?* A hypothesis is developed to identify the nature (positive or negative) of the relationship between the variables being studied. Examples of hypotheses that are answered with correlation statistics are: *Lower amounts of weight loss are associated with higher levels of depression* and *Higher levels of patient satisfaction are associated with increased health status.*

The **Pearson product-moment correlation** was the first of the correlation measures developed and is the most commonly used. As is explained in Exercise 13, this coefficient (statistic) is represented by the letter r, and the value of r is always between -1.00 and $+1.00$. A value of zero indicates no relationship between the two variables. A positive correlation indicates that higher values of x are associated with higher values of y. A negative or inverse correlation indicates that higher values of x are associated with lower values of y. The r value is indicative of the slope of the line (called a regression line) that can be drawn through a standard scatterplot of the two variables (see Exercise 11). The strengths of different relationships are identified in Table 29.1 (Cohen, 1988).

RESEARCH DESIGNS APPROPRIATE FOR THE PEARSON *r*

Research designs that may use the Pearson r include any associational design (Gliner et al., 2017; Kazdin, 2022). The variables involved in the design are often attributional, meaning the variables are characteristics of the participant, such as health status, blood pressure, gender, diagnosis, or race/ethnicity. Regardless of the nature of variables, the variables submitted to a Pearson correlation calculation must be measured at the interval or ratio level and in certain circumstances, ordinal level, explained below.

TABLE 29.1   STRENGTH OF ASSOCIATION FOR PEARSON *r*

Strength of Association	Positive Association	Negative Association
Weak association	0.00 – <0.30	0.00 – < −0.30
Moderate association	0.30 – 0.49	−0.49 to −0.30
Strong association	≥0.50	−1.00 to −0.50

STATISTICAL FORMULA AND ASSUMPTIONS

Use of the Pearson correlation coefficient involves the following assumptions:

1. Interval or ratio measurement of both variables (e.g., age, income, blood pressure, cholesterol levels); however, if the variables are measured with a Likert scale, and the frequency distribution is approximately normally distributed, these data are usually treated as interval-level measurements and are appropriate for the Pearson r (de Winter & Dodou, 2010; Rasmussen, 1989).
2. There is normal distribution of at least one variable.
3. There is independence of observational pairs.
4. Homoscedasticity is present.

Data that are **homoscedastic** are evenly dispersed both above and below a line of perfect prediction when variable x predicts variable y (see Exercise 30 for illustrations of homoscedasticity and heteroscedasticity). Homoscedasticity reflects equal variance of both variables. In other words, for every value of x, the distribution of y values should have equal variability. If the data for the two variables being correlated are not homoscedastic, inferences made during significance testing could be invalid (Cohen & Cohen, 1983).

The Pearson product-moment correlation coefficient is computed using one of several formulas—the one here is considered the *computational formula* because it makes computation by hand easier (Zar, 2010):

$$r = \frac{n\sum xy - \sum x \sum y}{\sqrt{\left[n\sum x^2 - (\sum x)^2 \right]\left[n\sum y^2 - (\sum y)^2 \right]}}$$

where
 r = Pearson correlation coefficient
 n = total number of subjects
 x = value of the first variable
 y = value of the second variable
 xy = x multiplied by y

HAND CALCULATIONS

This example includes data collected from a survey study by Urban et al. (2022). Newly licensed registered nurses (RNs) were surveyed and administered several questionnaires. Two of these were the Perceived Stress Scale (PSS) and the Brief Resilience Scale (BRS). Scores on the PSS range from 0 to 40, with higher scores indicating increased (worse) self-reported stress levels. Scores on the BRS range from 1 to 5, with higher scores indicating greater (better) self-reported resilience levels. These Likert-scale variables were normally distributed and therefore suitable for parametric statistics (de Winter & Dodou, 2010; Rasmussen, 1989).

The null hypothesis is: *There is no correlation between stress levels and resilience levels among new RNs.* A simulated subset of 20 students was created for this example so that the computations would be small and manageable. In actuality, studies involving Pearson correlations need to be adequately powered (Cohen, 1988; Taylor & Spurlock, 2018). Observe that the data in Table 29.2 are arranged in columns that correspond to the elements of the formula. The summed values in the last row of Table 29.2 are inserted into the appropriate place in the Pearson r formula.

TABLE 29.2		SELF-REPORTED STRESS AND RESILIENCE LEVELS AMONG NEWLY LICENSED NURSES			
Participant Number	**x (Stress)**	**y (Resilience)**	**x²**	**y²**	**xy**
1	24.00	4.17	576.00	17.39	100.08
2	7.00	4.50	49.00	20.25	31.50
3	10.00	3.17	100.00	10.05	31.70
4	24.00	3.83	576.00	14.67	91.92
5	24.00	3.17	576.00	10.05	76.08
6	19.00	1.83	361.00	3.35	34.77
7	25.00	4.67	625.00	21.81	116.75
8	30.00	2.67	900.00	7.13	80.10
9	34.00	3.00	1156.00	9.00	102.00
10	31.00	2.83	961.00	8.01	87.73
11	28.00	2.17	784.00	4.71	60.76
12	24.00	2.17	576.00	4.71	52.08
13	13.00	4.67	169.00	21.81	60.71
14	21.00	3.17	441.00	10.05	66.57
15	10.00	4.00	100.00	16.00	40.00
16	7.00	4.67	49.00	21.81	32.69
17	15.00	2.50	225.00	6.25	37.50
18	21.00	3.33	441.00	11.09	69.93
19	14.00	4.00	196.00	16.00	56.00
20	15.00	3.50	225.00	12.25	52.50
sum Σ	**396.00**	**68.02**	**9,086.00**	**246.3746**	**1,281.37**

The computations for the Pearson r are as follows:

Step 1: Plug the values from the bottom row of Table 29.2 into the Pearson r formula.

$$r = \frac{n\sum xy - \sum x \sum y}{\sqrt{\left[n\sum x^2 - (\sum x)^2\right]\left[n\sum y^2 - (\sum y)^2\right]}}$$

$$r = \frac{20(1,281.37) - (396)(68.02)}{\sqrt{\left[(20)(9,086.00) - 396.00^2\right]\left[(20)(246.37) - 68.02^2\right]}}$$

Step 2: Solve for r.

$$r = \frac{20(1,281.37) - (396.00)(68.02)}{\sqrt{[24,904.00][300.77]}}$$

$$r = \frac{25,627.40 - 26,935.92}{\sqrt{[24,904.00][300.77]}}$$

$$r = \frac{-1,308.52}{2,736.86} = -0.48$$

Step 3: Compute the degrees of freedom (df).

$$df = n - 2$$

$$df = 20 - 2$$

$$df = 18$$

Step 4: Locate the critical r value in the r distribution table (Appendix B) and compare it to our obtained r value.

The r is -0.48, indicating a moderate negative (inverse) correlation between stress and resilience among new RNs. To determine whether this relationship is improbable to have been caused by chance alone, we consult the r probability distribution table in Appendix B. The formula for df

for a Pearson r is $n - 2$. With r of -0.48 and $df = 18$, the critical r value at $\alpha = 0.05$, $df = 18$ is 0.4438, rounded to 0.444, for a two-tailed test. Our obtained r was -0.48, which in absolute value exceeds the critical value in the table. Thus the r value of -0.48 is considered statistically significant. It should be noted that the absolute value of the obtained r is compared with the critical r value. The sign of the r is only used to indicate whether the association is positive or negative.

SPSS COMPUTATIONS

This is how our dataset looks in SPSS.

	ID	PSS	BRS
9	9	34.00	3.00
10	10	31.00	2.83
11	11	28.00	2.17
12	12	24.00	2.17
13	13	13.00	4.67
14	14	21.00	3.17
15	15	10.00	4.00
16	16	7.00	4.67
17	17	15.00	2.50
18	18	21.00	3.33
19	19	14.00	4.00
20	20	15.00	3.50
21			

Step 1: From the "Analyze" menu, choose "Correlate" and "Bivariate."
Step 2: Move the two variables, PSS and BRS, over to the right, as shown. Click "OK."

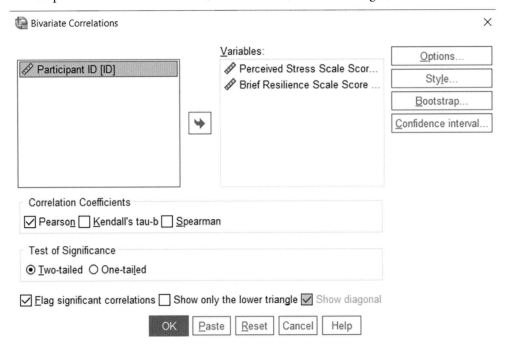

INTERPRETATION OF SPSS OUTPUT

The following table is generated from SPSS. The table contains a correlation matrix that includes the Pearson r between stress and resilience, along with the p value and df. The r is listed as -0.478 rounded to -0.48, and the p is 0.033.

Correlations

Correlations

		Perceived Stress Scale Score	Brief Resilience Scale Score
Perceived Stress Scale Score	Pearson Correlation	1	-.478*
	Sig. (2-tailed)		.033
	N	20	20
Brief Resilience Scale Score	Pearson Correlation	-.478*	1
	Sig. (2-tailed)	.033	
	N	20	20

*. Correlation is significant at the 0.05 level (2-tailed).

Observe that the upper diagonal is a mirror image of the lower diagonal

The exact p value is 0.033

FINAL INTERPRETATION IN AMERICAN PSYCHOLOGICAL ASSOCIATION FORMAT

The following interpretation is written as it might appear in a research article, formatted according to American Psychological Association (APA) guidelines (APA, 2020). It should be noted that all statistical values reported here are rounded to two decimal places, with the exception of the p value, which is rounded to three decimal places.

A Pearson correlation analysis indicated that there was a significant correlation between stress and resilience among new RNs, $r(18) = -0.48$, $p = 0.033$. Higher levels of stress were associated with lower levels of resilience and vice versa, lower levels of stress were associated with higher resilience.

EFFECT SIZE

After establishing the statistical significance of the r value, it must subsequently be examined for clinical importance. There are ranges for strength of association suggested by Cohen (1988), as displayed in Table 29.1. One can also assess the magnitude of association by obtaining the **coefficient of determination** for the Pearson correlation. Computing the coefficient of determination simply involves squaring the r value. The r^2 multiplied by 100% represents the percentage of variance shared between the two variables (Cohen & Cohen, 1983). In our example, the r was -0.48, and therefore the r^2 was 0.2304. This indicates that stress and resilience shared 23.04% ($0.2304 \times 100\%$) of the same variance. More specifically, 23.04% of the variance in stress can be explained by knowing the nurse's resilience level, and vice versa—23.04% of the variance in resilience can be explained by knowing the nurse's level of stress.

STUDY QUESTIONS

1. If you have access to SPSS, compute the Shapiro-Wilk test of normality for the variables of stress (PSS) and resilience (BRS) (as demonstrated in Exercise 27). If you do not have access to SPSS, plot the frequency distributions by hand. What do the results indicate with regard to the normality of the distributions?

2. What is the null hypothesis in the example?

3. What was the exact likelihood of obtaining an r value at least as extreme or close to the one that was actually observed, assuming that the null hypothesis is true?

4. How would you characterize the magnitude of the effect between stress and resilience? Provide a rationale for your answer.

5. In the study of newly licensed nurses, depression levels were also measured. If the Pearson correlation between resilience and depression is $r = -0.609$, how much variance in resilience levels is explained by knowing the new RN's level of depression? Show your calculations for this value.

6. What kind of design was used in the example? Provide a rationale for your answer.

7. Was the sample size adequate to detect a significant correlation in this example? Provide a rationale for your answer.

8. A researcher computed a Pearson r and obtained an r of 0.57. How would you characterize the magnitude of the r value? What is the percentage of variance explained by this r value? Show your calculations.

9. A researcher computed a Pearson r and obtained an r of 0.12. How would you characterize the magnitude of the r value? Provide a rationale for your answer.

10. A researcher computed a Pearson r on two different samples, one with $n = 15$, and the other with $n = 40$. In both samples, she obtained an r of 0.50. What is the critical tabled r for each sample at $\alpha = 0.05$, two-tailed? Discuss the meaning of the critical table values of r for the samples of different sizes.

Answers to Study Questions

1. As shown in the SPSS output here, the Shapiro-Wilk p values for stress and resilience were 0.456 and 0.357, respectively, indicating that the frequency distributions did not significantly deviate from normality. Moreover, visual inspection of the frequency distributions indicates that the variables are approximately normally distributed, although the distribution for resilience appears to be very slightly negatively skewed.

Tests of Normality

	Kolmogorov-Smirnov[a]			Shapiro-Wilk		
	Statistic	Df	Sig.	Statistic	df	Sig.
Perceived Stress Scale Score	.148	20	.200*	.955	20	.456
Brief Resilience Scale Score	.102	20	.200*	.949	20	.357

*. This is a lower bound of the true significance.

a. Lilliefors Significance Correction

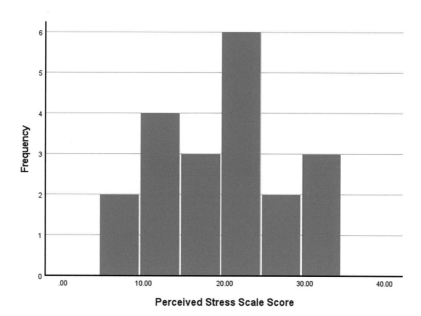

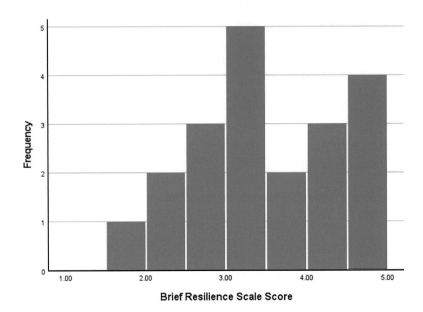

2. The null hypothesis is: *There is no correlation between stress levels and resilience levels among new RNs.*

3. The exact likelihood of obtaining an *r* value at least as extreme or close to the one that was actually observed, assuming that the null hypothesis is true, was 3.30%. This value was obtained by taking the *p* value listed in the SPSS output table titled "Correlations" in the row labeled "Sig. (2-tailed)" and multiplying by 100%: $0.033 \times 100\% = 3.30\%$.

4. The magnitude of the effect between stress and resilience would be considered a moderate effect according to the effect size tables in Exercises 24 and 25 and Table 29.1 in this exercise. Although the absolute value of the *r* is |0.48| and is close to the threshold of a large effect size, it is less than |0.50| and therefore is considered moderate.

5. The *r* is −0.609, and therefore the r^2 is 0.3709. This indicates that depression and resilience shared 37.09% ($0.3709 \times 100\%$) of the same variance. Therefore 37.09% of the variance in depression levels is explained by knowing the RN's resilience level, and vice versa.

6. The study design was associational or correlational (Gliner et al., 2017; Kazdin, 2022).

7. The sample size was indeed adequate to detect a significant correlation because $p = 0.033$, which is less than the alpha of 0.05.

8. An *r* of 0.57 is considered a large effect according to the effect size tables in Exercises 24 and 25 and Table 29.1 in this exercise.

9. An *r* of 0.12 is considered a small effect according to the effect size tables in Exercises 24 and 25 and Table 29.1 in this exercise.

10. For the sample of 15, the *df* is 13 and the critical tabled *r* for 13 *df* at $\alpha = 0.05$ is 0.514 for a two-tailed test. For the sample of 40, the *df* is 38 and the critical tabled *r* for 38 *df* at $\alpha = 0.05$ is 0.312 for a two-tailed test. Therefore the *r* in the smaller sample would not have been considered statistically significant, but the *r* in the larger sample would have been considered statistically significant. This example demonstrates the importance of having an adequate sample size for a study to prevent a Type II error (Aberson, 2019; Cohen, 1988; Taylor & Spurlock, 2018).

DATA FOR ADDITIONAL COMPUTATIONAL PRACTICE

This example includes additional data collected from the same survey study of newly licensed RNs by Urban et al. (2022). Two of the questionnaires administered were the PSS and the General Anxiety Disorder-7 Scale (GAD). Scores on the PSS range from 0 to 40, with higher scores indicating increased (worse) self-reported stress levels. Scores on the GAD range from 1 to 21, with higher scores indicating increased (worse) self-reported anxiety levels.

The null hypothesis is: *There is no correlation between stress levels and anxiety levels among new RNs.* A simulated subset of 20 students was created for this example so that the computations would be small and manageable. In actuality, studies involving Pearson correlations need to be adequately powered (Cohen, 1988; Taylor & Spurlock, 2018).

The data are presented in Table 29.3.

TABLE 29.3 SELF-REPORTED STRESS AND ANXIETY LEVELS AMONG NEWLY LICENSED NURSES

Participant Number	x (Stress)	y (Anxiety)	x^2	y^2	xy
1	24.00	6.00	576.00	36.00	144.00
2	7.00	1.00	49.00	1.00	7.00
3	10.00	10.00	100.00	100.00	100.00
4	24.00	5.00	576.00	25.00	120.00
5	24.00	13.00	576.00	169.00	312.00
6	19.00	17.00	361.00	289.00	323.00
7	25.00	9.00	625.00	81.00	225.00
8	30.00	20.00	900.00	400.00	600.00
9	34.00	16.00	1156.00	256.00	544.00
10	31.00	20.00	961.00	400.00	620.00
11	28.00	13.00	784.00	169.00	364.00
12	24.00	12.00	576.00	144.00	288.00
13	13.00	5.00	169.00	25.00	65.00
14	21.00	3.00	441.00	9.00	63.00
15	10.00	0.00	100.00	0.00	0.00
16	7.00	7.00	49.00	49.00	49.00
17	15.00	5.00	225.00	25.00	75.00
18	21.00	4.00	441.00	16.00	84.00
19	14.00	3.00	196.00	9.00	42.00
20	15.00	4.00	225.00	16.00	60.00
sum Σ	**396.00**	**173.00**	**9,086.00**	**2,219.00**	**4,085.00**

Questions for Additional Study

Name: _____ Class: _____

Date: _____

Answer the following questions with hand calculations using the data presented in Table 29.3 or the SPSS dataset called "Exercise 29 Example 2.sav" available on the Evolve website. Follow your instructor's directions to submit your answers to the following questions for additional study. Your instructor may ask you to write your answers below and submit them as a hard copy for evaluation. Alternatively, your instructor may ask you to submit your answers online.

1. If you have access to SPSS, compute the Shapiro-Wilk test of normality for the variables of stress (Perceived Stress Scale: *PSS*) and anxiety (General Anxiety Disorder-7 Scale: *GAD*) as demonstrated in Exercise 27. If you do not have access to SPSS, plot the frequency distributions by hand. What do the results indicate?

2. What is the null hypothesis in the example?

3. What is the Pearson r between the variables of stress and anxiety?

4. Is the r significant at $\alpha = 0.05$? Provide a rationale for your answer.

5. If using SPSS, what is the exact likelihood of obtaining an r value at least as extreme or close to the one that was actually observed, assuming that the null hypothesis is true? Show your calculations.

6. How would you characterize the magnitude of the effect between the variables of stress and anxiety? Provide a rationale for your answer.

7. What was the research design of this example?

8. Write your interpretation of the results for stress and anxiety in newly licensed RNs, as you would in an APA-formatted journal (American Psychological Association, 2020).

9. How much variance in anxiety is explained by knowing stress levels and vice versa? Show your calculations.

10. Can the researchers make a statement regarding the extent to which stress caused newly licensed RNs' anxiety to increase? Provide a rationale for your answer.

Calculating Simple Linear Regression

Simple linear regression is a procedure that provides an estimate of the value of a dependent variable (outcome) based on the value of an independent variable (predictor). Knowing that estimate with some degree of accuracy, we can use regression analysis to predict the value of one variable if we know the value of the other variable (Cohen & Cohen, 1983). The regression equation is a mathematical expression of the influence that a predictor has on a dependent variable, based on a theoretical proposition or framework (Gray & Grove, 2021). For example, in Exercise 14, Fig. 14.2 illustrates the linear relationship between gestational age and birth weight. As shown in the scatterplot, there is a strong positive relationship between the two variables. Advanced gestational ages predict higher birth weights.

A regression equation can be generated with a dataset containing study participants' x and y values. Once this equation is generated, it can be used to predict future participants' y values, given only their x values. In simple or bivariate regression, predictions are made in cases with two variables. The score on variable y (dependent variable, or outcome) is predicted from the same individual's known score on variable x (independent variable, or predictor; Gray & Grove, 2021).

RESEARCH DESIGNS APPROPRIATE FOR SIMPLE LINEAR REGRESSION

Research designs that may use simple linear regression include any associational design (Gliner et al., 2017; Kazdin, 2022). The variables involved in the design are attributional, meaning the variables are characteristics of the participant, such as health status, blood pressure, gender, diagnosis, or ethnicity. Regardless of the nature of variables, the dependent variable submitted to simple linear regression must be measured at the interval or ratio level (see Exercise 1).

STATISTICAL FORMULA AND ASSUMPTIONS

Use of simple linear regression involves the following assumptions (Zar, 2010):

1. Normal distribution of the dependent (y) variable
2. Linear relationship between x and y
3. Independent observations
4. No (or little) multicollinearity
5. Homoscedasticity

Data that are **homoscedastic** are evenly dispersed both above and below a plotted line of perfect prediction when variable x predicts variable y. If the data for the predictor and dependent variable are not homoscedastic, inferences made during significance testing could be invalid (Cohen & Cohen, 1983; Zar, 2010). Visual examples of homoscedasticity and heteroscedasticity are presented in Exercise 31.

In simple linear regression, the dependent variable is measured as interval or ratio. However, if the variable is measured with a Likert scale, and the frequency distribution is approximately normally distributed, these data are usually considered interval-level measurements and are appropriate to serve as the outcome in a linear regression model (Rasmussen, 1989; Waltz et al., 2017). The predictor can be any scale of measurement; however, if the predictor is nominal, it must be correctly coded. Once the data are ready, the parameters a and b are computed to obtain a regression equation. To understand the mathematical process, recall the algebraic equation for a straight line:

$$y = bx + a$$

where

$$y = \text{the dependent variable (outcome)}$$

$$x = \text{the independent variable (predictor)}$$

$$b = \text{the slope of the line, also referred to as unstandardized beta}$$

$$a = y\text{-intercept (the point where the regression line intersects the } y\text{-axis)}$$

No single regression line can be used to predict with complete accuracy every y value from every x value. In fact, you could draw an infinite number of lines through the scattered paired values (Zar, 2010). However, the purpose of the regression equation is to develop the line to allow the highest degree of prediction possible—the line of best fit. The procedure for developing the line of best fit is the **method of least squares** (Tabachnick & Fidell, 2019). The formulas for the unstandardized beta (b) and y-intercept (a) of the regression equation are computed as follows. Note that once the b is calculated, the value is inserted into the formula for a.

$$b = \frac{n \sum xy - \sum x \sum y}{n \sum x^2 - \left(\sum x \right)^2}$$

$$a = \frac{\sum y - b \sum x}{n}$$

HAND CALCULATIONS

This example includes data collected from a survey study by Urban et al. (2022). Newly licensed registered nurses (RNs) were surveyed and administered several questionnaires. Two of these were the Patient Health Questionnaire (PHQ-9) and the Brief Resilience Scale (BRS). Scores on the PHQ-9 range from 0 to 27, with higher scores indicating increased (worse) self-reported depression levels. Scores on the BRS range from 1 to 5, with higher scores indicating greater (better) self-reported resilience levels.

The null hypothesis is: *Self-reported depression levels do not predict resilience levels among newly licensed RNs.* A simulated subset of 20 participants was created for this example so that the computations would be small and manageable. In actuality, studies involving linear regression need to be adequately powered (Aberson, 2019; Gaskin & Happell, 2014; Taylor & Spurlock, 2018;). Observe that the data in Table 30.1 are arranged in columns that correspond to the elements of the formula. The summed values in the last row of Table 30.1 are inserted into the appropriate place in the formula for b.

TABLE 30.1   SELF-REPORTED DEPRESSION AND RESILIENCE LEVELS AMONG NEWLY LICENSED NURSES

Participant Number	x (Depression)	y (Resilience)	x^2	xy
1	6.00	4.17	36.00	25.02
2	5.00	4.50	25.00	22.50
3	8.00	3.17	64.00	25.36
4	10.00	3.83	100.00	38.30
5	10.00	3.17	100.00	31.70
6	11.00	1.83	121.00	20.13
7	11.00	4.67	121.00	51.37
8	12.00	2.67	144.00	32.04
9	13.00	3.00	169.00	39.00
10	15.00	2.83	225.00	42.45
11	18.00	2.17	324.00	39.06
12	19.00	2.17	361.00	41.23
13	1.00	4.67	1.00	4.67
14	2.00	3.17	4.00	6.34
15	3.00	4.00	9.00	12.00
16	4.00	4.67	16.00	18.68
17	4.00	2.50	16.00	10.00
18	4.00	3.33	16.00	13.32
19	5.00	4.00	25.00	20.00
20	6.00	3.50	36.00	21.00
Sum Σ	**167.00**	**68.02**	**1,913.00**	**514.17**

The computations for the _b_ and _a_ are as follows:

Step 1: Calculate _b_.

From the values in Table 30.1, we know that $n = 20$, $\Sigma x = 167.00$, $\Sigma y = 68.02$, $\Sigma x^2 = 1,913.00$, and $\Sigma xy = 514.17$. These values are inserted into the formula for _b_, as follows:

$$b = \frac{20(514.17) - (167.00)(68.02)}{20(1913.00) - 167.00^2}$$

$$b = \frac{-1,075.94}{10,371.00}$$

$$b = -0.104$$

Step 2: Calculate _a_.

From Step 1, we now know that $b = -0.104$, and we plug this value into the formula for _a_. Note that the three decimal places in _b_ are being retained so that the resulting values for the remaining steps will be more accurate.

$$a = \frac{68.020 - (-0.104)(167.000)}{20}$$

$$a = \frac{85.388}{20}$$

$$a = 4.269$$

Step 3: Write the new regression equation:

$$y = -0.104x + 4.269$$

Step 4: Calculate *R*.

The multiple *R* is defined as the correlation between the actual *y* values and the predicted *y* values using the new regression equation. The predicted *y* value using the new equation is represented by the symbol $\hat{y}$ to differentiate from *y*, which represents the actual *y* values in the dataset. We can use our new regression equation from Step 3 to compute predicted resilience levels for each RN, using their self-reported level of depression. For example, participant #1 had a PHQ (depression) score of 6.00, and their predicted level of resilience is calculated as:

$$\hat{y} = -0.104(6) + 4.269$$

$$\hat{y} = 3.645, \text{ rounded to } 3.65$$

Thus the predicted $\hat{y}$ is 3.65. This procedure would be continued for the rest of the participants, and the Pearson correlation between the resilience score (*y*) and the predicted resilience score ($\hat{y}$) would yield the multiple *R* value. In this example, the *R* = 0.609, rounded to 0.61. The higher the *R*, the more likely that the new regression equation accurately predicts *y*, because the higher the correlation, the closer the actual *y* values are to the predicted $\hat{y}$ values. Fig. 30.1 displays the regression line where the *x*-axis represents possible depression scores, and the *y*-axis represents the predicted resilience scores ($\hat{y}$ values).

Step 5: Determine whether the predictor significantly predicts *y*.

$$t = R\sqrt{\frac{n-2}{1-R^2}}$$

To know whether the predictor significantly predicts *y*, the *b* must be tested against zero. In simple regression, this is most easily accomplished by using the *R* value from Step 4:

$$t = 0.61\sqrt{\frac{20-2}{1-0.371}}$$

$$t = 0.61(5.35)$$

$$t = 3.26$$

The *t* value is then compared with the *t* probability distribution table (see Appendix A). The degrees of freedom (*df*) for this *t* statistic is *n* − 2. The critical *t* value at alpha (α) = 0.05, *df* = 18 is 2.101, rounded to 2.10 for a two-tailed test. Our obtained *t* was 3.26, which exceeds the critical value in the table, thereby indicating a significant association between the predictor (*x*) and outcome (*y*).

Step 6: Calculate R^2.

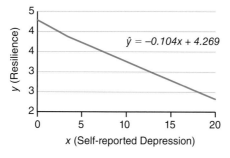

FIG. 30.1 ▪ REGRESSION LINE REPRESENTED BY NEW REGRESSION EQUATION.

After establishing the statistical significance of the R value, it must subsequently be examined for clinical importance. This is accomplished by obtaining the coefficient of determination for regression—which simply involves squaring the R value. The R^2 represents the percentage of variance explained in y by the predictor. Cohen describes R^2 values of 0.02 as small, 0.13 as moderate, and 0.26 or higher as large effect sizes (Cohen, 1988). In our example, the R was 0.609, and, therefore, the R^2 was 0.371. Multiplying 0.371 × 100% indicates that 37.10% of the variance in resilience levels can be explained by knowing the participant's depression score (Cohen & Cohen, 1983).

The R^2 can be very helpful in testing more than one predictor in a regression model. Unlike R, the R^2 for one regression model can be compared with another regression model that contains additional predictors (Cohen & Cohen, 1983). The R^2 is discussed further in Exercise 31.

The standardized beta (β) is another statistic that represents the magnitude of the association between x and y. The standardized beta has limits just like a Pearson r, meaning that the standardized beta cannot be lower than -1.00 or higher than $+1.00$. This value can be calculated by hand but is best computed with statistical software. The standardized beta is calculated by converting the x and y values to z scores and then correlating the x and y value using the Pearson r formula, located in Exercise 29. The standardized beta (β) is often reported in the literature instead of the unstandardized beta (b), because the unstandardized beta does not have lower or upper limits and therefore the magnitude of the unstandardized beta cannot be judged. The standardized beta, on the other hand, is interpreted as a Pearson r and the descriptions of the magnitude of the standardized beta can be applied, as recommended by Cohen (1988). In this example, the standardized beta is -0.609. Thus the magnitude of the association between x and y in this example is considered a large predictive association (Cohen, 1988; Tabachnick & Fidell, 2019).

SPSS COMPUTATIONS

This is how our dataset looks in SPSS.

	ID	PHQ	BRS
1	1	6.00	4.17
2	2	5.00	4.50
3	3	8.00	3.17
4	4	10.00	3.83
5	5	10.00	3.17
6	6	11.00	1.83
7	7	11.00	4.67
8	8	12.00	2.67
9	9	13.00	3.00
10	10	15.00	2.83
11	11	18.00	2.17
12	12	19.00	2.17
13	13	1.00	4.67
14	14	2.00	3.17
15	15	3.00	4.00
16	16	4.00	4.67

Step 1: From the "Analyze" menu, choose "Regression" and "Linear."

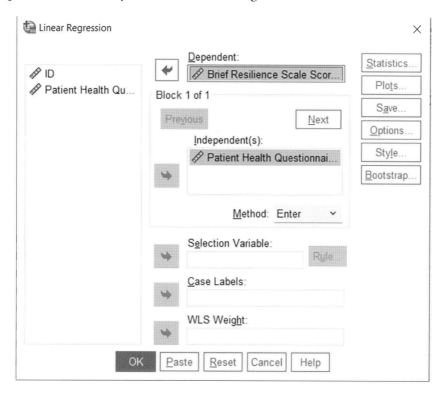

Step 2: Move the predictor, PHQ (depression), to the space labeled "Independent(s)." Move the dependent variable, BRS (resilience), to the space labeled "Dependent." Click "OK."

INTERPRETATION OF SPSS OUTPUT

The following tables are generated from SPSS. The first table contains the multiple R and the R^2 values. The multiple R is 0.609, indicating that the correlation between the actual y values and the predicted y values using the new regression equation is 0.609. The R^2 is 0.371, indicating that 37.10% of the variance in resilience levels can be explained by knowing the participant's depression score.

Regression

Model Summary

Model	R	R Square	Adjusted R Square	Std. Error of the Estimate
1	.609ᵃ	.371	.336	.72485

a. Predictors: (Constant), Patient Health Questionnaire (Depression) Score

The second table contains the analysis of variance (ANOVA) table. As presented in Exercises 18 and 35, the ANOVA is usually performed to test for differences between group means. However, ANOVA can also be performed for regression, where the null hypothesis is that *knowing the value of x explains no information about y.* This table indicates that knowing the value of x explains a significant amount of variance in y. The contents of the ANOVA table are rarely reported in published articles, because the significance of each predictor is presented in the last SPSS table titled "Coefficients" (see below).

ANOVA[a]

Model		Sum of Squares	df	Mean Square	F	Sig.
1	Regression	5.581	1	5.581	10.622	.004[b]
	Residual	9.457	18	.525		
	Total	15.039	19			

a. Dependent Variable: Brief Resilience Scale Score

b. Predictors: (Constant), Patient Health Questionnaire (Depression) Score

The third table contains the unstandardized beta and *a* values, standardized beta, *t,* and exact *p* value. The *a* is listed in the first row, next to the label "Constant." The standardized beta is listed in the second row, next to the name of the predictor. The remaining information that is important to extract when interpreting regression results can be found in the second row. The standardized beta is −0.609. This value has limits just like a Pearson *r,* meaning that the standardized beta cannot be lower than −1.00 or higher than +1.00. The *t* value is −3.259, and the exact *p* value is 0.004.

Coefficients[a]

Model		Unstandardized Coefficients		Standardized Coefficients		
		B	Std. Error	Beta	t	Sig.
1	(Constant)	4.267	.311		13.707	<.001
	Patient Health Questionnaire (Depression) Score	-.104	.032	-.609	-3.259	.004

a. Dependent Variable: Brief Resilience Scale Score

FINAL INTERPRETATION IN AMERICAN PSYCHOLOGICAL ASSOCIATION FORMAT

The following interpretation is written as it might appear in a research article, formatted according to American Psychological Association (APA) guidelines (APA, 2020). It should be noted that all statistical values reported here are rounded to two decimal places, with the exception of the *p* value, which is rounded to three decimal places.

Simple linear regression was performed with newly licensed RNs' level of depression as the predictor and resilience as the dependent variable. The nurses' depression levels significantly predicted their levels of resilience, $\beta = -0.61$, $p = 0.004$, and $R^2 = 37.10\%$. Higher levels of depression significantly predicted lower levels of resilience among newly licensed RNs.

STUDY QUESTIONS

1. If you have access to SPSS, compute the Shapiro-Wilk test of normality for BRS (resilience) as demonstrated in Exercise 27. If you do not have access to SPSS, plot the frequency distributions by hand. What do the results indicate?

2. State the null hypothesis for the example where depression levels were tested as a predictor of resilience among newly licensed RNs.

3. In the formula $y = bx + a$, what does b represent?

4. In the formula $y = bx + a$, what does a represent?

5. Using the new regression equation, $\hat{y} = -0.104x + 4.27$, compute the predicted BRS (resilience) score if a RN's PHQ (depression) score is 1. Show your calculations.

6. Using the new regression equation, $\hat{y} = -0.104x + 4.27$, compute the predicted BRS (resilience) score if a RN's PHQ (depression) score is 13. Show your calculations.

7. What is the correlation between the actual y values and the predicted $\hat{y}$ values using the new regression equation in the example?

8. What is the exact likelihood of obtaining a t value at least as extreme as or as close to the one that was actually observed, assuming that the null hypothesis is true?

9. How much variance in resilience levels is explained by knowing the participant's depression score?

10. How would you characterize the magnitude of the R^2 in the example? Provide a rationale for your answer.

Answers to Study Questions

1. The Shapiro-Wilk *p* value for resilience was 0.357, indicating that the frequency distribution did not significantly deviate from normality. Moreover, visual inspection of the frequency distribution indicates that the resilience scores are approximately normally distributed. See SPSS output for the histogram of the distribution and the test of normality table.

Tests of Normality

	Kolmogorov-Smirnov[a]			Shapiro-Wilk		
	Statistic	df	Sig.	Statistic	df	Sig.
Brief Resilience Scale Score	.102	20	.200*	.949	20	.357

*. This is a lower bound of the true significance.

a. Lilliefors Significance Correction

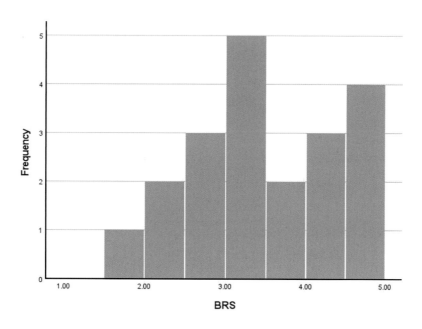

2. The null hypothesis is: *Self-reported depression levels do not predict resilience levels among newly licensed RNs.*

3. In the formula $y = bx + a$, *b* represents the slope of the regression line.

4. In the formula $y = bx + a$, *a* represents the *y*-intercept, or the point at which the regression line intersects the *y*-axis.

5. The predicted *BRS* (resilience) score if a RN's *PHQ* (depression) score is 1 is calculated as: $\hat{y} = -0.104(1) + 4.27 = 4.166$, rounded to 4.17.

6. The predicted *BRS* (resilience) score if a RN's *PHQ* (depression) score is 13 is calculated as: $\hat{y} = -0.104(13) + 4.27 = 2.918$, rounded to 2.92.

7. The correlation between the actual *y* values and the predicted *y* values using the new regression equation in the example, also known as the multiple *R*, is 0.609, rounded to 0.61.

8. The exact likelihood of obtaining a standardized beta value at least as extreme as or as close to the one that was actually observed, assuming that the null hypothesis is true, is 0.40%. This value was obtained by taking the *p* value listed in the SPSS output table titled "Coefficients" in the column labeled "Sig" and multiplying by 100%: $0.004 \times 100\% = 0.40\%$.

9. Of the variance in resilience levels, 37.10% can be explained by knowing the participant's depression score. This value is seen in the Model Summary Table under the column labeled R^2. The value is multiplied by 100% to report as a percentage.

10. The magnitude of the R^2 in this example, 0.371, would be considered a large effect according to the effect size tables in Exercises 24 and 25 of this text.

DATA FOR ADDITIONAL COMPUTATIONAL PRACTICE

This example includes additional data collected from the same survey study of newly licensed RNs by Urban and colleagues (2023). Two of the questionnaires administered were the General Anxiety Disorder-7 Scale (GAD) and the BRS. Scores on the GAD range from 1 to 21, with higher scores indicating increased (worse) self-reported anxiety levels. Scores on the BRS range from 1 to 5, with higher scores indicating greater (better) self-reported resilience levels.

The null hypothesis is: *Self-reported anxiety levels do not predict resilience levels among newly licensed RNs*. A simulated subset of 20 participants was created for this example so that the computations would be small and manageable. In actuality, studies involving linear regression need to be adequately powered (Cohen, 1988; Taylor & Spurlock, 2018). The data are presented in Table 30.2.

TABLE 30.2   SELF-REPORTED ANXIETY AND RESILIENCE LEVELS AMONG NEWLY LICENSED NURSES

Participant Number	x (Anxiety)	y (Resilience)	x^2	xy
1	6	4.17	36.00	25.02
2	1	4.5	1.00	4.50
3	10	3.17	100.00	31.70
4	5	3.83	25.00	19.15
5	13	3.17	169.00	41.21
6	17	1.83	289.00	31.11
7	9	4.67	81.00	42.03
8	20	2.67	400.00	53.40
9	16	3	256.00	48.00
10	20	2.83	400.00	56.60
11	13	2.17	169.00	28.21
12	12	2.17	144.00	26.04
13	5	4.67	25.00	23.35
14	3	3.17	9.00	9.51
15	0	4	0.00	0.00
16	7	4.67	49.00	32.69
17	5	2.5	25.00	12.50
18	4	3.33	16.00	13.32
19	3	4	9.00	12.00
20	4	3.5	16.00	14.00
sum Σ	173.00	68.02	2,219.00	524.34

Questions for Additional Study

Name: _____ Class: _____

Date: _____

Answer the following questions with hand calculations using the data presented in Table 30.2 or the SPSS dataset called "Exercise 30 Example 2.sav" available on the Evolve website. Follow your instructor's directions to submit your answers to the following questions for additional study. Your instructor may ask you to write your answers below and submit them as a hard copy for evaluation. Alternatively, your instructor may ask you to submit your answers online.

1. State the null hypothesis where self-reported anxiety is tested as a predictor of levels of resilience among newly licensed registered nurses (RNs).

2. What is the exact likelihood of obtaining a standardized beta value at least as extreme or close to the one that was actually observed, assuming that the null hypothesis is true?

3. Calculate the unstandardized beta (b) by hand or using SPSS.

4. Calculate the *y*-intercept (*a*) by hand or using SPSS.

5. Write the new regression equation.

6. How would you characterize the magnitude of the obtained R^2 value? Provide a rationale for your answer.

7. How much variance in resilience levels is explained by knowing the participant's anxiety score?

8. What was the correlation between the actual *y* values and the predicted $\hat{y}$ values using the new regression equation in the example?

9. Write your interpretation of the results as you would in an APA-formatted journal (American Psychological Association, 2020).

10. Given the results of your analyses, would you use the calculated regression equation to predict future RNs' resilience levels by using anxiety scores as *x*? Provide a rationale for your answer.

Calculating Multiple Linear Regression

Multiple linear regression analysis is an extension of simple linear regression in which more than one independent variable is entered into the analysis. Interpretations of multiple regression findings are much the same as with simple linear regression, which is reviewed in Exercise 30. The beta values of each predictor are tested for significance, and a multiple R and R^2 are computed. In multiple linear regression, however, when all predictors are tested simultaneously, each beta has been adjusted for every other predictor in the regression model. The beta represents the independent relationship between that predictor and y, even after controlling for (or accounting for) the presence of every other predictor in the model (Stevens, 2009; Tabachnick & Fidell, 2019).

In multiple linear regression, relationships between multiple predictors and y are tested simultaneously with a series of matrix algebra calculations. Therefore multiple linear regression is best conducted using a statistical software package; however, full explanations and examples of the matrix algebraic computations of multiple linear regression are presented in Stevens (2009) and Tabachnick and Fidell (2019).

RESEARCH DESIGNS APPROPRIATE FOR MULTIPLE LINEAR REGRESSION

Research designs that may use multiple linear regression include any associational design (Gliner et al., 2017; Kazdin, 2022). The variables involved in the design are usually attributional, meaning the variables are characteristics of the participant, such as health status, blood pressure, gender, diagnosis, or ethnicity. Regardless of the nature of the predictor variables, the dependent variable submitted to multiple linear regression must be measured as interval or ratio level (see Exercise 1; Gray & Grove, 2021). Although the predictor can be any scale of measurement, if it is nominal, it must be correctly coded, which is described later in this exercise.

STATISTICAL ASSUMPTIONS

Use of multiple linear regression involves the following assumptions (Tabachnick & Fidell, 2019; Zar, 2010):

1. Normal distribution of the dependent (y) variable
2. Linear relationship between x and y
3. Independent observations
4. Homoscedasticity (discussed later in this exercise)
5. Interval or ratio measurement of the dependent variable; however, if the dependent variable is measured with a Likert scale, and the frequency distribution is approximately normally distributed, these data are usually considered interval-level measurement and are appropriate to serve as the outcome in a linear regression model (Rasmussen, 1989; Waltz et al., 2017).

Multiple Linear Regression Equation

The parameters a and b (a beta is computed for each predictor) are computed to obtain a regression equation. The equation looks similar to that of the simple linear regression equation presented in Exercise 30, but has been expanded to reflect the presence of multiple predictors:

$$y = b_1 x_1 + b_2 x_2 + b_3 x_3 \cdots + a$$

where

y = **the dependent variable**

x_1, x_2, x_3, etc. = **the independent variables (predictors)**

b_1, b_2, b_3, etc. = **the slopes of the line for each predictor**

a = **y-intercept (the point where the regression line intersects the y-axis)**

As mentioned earlier, multiple linear regression can be computed by hand but requires knowledge of matrix algebra. Therefore we will use SPSS to compute the regression equation and other important parameters such as the R and R^2.

Homoscedasticity and Heteroscedasticity

Data that are **homoscedastic** are evenly dispersed both above and below a plotted line of perfect prediction when variable x predicts variable y. Homoscedasticity reflects equal variance of both variables. In other words, for every value of x, the distribution of y values should have equal variability. If the data for the predictor and dependent variable are not homoscedastic, inferences made during significance testing could be invalid (Cohen & Cohen, 1983; Tabachnick & Fidell, 2019).

The assumption of homoscedasticity can be checked by visual examination of a plot of the standardized residuals (the errors) by the regression standardized predicted value. Ideally, residuals are randomly scattered around zero (the horizontal line representing perfectly accurate prediction), providing a relatively even distribution. **Heteroscedasticity** is indicated when the residuals are not evenly scattered around the line. Heteroscedasticity manifests itself in all kinds of uneven shapes. When the plot of residuals appears to deviate substantially from normal, more formal tests for heteroscedasticity should be performed. Formal tests for heteroscedasticity include the Breusch-Pagan Test (Breusch & Pagan, 1979) and the White Test (White, 1980).

Take for example the plots in Figs. 31.1 and 31.2 that follow. Two multiple linear regression analyses were performed, and the predicted y values were plotted against the residuals (actual y − predicted $\hat{y}$). Homoscedasticity occurs when the observations (seen as dots) are equally distributed above the line and below the line. It should look like a "bird's nest," such as the shape exhibited in Fig. 31.1, and not a cone or triangle, such as the shape in Fig. 31.2.

Multicollinearity

Multicollinearity occurs when the predictors in a multiple regression equation are strongly correlated (Cohen & Cohen, 1983). Multicollinearity is minimized by carefully selecting the predictors and thoroughly determining the interrelationships among predictors before the regression analysis. Multicollinearity does not affect predictive power (the capacity of the predictors to predict values of the dependent variable in that specific sample); rather it causes problems related to generalizability (Tabachnick & Fidell, 2019). If multicollinearity is present, the equation will not have predictive validity. The amount of variance explained by each variable in the equation will be inflated. The beta values will not remain consistent across

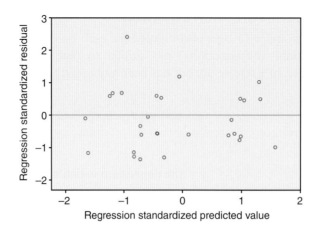

FIG. 31.1 ■ **EXAMPLE OF HOMOSCEDASTICITY.**

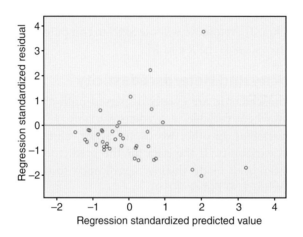

FIG. 31.2 ■ **EXAMPLE OF HETEROSCEDASTICITY.**

samples when crossvalidation (the process of testing a new regression equation's ability to predict new data) is performed (Cohen & Cohen, 1983; Tabachnick & Fidell, 2019).

The first step in identifying multicollinearity is to examine the correlations among the predictor variables. The correlation matrix is carefully examined for evidence of multicollinearity. SPSS provides two statistics (tolerance and variance inflation factor [VIF]) that describe the extent to which your model has a multicollinearity problem. A tolerance of less than 0.20 or 0.10 and/or a VIF of 5 or 10 and above indicates a multicollinearity problem (Allison, 1999).

Dummy Coding of Nominal Predictors

As discussed earlier, a predictor can be any scale of measurement; however, if the predictor is nominal, it must be correctly coded. To use categorical predictors in regression analysis, a coding system is developed to represent group membership. Categorical variables of interest in nursing that might be used in regression analysis include gender, income, ethnicity, social status, level of education, and diagnosis. If the variable is dichotomous, such as gender, members of one category are assigned the number 1, and all others are assigned the number 0. In this case for gender the coding could be:

1 = female, 0 = male

The process of creating dichotomous variables from categorical variables is called **dummy coding**. If the categorical variable has three values, two dummy variables are used; for example, social class could be classified as lower class, middle class, or upper class. The first dummy variable (x_1) would be classified as:

1 = lower class

0 = not lower class

The second dummy variable (x_2) would be classified as

1 = middle class

0 = not middle class

The three social classes would then be specified in the equation in the following manner:

Lower class $x_1 = 1, x_2 = 0$

Middle class $x_1 = 0, x_2 = 1$

Upper class $x_1 = 0, x_2 = 0$

When more than three categories define the values of the variable, increased numbers of dummy variables are used. The number of dummy variables is always one less than the number of categories (Aiken & West, 1991)—otherwise multicollinearity will be very high.

SPSS COMPUTATIONS

This example includes data collected from a survey study by Urban et al. (2022). Newly licensed registered nurses (RNs) were surveyed and administered several questionnaires: Patient Health Questionnaire (PHQ-9), General Anxiety Disorder-7 Scale (GAD), Perceived Stress Scale (PSS), and the Brief Resilience Scale (BRS). Higher scores on the PHQ-9, GAD, and PSS are indicative of increased (worse) depression, anxiety, and stress levels, respectively. Scores on the BRS range from 1 to 5, with higher scores indicating greater (better) self-reported resilience levels.

The null hypothesis is: *Self-reported depression, anxiety, and stress do not predict resilience levels among newly licensed RNs.* A simulated subset of 45 students was created for this example. In actuality, studies involving linear regression need to be adequately powered (Aberson, 2019; Gaskin & Happell, 2014; Taylor & Spurlock, 2018). See Exercises 24 and 25 for more information regarding statistical power. The data are presented in Table 31.1.

TABLE 31.1 PREDICTORS OF RESILIENCE IN NEWLY LICENSED NURSES

Participant ID	x_1 (Depression)	x_2 (Anxiety)	x_3 (Stress)	y (Resilience)
1	6.00	6.00	24.00	4.17
2	5.00	3.00	14.00	4.00
3	3.00	4.00	10.00	4.00
4	7.00	7.00	7.00	4.67
5	6.00	6.00	15.00	2.50
6	6.00	5.00	15.00	2.50
7	10.00	13.00	24.00	3.17
8	10.00	13.00	24.00	3.17
9	12.00	20.00	30.00	2.67
10	10.00	5.00	24.00	3.83
11	5.00	1.00	7.00	4.50
12	10.00	5.00	24.00	3.83
13	13.00	16.00	34.00	3.00
14	19.00	12.00	24.00	2.17
15	6.00	4.00	15.00	3.50
16	15.00	15.00	29.00	2.83
17	8.00	10.00	10.00	3.17
18	1.00	5.00	13.00	4.50
19	10.00	13.00	24.00	3.17
20	6.00	6.00	24.00	4.17
21	18.00	13.00	28.00	2.17
22	18.00	13.00	28.00	2.17
23	11.00	17.00	19.00	1.83
24	11.00	9.00	25.00	3.00
25	5.00	3.00	14.00	4.00
26	2.00	3.00	21.00	3.17
27	11.00	17.00	19.00	1.83
28	7.00	7.00	7.00	2.00
29	11.00	17.00	19.00	1.83
30	5.00	1.00	7.00	4.50
31	8.00	10.00	10.00	3.17
32	2.00	3.00	21.00	3.17
33	6.00	6.00	24.00	4.17
34	5.00	1.00	7.00	4.50
35	6.00	4.00	15.00	3.50
36	10.00	5.00	24.00	3.83
37	5.00	4.00	11.00	3.33
38	5.00	4.00	11.00	3.33
39	12.00	20.00	30.00	2.67
40	13.00	16.00	34.00	3.00
41	11.00	9.00	25.00	3.00
42	8.00	10.00	10.00	3.17
43	19.00	12.00	24.00	2.17
44	15.00	15.00	29.00	2.83
45	4.00	4.00	10.00	3.80

This is how the dataset looks in SPSS.

	ID	PHQ	GAD	PSS	BRS
1	1	6.00	6.00	24.00	4.17
2	2	5.00	3.00	14.00	4.00
3	3	3.00	4.00	10.00	4.00
4	4	7.00	7.00	7.00	4.67
5	5	6.00	6.00	15.00	2.50
6	6	6.00	5.00	15.00	2.50
7	7	10.00	13.00	24.00	3.17
8	8	10.00	13.00	24.00	3.17
9	9	12.00	20.00	30.00	2.67
10	10	10.00	5.00	24.00	3.83
11	11	5.00	1.00	7.00	4.50
12	12	10.00	5.00	24.00	3.83
13	13	13.00	16.00	34.00	3.00
14	14	19.00	12.00	24.00	2.17
15	15	6.00	4.00	15.00	3.50
16	16	15.00	15.00	29.00	2.83

Step 1: From the "Analyze" menu, choose "Regression" and "Linear."

Step 2: Move the predictors PHQ (depression), GAD (anxiety), and PSS (stress) to the space labeled "Independent(s)." Move the dependent variable, BRS (resilience), to the space labeled "Dependent."

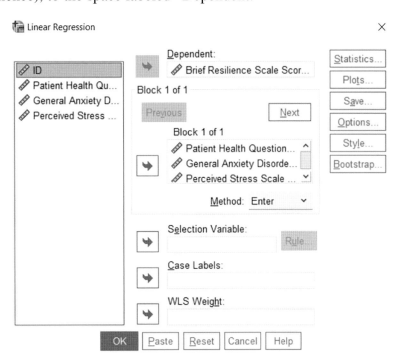

Step 3: Click "Statistics." Check the box labeled "Collinearity diagnostics." Click "Continue."

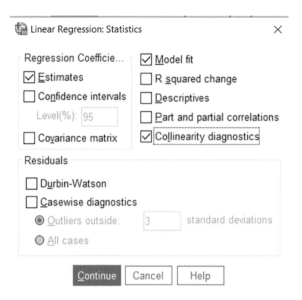

Step 4: Click "Plots." Move the variable "ZPRED" (standardized predictor values) to the box labeled "X." Move the variable "ZRESID" (standardized residual values) to the box labeled "Y." Click "Continue" and "OK."

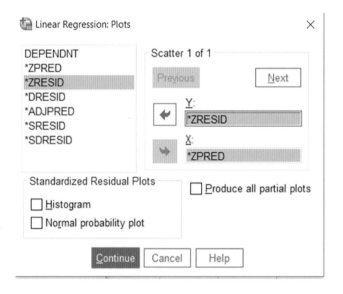

INTERPRETATION OF SPSS OUTPUT

The following tables and figure are generated from SPSS. The first table contains the multiple R and the R^2 values. The multiple R is 0.736, indicating that the correlation between the actual y values and the predicted $\hat{y}$ values using the new regression equation is 0.736. The R^2 is 0.542, indicating that 54.20% of the variance in resilience levels can be explained by knowing the nurse's depression, anxiety, and stress levels. The adjusted R^2 is 0.509, which is slightly lower because it reflects an elimination of increases in R^2 that occurred because of chance by simply adding predictors to the model (Allison, 1999).

Regression

Model Summary[b]

Model	R	R Square	Adjusted R Square	Std. Error of the Estimate
1	.736[a]	.542	.509	.56575

a. Predictors: (Constant), Perceived Stress Scale Score, General Anxiety Disorder Scale Score, Patient Health Questionnaire (Depression) Score

b. Dependent Variable: Brief Resilience Scale Score

The second table contains the analysis of variance (ANOVA) table. As presented in Exercise 35, the ANOVA is usually performed to test for differences between group means; however, ANOVA can also be performed for regression, where the null hypothesis is that *knowing the value of x explains no information about y.* This table indicates that knowing the value of *x* explains a significant amount of variance in *y.* The contents of the ANOVA table are rarely reported in published manuscripts, because the significance of each predictor is presented in the last SPSS table titled "Coefficients" (see below).

ANOVA[a]

Model		Sum of Squares	df	Mean Square	F	Sig.
1	Regression	15.541	3	5.180	16.185	<.001[b]
	Residual	13.123	41	.320		
	Total	28.664	44			

a. Dependent Variable: Brief Resilience Scale Score

b. Predictors: (Constant), Perceived Stress Scale Score, General Anxiety Disorder Scale Score, Patient Health Questionnaire (Depression) Score

The third table contains the *b* and *a* values, standardized beta (β), *t*, exact *p* values, and collinearity diagnostics. The *a* is listed in the first row, next to the label "Constant." The *b* is listed in the following rows, next to the name of each predictor. The remaining information that is important to extract when interpreting regression results can be found in the second through fourth rows, which list the standardized beta and the *p* values. It should be noted that in some versions of SPSS, a very low *p* value might display as ". 000." However, *p* is never zero and should more accurately be written as less than 0.001 or <0.001. Finally, the collinearity diagnostics, tolerance, and VIF are listed for each predictor. A tolerance of less than 0.20 or 0.10 and/or a VIF of 5 or 10 and above indicates a multicollinearity problem (Allison, 1999). Here, there does not appear to be a multicollinearity problem, as the tolerance values are greater than 0.20, and the VIF values are less than 5.0.

Coefficients[a]

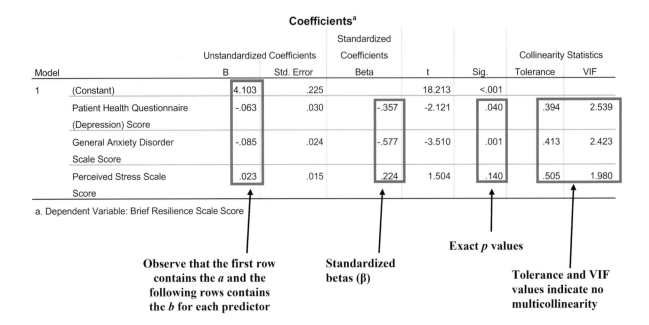

Model		Unstandardized Coefficients B	Std. Error	Standardized Coefficients Beta	t	Sig.	Collinearity Statistics Tolerance	VIF
1	(Constant)	4.103	.225		18.213	<.001		
	Patient Health Questionnaire (Depression) Score	-.063	.030	-.357	-2.121	.040	.394	2.539
	General Anxiety Disorder Scale Score	-.085	.024	-.577	-3.510	.001	.413	2.423
	Perceived Stress Scale Score	.023	.015	.224	1.504	.140	.505	1.980

a. Dependent Variable: Brief Resilience Scale Score

Observe that the first row contains the *a* and the following rows contains the *b* for each predictor

Standardized betas (β)

Exact *p* values

Tolerance and VIF values indicate no multicollinearity

The last figure in the output is the scatterplot that assists us in identifying heteroscedasticity. Recall that homoscedasticity occurs when the observations (seen as dots in the figure) are equally distributed above a horizontal line representing perfectly accurate prediction drawn at $y = 0$ and below the line at $y = 0$. In this example, our data appear to have met the homoscedasticity assumption, because the values appear to be evenly dispersed above and below the line.

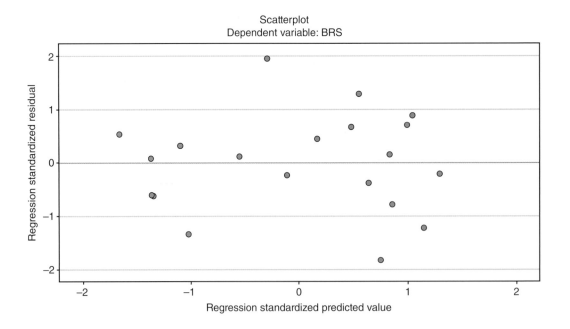

Scatterplot
Dependent variable: BRS

FINAL INTERPRETATION IN AMERICAN PSYCHOLOGICAL ASSOCIATION FORMAT

The following interpretation is written as it might appear in a research article, formatted according to the American Psychological Association (APA) guidelines (APA, 2020). It should be noted that all statistical values reported here are rounded to two decimal places, with the exception of the p value, which is rounded to three decimal places.

Multiple linear regression was performed with newly licensed RNs' levels of self-reported depression, anxiety, stress as the predictors and resilience as the dependent variable. Collinearity diagnostics indicated no multicollinearity, and visual inspection of the scatterplot of the residuals revealed no heteroscedasticity. The nurses' depression and anxiety levels significantly predicted their levels of resilience, $R^2 = 54.20\%$, adjusted $R^2 = 50.90\%$. Higher levels of depression significantly predicted lower levels of resilience ($\beta = -0.36$, $p = 0.040$). Higher levels of anxiety also significantly predicted lower levels of resilience ($\beta = -0.58$, $p = 0.001$). However, stress levels did not significantly predict resilience among the newly licensed RNs after controlling for self-reported depression and anxiety.

STUDY QUESTIONS

1. State the null hypothesis for this study where depression, anxiety, and stress are tested as predictors of resilience among newly licensed nurses.

2. If you have access to SPSS, compute the Pearson correlation between stress and resilience. Note the differences between the Pearson r results and the β (standardized beta) in the multiple regression output. Provide an explanation for the differences in findings between the two sets of results.

3. Write the newly computed regression equation, predicting resilience.

4. Using the new regression equation, compute the predicted resilience score if the nurse's PHQ score is 5, GAD score is 1, and PSS score is 7. Show your calculations.

5. Using the new regression equation, compute the predicted resilience score if the nurse's PHQ score is 12, GAD score is 20, and PSS score is 30. Show your calculations.

6. What was the correlation between the actual y values and the predicted $\hat{y}$ values using the new regression equation in the example?

7. What was the exact likelihood of obtaining a β value for PSS (stress) that is at least as extreme or as close to the one that was actually observed, assuming that the null hypothesis is true and after controlling for the other two predictors?

8. Which predictor has the strongest association with y? Provide a rationale for your answer.

9. How much variance in resilience is explained by the three model predictors?

10. How would you characterize the magnitude of the R^2 in the example? Provide a rationale for your answer.

Answers to Study Questions

1. The null hypothesis is: *Self-reported depression, anxiety, and stress do not predict resilience levels among newly licensed RNs.*

2. The Pearson correlation between stress and resilience is $r(43) = -0.386, p = 0.009$. The β (standardized beta) between stress and resilience in the multiple linear regression model with three predictors is 0.224, $p = 0.14$. When predictors in a regression model are being adjusted for the presence of other predictors in the model, the β values can change substantially depending on the extent to which the other predictors are associated with y and with one another (Tabachnick & Fidell, 2019). This explains why the Pearson r is significant but the β is not significant.

3. The newly computed regression equation is: $\hat{y} = -0.063x_1 + -0.085x_2 + 0.023x_3 + 4.103$, where x_1 = PHQ (depression), x_2 = GAD (anxiety), x_3 = PSS (stress), and $a = 4.103$.

4. The predicted resilience score if the nurse's PHQ score is 5, GAD score is 1, and PSS score is 7 is:
   $\hat{y} = -0.063(5) + -0.085(1) + 0.023(7) + 4.103 = -0.315 + -0.085 + 0.161 + 4.103$
   $\hat{y} = 3.864$, rounded to 3.86.

5. The predicted resilience score if the nurse's PHQ score is 12, GAD score is 20, and PSS score is 30 is:
   $\hat{y} = -0.063(12) + -0.085(20) + 0.023(30) + 4.103 = -0.756 + -1.70 + 0.69 + 4.103$
   $\hat{y} = 2.337$, rounded to 2.34

6. The multiple R is 0.736. This value can be observed in the "Model Summary" table of the SPSS output.

7. The exact likelihood of obtaining a β value for PSS (stress) at least as extreme as or as close to the one that was actually observed, assuming that the null hypothesis is true and after controlling for the other two predictors, is 14.00%. This value was obtained by taking the p value listed in the SPSS output table titled "Coefficients" in the column labeled "Sig." and multiplying by 100%: $0.14 \times 100\%$ = 14.00%. Because this value is greater than the study alpha of 0.05 or 5%, stress is not a significant predictor of resilience after controlling for the other two predictors.

8. The predictor GAD (anxiety) has the strongest association with y, with a standardized β of -0.577. The other two predictors had lower standardized beta values, as presented in the "Coefficients" Table.

9. Of the variance in resilience, 54.20% is explained by the three model predictors. This value ($\times 100\%$) is located in the "Model Summary" table.

10. The magnitude of the R^2, 0.542 or 54.20%, is considered a large effect according to the effect size tables in Exercises 24 and 25 (Tables 24.1 and 25.1 respectively).

DATA FOR ADDITIONAL COMPUTATIONAL PRACTICE

Using the same example from Urban and colleagues (2022), the following data include only the two significant predictors from the previous analysis. The significant predictors were PHQ (depression) and GAD (anxiety) and the dependent variable was BRS (resilience). The data are presented in Table 31.2.

TABLE 31.2   PREDICTORS OF RESILIENCE IN NEWLY LICENSED NURSES

Participant ID	x_1 (Depression)	x_2 (Anxiety)	y (Resilience)
1	6.00	6.00	4.17
2	5.00	3.00	4.00
3	3.00	4.00	4.00
4	7.00	7.00	4.67
5	6.00	6.00	2.50
6	6.00	5.00	2.50
7	10.00	13.00	3.17
8	10.00	13.00	3.17
9	12.00	20.00	2.67
10	10.00	5.00	3.83
11	5.00	1.00	4.50
12	10.00	5.00	3.83
13	13.00	16.00	3.00
14	19.00	12.00	2.17
15	6.00	4.00	3.50
16	15.00	15.00	2.83
17	8.00	10.00	3.17
18	1.00	5.00	4.50
19	10.00	13.00	3.17
20	6.00	6.00	4.17
21	18.00	13.00	2.17
22	18.00	13.00	2.17
23	11.00	17.00	1.83
24	11.00	9.00	3.00
25	5.00	3.00	4.00
26	2.00	3.00	3.17
27	11.00	17.00	1.83
28	7.00	7.00	2.00
29	11.00	17.00	1.83
30	5.00	1.00	4.50
31	8.00	10.00	3.17
32	2.00	3.00	3.17
33	6.00	6.00	4.17
34	5.00	1.00	4.50
35	6.00	4.00	3.50
36	10.00	5.00	3.83
37	5.00	4.00	3.33
38	5.00	4.00	3.33
39	12.00	20.00	2.67
40	13.00	16.00	3.00
41	11.00	9.00	3.00
42	8.00	10.00	3.17
43	19.00	12.00	2.17
44	15.00	15.00	2.83
45	4.00	4.00	3.80

Name:	Class:
Date:	

Answer the following questions with hand calculations using the data presented in Table 31.2 or the SPSS dataset called "Exercise 31 Example 2.sav" available on the Evolve website. Follow your instructor's directions to submit your answers to the following questions for additional study. Your instructor may ask you to write your answers below and submit them as a hard copy for evaluation. Alternatively, your instructor may ask you to submit your answers online.

1. Write the newly computed regression equation, predicting levels of resilience among newly licensed RNs. Include the table titled "Coefficients" from the SPSS output.

2. Why have the values in the equation changed slightly from the first example that included three predictors?

3. Using SPSS, create the scatterplot of predicted values and residuals that assists us in identifying heteroscedasticity. Do the data meet the homoscedasticity assumption? Provide a rationale for your answer.

4. Using the new regression equation, compute the predicted resilience score if the nurse's PHQ score is 3 and GAD score is 4. Show your calculations.

5. Using the new regression equation, compute the predicted resilience score if the nurse's PHQ score is 20 and GAD score is 12. Show your calculations.

6. What was the correlation between the actual y values and the predicted $\hat{y}$ values using the new regression equation in the example?

7. Which predictor has the strongest association with y? Provide a rationale for your answer.

8. How much variance in resilience is explained by the two model predictors?

9. Write your interpretation of the results as you would in an APA-formatted journal (American Psychological Association, 2020).

10. Given the results of your analyses, would you use the calculated regression equation to predict future newly licensed nurses' resilience levels by using depression and anxiety scores as the predictors?

Calculating *t*-Tests for Independent Samples

One of the most common statistical tests chosen to investigate significant differences between two independent samples is the independent samples *t*-test. The samples are independent if the study participants in one group are unrelated or different participants than those in the second group (see Exercise 16 for an introduction to the independent samples *t*-test). The dependent variable in an independent samples *t*-test must be scaled as interval or ratio. If the dependent variable is measured with a Likert scale, and the frequency distribution is approximately normally distributed, these data are usually considered interval-level measurement and are appropriate for an independent samples *t*-test (see Exercise 1; de Winter & Dodou, 2010; Rasmussen, 1989; Waltz et al., 2017).

RESEARCH DESIGNS APPROPRIATE FOR THE INDEPENDENT SAMPLES *t*-TEST

Research designs that may use the independent samples *t*-test include the randomized experimental, quasi-experimental, and comparative designs (Gliner et al., 2017; Gray & Grove, 2021; Kazdin, 2022). The independent variable (the grouping variable for the *t*-test) may be active or attributional. An **active independent variable** refers to an intervention, treatment, or program. An **attributional independent variable** refers to a characteristic of the participant, such as gender, diagnosis, or ethnicity. Regardless of the nature of the independent variable, the independent samples *t*-test only compares two groups at a time.

Example 1: Researchers conduct a randomized experimental study where the participants are randomized to either a novel weight loss intervention or a placebo. The number of pounds lost from baseline to posttreatment for both groups is measured. The research question is: *Is there a difference between the two groups in weight loss?* The active independent variable is the weight loss intervention, and the dependent variable is the number of pounds lost over the treatment span.

Null hypothesis: *There is no difference between the intervention and the control (placebo) groups in weight loss.*

Example 2: Researchers conduct a retrospective comparative descriptive study where a chart review of patients is done to identify patients who recently underwent a colonoscopy. The patients were divided into two groups: those who used statins continuously in the past year, and those who did not. The dependent variable is the number of polyps found during the colonoscopy, and the independent variable is statin use. The research question is: *Is there a significant difference between the statin users and nonusers in number of colon polyps found?*

Null hypothesis: *There is no difference between the group taking statins versus the group not taking statins (control) in number of colon polyps found.*

STATISTICAL FORMULA AND ASSUMPTIONS

Use of the independent samples *t*-test involves the following assumptions (Zar, 2010):

1. Sample means from the population are normally distributed.
2. The dependent variable is measured at the interval/ratio level.
3. The two samples have equal variance.
4. All observations within each sample are independent.

The formula and calculation of the independent samples *t*-test are presented in this exercise. The formula for the independent samples *t*-test (*t*) is:

$$t = \frac{\overline{X}_1 - \overline{X}_2}{s_{X1-X2}}$$

where

$$\overline{X}_1 = \textbf{mean of group 1}$$

$$\overline{X}_2 = \textbf{mean of group 2}$$

$$s_{X_1-X_2} = \textbf{standard error of the difference between the two groups}$$

To compute the *t*-test, one must compute the denominator in the formula, which is the standard error of the difference between the means. If the two groups have different sample sizes, then one must use this formula:

$$s_{\overline{X}_1-\overline{X}_2} = \sqrt{\frac{(n_1-1)s_1^2 + (n_2-1)s_2^2}{n_1+n_2-2}\left(\frac{1}{n_1}+\frac{1}{n_2}\right)}$$

where

$$n_1 = \textbf{group 1 sample size}$$

$$n_2 = \textbf{group 2 sample size}$$

$$s_1 = \textbf{group 1 variance}$$

$$s_2 = \textbf{group 2 variance}$$

If the two groups have the same number of participants in each group, then one can use this simplified formula:

$$s_{\overline{X}_1-\overline{X}_2} = \sqrt{\frac{s_1^2 + s_2^2}{n}}$$

where

$$n = \textbf{the sample size in each group and not the total sample of both groups}$$

HAND CALCULATIONS

A randomized experimental study examined the effect of the discontinuation of proton pump inhibitors (PPIs) on gastrointestinal symptoms among those with gastroesophageal reflux disease (GERD; Hendricks et al., 2021). The researchers followed two randomized groups of participants over time: those who underwent abrupt PPI discontinuation and those who underwent tapered PPI discontinuation.

The data from this study are presented in Table 32.1. A simulated subset was selected for this example so that the computations would be small and manageable. In actuality, studies involving independent samples *t*-tests need to be adequately powered (Aberson, 2019; Cohen, 1988. See Exercises 24 and 25 for more information regarding statistical power).

The independent variable in this example is the type of PPI discontinuation (abrupt versus tapered). The dependent variable was the score on the Dyspepsia Symptom Severity Index (DSSI) assessed at a follow-up assessment 14 weeks postdiscontinuation. The items on the DSSI are rated on a 5-point Likert scale ranging from 0 (absent) to 4 (very severe). The null hypothesis is: *There is no difference between the abrupt and tapered discontinuation groups on the severity of dyspepsia symptoms among persons with GERD.*

The computations for the independent samples *t*-test are as follows:

Step 1: Compute means for both groups, which involves the sum of scores for each group divided by the number in the group.

$$\text{The mean for Group 1, Abrupt Discontinuation Group: } \bar{X}_1 = 3.43$$

$$\text{The mean for Group 2, Tapered Discontinuation Group: } \bar{X}_2 = 2.95$$

Step 2: Compute the numerator of the *t*-test:
$$3.43 - 2.95 = \mathbf{0.48}$$

It does not matter which group is designated as "group 1" or "group 2."

Another possible correct method for Step 2 is to subtract group 1's mean from group 2's mean, such as: $\bar{X}_2 - \bar{X}_1$: $2.95 - 3.43 = \mathbf{-0.48}$

Step 3: Compute the standard error of the difference.

a. Compute the variances for each group:

$$s^2 \text{ for group 1} = 0.20$$

$$s^2 \text{ for group 2} = 0.10$$

TABLE 32.1	DSSI SCORES BY GROUP		
Abrupt Discontinuation Group		**Tapered Discontinuation Group**	
Participant #	**DSSI Score (Dyspepsia Symptoms)**	**Participant #**	**DSSI Score (Dyspepsia Symptoms)**
1	3.20	11	3.30
2	4.10	12	2.70
3	3.90	13	2.90
4	3.60	14	2.60
5	3.80	15	3.10
6	3.70	16	3.20
7	2.90	17	3.40
8	2.80	18	2.90
9	3.10	19	3.00
10	3.20	20	2.40

DSSI, Dyspepsia Symptom Severity Index.

b. Plug into the standard error of the difference formula:

$$s_{\bar{X}_1 - \bar{X}_2} = \sqrt{\frac{s^2_1 + s^2_2}{n}}$$

$$s_{\bar{X}_1 - \bar{X}_2} = \sqrt{\frac{0.20 + 0.10}{10}}$$

$$s_{\bar{X}_1 - \bar{X}_2} = \sqrt{.030}$$

$$s_{\bar{X}_1 - \bar{X}_2} = 0.1732$$

Step 4: Compute *t* value:

$$t = \frac{\bar{X}_1 - \bar{X}_2}{s_{\bar{X}_1 - \bar{X}_2}}$$

$$t = \frac{0.48}{0.1732}$$

$$t = 2.77$$

Step 5: Compute the degrees of freedom *(df):*

$$df = n_1 + n_2 - 2$$

$$df = 10 + 10 - 2$$

$$df = 18$$

Step 6: Locate the critical *t* value in the *t* distribution table (Appendix A) and compare it to the obtained *t* value.

The critical *t* value for a two-tailed test with 18 *df* at alpha (α) = 0.05 is 2.101, rounded to 2.10. This means that if we viewed the *t* distribution for *df* = 18, the middle 95% of the distribution would be marked by −2.10 and 2.10. The obtained *t* is 2.77, exceeding the critical value, which means our *t*-test is statistically significant and represents a real difference between the two groups. Therefore we can reject our null hypothesis. It should be noted that if the obtained *t* was −2.77, it would also be considered statistically significant, because the absolute value of the obtained *t* is compared with the critical *t* tabled value (Kim et al., 2022).

SPSS COMPUTATIONS

This is how our dataset looks in SPSS.

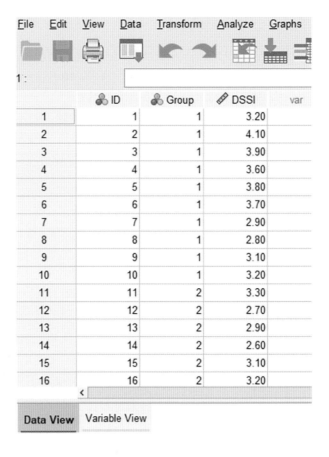

Step 1: From the "Analyze" menu, choose "Compare Means" and "Independent-Samples T Test." Move the dependent variable, "DSSI" (dyspepsia symptoms), over to the right, like the window below and click OK.

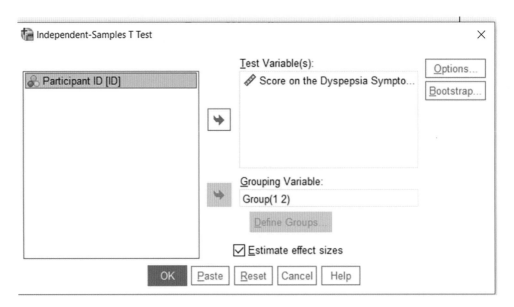

Step 2: Move the independent variable, "Group," into the space titled "Grouping Variable." Click "Define Groups" and enter 1 and 2 to represent the coding chosen to differentiate between the two groups. Click "Continue" and "OK."

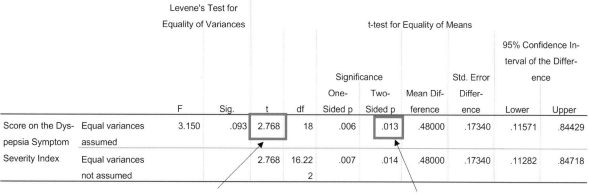

INTERPRETATION OF SPSS OUTPUT

The following tables are generated from SPSS. The first table contains descriptive statistics for dyspepsia symptom scores, separated by the two groups. The second table contains the *t*-test results.

T-Test

Group Statistics

	Abrupt or Tapered Discontinuation	N	Mean	Std. Deviation	Std. Error Mean
Score on the Dyspepsia	Abrupt	10	3.4300	.44734	.14146
Symptom Severity Index	Tapered	10	2.9500	.31710	.10028

Observe the means for the two groups

The first table displays descriptive statistics that allow us to observe the means for both groups. This table is important because it indicates that the participants in the abrupt discontinuation group had a mean DSSI score of 3.43, and the participants in the tapered discontinuation group had a mean DSSI score of 2.95.

Independent Samples Test

		Levene's Test for Equality of Variances		t-test for Equality of Means						95% Confidence Interval of the Difference	
						Significance					
						One-Sided p	Two-Sided p	Mean Difference	Std. Error Difference	Lower	Upper
		F	Sig.	t	df						
Score on the Dyspepsia Symptom Severity Index	Equal variances assumed	3.150	.093	2.768	18	.006	.013	.48000	.17340	.11571	.84429
	Equal variances not assumed			2.768	16.222	.007	.014	.48000	.17340	.11282	.84718

The *t* value is 2.768   The exact two-tailed *p* value is .013

The last table contains the actual *t*-test value, the *p* value, along with the values that compose the *t*-test formula. The first value in the table is the Levene test for equality of variances. The Levene test is a statistical test of the equal variances assumption (Field, 2013; Tabachnick & Fidell, 2019). The *p* value is 0.093, indicating there was no significant difference between the two groups' variances. If there had been a significant difference, the second row of the table, titled "Equal variances not assumed," would be reported in the results.

Following the Levene test results are the *t*-test value of 2.768 and the two-sided *p* value of 0.013, otherwise known as the probability of obtaining a statistical value at least as extreme or as close to the one that was actually observed, assuming that the null hypothesis is true. In this example, the two-sided *p* value (also known as *two-tailed p value*) is being reported instead of the one-sided *p* value. This is because the one-sided *p* value only allows for a one-sided or directional hypothesis, where the hypothesized difference is only tested in one direction or one tail of the normal curve. For a two-sided test, we allow for the possibility that one group could either be higher or lower than the other group on the dependent variable.

Following the *t*-test value, the next value in the table is 0.48, which is the mean difference that we computed in Step 2 of our hand calculations. The next value in the table is 0.1734, similar to the value we computed in Steps 3a and 3b of our hand calculations.

FINAL INTERPRETATION IN AMERICAN PSYCHOLOGICAL ASSOCIATION FORMAT

The following interpretation is written as it might appear in a research article, formatted according to American Psychological Association (APA) guidelines (APA, 2020). It should be noted that all statistical values reported here are rounded to two decimal places, with the exception of the *p* value, which is rounded to three decimal places.

An independent samples *t*-test revealed that participants in the abrupt discontinuation group reported significantly more dyspepsia symptoms at the 14-week follow-up assessment than the participants in the tapered discontinuation group, $t(18) = 2.77$, $p = 0.013$; $\bar{X} = 3.43$ versus 2.95, respectively. Thus the particular type of discontinuation that was implemented appears to have had an impact on GERD symptoms several months after the participants stopped taking PPIs.

STUDY QUESTIONS

1. If you have access to SPSS, compute the Shapiro-Wilk test of normality for the dependent variable of DSSI (dyspepsia symptoms; as demonstrated in Exercise 27). What do the results indicate?

2. Do the data meet criteria for the equality of variances assumption? Provide a rationale for your answer.

3. Do the data meet criteria for independent samples? Provide a rationale for your answer.

4. What is the null hypothesis in the example?

5. What was the exact likelihood of obtaining a *t*-test value at least as extreme or as close to the one that was actually observed, assuming that the null hypothesis is true?

6. If Levene's test for equality of variances was significant at $p \leq 0.05$, what SPSS output would the researcher need to report?

7. What does the numerator of the independent samples *t*-test represent?

8. What does the denominator of the independent samples *t*-test represent?

9. What kind of design was implemented in the example?

10. Was the sample size adequate to detect differences between the two groups in this example? Provide a rationale for your answer.

Answers to Study Questions

1. As shown below, the Shapiro-Wilk p value for DSSI score was 0.807, indicating that the frequency distribution did not significantly deviate from normality.

Tests of Normality

	Kolmogorov-Smirnov[a]			Shapiro-Wilk		
	Statistic	df	Sig.	Statistic	df	Sig.
Score on the Dyspepsia Symptom Severity Index	.141	20	.200*	.973	20	.807

*. This is a lower bound of the true significance.

a.　Lilliefors Significance Correction

2. The two groups' variances did not significantly differ, as evidenced by the nonsignificant Levene test result, $p = 0.093$. This value is found on the top row in the column labeled "Sig." of the "Independent Samples t-Test" table, indicating that there was no significant difference between the two groups' variances.

3. Yes, the data meet criteria for independent samples because the dependent variable data were collected from two mutually exclusive groups of study participants. In addition, the study participants were randomly assigned to either the abrupt or tapered discontinuation group, which makes the groups independent (Grove & Gray, 2023).

4. The null hypothesis is: *There is no difference between the abrupt and tapered discontinuation groups on the severity of dyspepsia symptoms.*

5. The exact likelihood of obtaining a t-test value at least as extreme or as close to the one that was actually observed, assuming that the null hypothesis is true, is 1.30%. This value can be found in the "Independent Samples t-Test" table in the SPSS output, where the exact p value is reported as 0.013. The value is calculated as follows: $0.013 \times 100\% = 1.30\%$.

6. If Levene's test for equality of variances was significant at $p \leq 0.05$, the researcher would need to report the second row of values from the "Independent Samples t-Test" table in the SPSS output, containing the t-test value that has been adjusted for unequal variances.

7. The numerator represents the mean difference between the two groups (see formula for the independent samples t-test).

8. The denominator represents the extent to which there is dispersion among the values of the dependent variable.

9. The study design in the example was a randomized experimental design, as evidenced by the fact that the participants were randomly assigned to receiving the abrupt or tapered discontinuation conditions (Gliner et al., 2017; Kazdin, 2022).

10. The sample size was adequate to detect differences between the two groups, because a significant difference was found, $p = 0.013$. However, this sample is considered small, and as emphasized in Exercises 24 and 25, it is strongly recommended that a power analysis be conducted prior to the study beginning in order to avoid the risk of Type II error (Taylor & Spurlock, 2018).

DATA FOR ADDITIONAL COMPUTATIONAL PRACTICE

This example involves additional data collected in the same study by Hendricks et al. (2021).

The researchers compared the two randomized groups, abrupt PPI discontinuation versus tapered PPI discontinuation, on the self-reported number (raw count) of GERD symptoms at the 14-week follow-up assessment. Examples of GERD symptoms include acid reflux, nausea, vomiting, abdominal pain, and early satiety. The null hypothesis is: *There is no difference between the abrupt and tapered discontinuation groups on the participants' number of GERD symptoms.*

A simulated subset of 20 observations was created for this example. The data are presented in Table 32.2 below.

TABLE 32.2   NUMBER OF GERD SYMPTOMS BY GROUP

Abrupt Discontinuation Group		Tapered Discontinuation Group	
Participant #	Number of GERD Symptoms	Participant #	Number of GERD Symptoms
1	6	11	6
2	7	12	4
3	8	13	2
4	7	14	3
5	7	15	6
6	3	16	5
7	6	17	5
8	6	18	3
9	5	19	6
10	6	20	5

GERD, gastroesophageal reflux disease.

Name: _____ Class: _____

Date: _____

Answer the following questions with hand calculations using the data presented in Table 32.2 or the SPSS dataset called "Exercise 32 Example 2.sav" available on the Evolve website. Follow your instructor's directions to submit your answers to the following questions for additional study. Your instructor may ask you to write your answers below and submit them as a hard copy for evaluation. Alternatively, your instructor may ask you to submit your answers online.

1. Do the example data meet the assumptions for the independent samples *t*-test? Provide a rationale for your answer.

2. If calculating by hand, draw the frequency distributions of the dependent variable of number of GERD symptoms. What is the shape of the distribution? If using SPSS, what is the result of the Shapiro-Wilk test of normality for the dependent variable?

3. List the mean number of GERD symptoms for the two groups. Which group had the highest mean number of GERD symptoms at the 14-week follow-up assessment?

4. Compute the independent samples *t*-test. What is the *t* value?

5. Is the *t*-test significant at $\alpha = 0.05$? Specify how you arrived at your answer.

6. If using SPSS, what is the exact likelihood of obtaining a *t*-test value at least as extreme or as close to the one that was actually observed, assuming that the null hypothesis is true?

7. Why are the mean group values important in the interpretation of the *t*-test results?

8. Write your interpretation of the results as you would in an APA-formatted journal (American Psychological Association, 2020).

9. What do the results indicate regarding the effect of the proton pump inhibitor (PPI) discontinuation approach used by persons suffering from GERD on their gastrointestinal symptoms?

10. Was the sample size adequate to detect significant differences between the two groups in this example? Provide a rationale for your answer.

Calculating *t*-Tests for Paired (Dependent) Samples

A **paired samples *t*-test** (also referred to as a dependent samples *t*-test) is a statistical procedure that compares two sets of data from one group of people. The paired samples *t*-test was introduced in Exercise 17, which is focused on understanding these results in research reports. This exercise focuses on calculating and interpreting the results from paired samples *t*-tests. When samples are related, the formula used to calculate the *t* statistic is different from the formula for the independent samples *t*-test (see Exercise 32).

RESEARCH DESIGNS APPROPRIATE FOR THE PAIRED SAMPLES *t*-TEST

The term *paired samples* refers to a research design that repeatedly assesses the same group of people, an approach commonly referred to as **repeated measures**. Paired samples can also refer to naturally occurring pairs, such as siblings or spouses. The most common research design that may use a paired samples *t*-test is the one-group pretest–posttest design, wherein a single group of participants is assessed at baseline and once again after receiving an intervention (Gliner et al., 2017; Gray & Grove, 2021). Another design that may use a paired samples *t*-test is where one group of participants is exposed to one level of an intervention and then those scores are compared with the same participants' responses to another level of the intervention, resulting in paired scores. This is called a **one-sample crossover design** (Gliner et al., 2017).

Example 1: A researcher conducts a one-sample pretest–posttest study wherein she assesses her sample for health status at baseline, and again posttreatment. Her research question is: *Is there a difference in health status from baseline to posttreatment?* The dependent variable is health status.

Null hypothesis: *There is no difference between the baseline and posttreatment health status scores.*

Example 2: A researcher conducts a crossover study wherein participants receive a randomly generated order of two medications. One is a standard Food and Drug Administration (FDA)-approved medication to reduce blood pressure, and the other is an experimental medication. The dependent variable is reduction in blood pressure (systolic and diastolic), and the independent variable is medication type. Her research question is: *Is there a difference between the experimental medication and the control medication in blood pressure reduction?*

Null hypothesis: *There is no difference between the two medication trials in blood pressure reduction.*

STATISTICAL FORMULA AND ASSUMPTIONS

Use of the paired samples *t*-test involves the following assumptions (Zar, 2010):

1. The distribution of values is normal or approximately normal.
2. The dependent variable(s) is (are) measured at interval or ratio levels.
3. Repeated measures data are collected from one group of participants, resulting in paired scores.
4. The differences between the paired scores are independent (Gray & Grove, 2021; Kazdin, 2022; Shadish et al., 2002).

The formula for the paired samples *t*-test is:

$$t = \frac{\bar{D}}{s_{\bar{D}}}$$

where:

$\bar{D}$ = the mean difference of the paired data

$s_{\bar{D}}$ = the standard error of the difference

To compute the *t*-test, one must calculate the denominator in the formula, the standard error of the difference:

$$s_{\bar{D}} = \frac{s_D}{\sqrt{n}}$$

where:

s_D = the standard deviation of the differences between the paired data

n = the number of participants in the sample (or number of paired scores in the case of sibling or spousal data)

HAND CALCULATIONS

Using an example from a study of adults with gastroesophageal reflux disease (GERD), symptoms of gastroesophageal reflux were examined over time (Dunbar et al., 2016). Twelve adults with GERD were followed over a period of 2 weeks while being required to be free of all proton pump inhibitor (PPI) medications (the intervention). A subset of these data ($n = 10$) is presented in Table 33.1. One of the dependent variables was esophageal impedance, which is an index of mucosal integrity, where higher numbers are more desirable and indicative of healthy esophageal functioning. Impedance was measured with a pH electrode

TABLE 33.1	**ESOPHAGEAL IMPEDANCE VALUES AT BASELINE AND 2-WEEK FOLLOW-UP**		
Participant #	**Esophageal Impedance, Baseline**	**Esophageal Impedance, 2-Week Follow-Up**	**Difference Scores**
1	2249	773	1476
2	3993	1329	2664
3	1422	1113	309
4	3676	1670	2006
5	2004	1231	773
6	3271	2660	611
7	2130	1784	346
8	2947	2000	947
9	2000	850	1150
10	3021	1674	1347

positioned 5 cm above the lower esophageal sphincter. For this example, the null hypothesis is: *There is no change in esophageal impedance from baseline to follow-up for patients with GERD who had stopped taking PPI medications.*

The computations for the paired *t*-test are as follows:

Step 1: Compute the difference between each participant's pair of data (see last column of Table 33.1).

Step 2: Compute the mean of the difference scores, which becomes the numerator of the *t*-test:

$$\bar{D} = 11{,}629.00 \div 10$$

$$\bar{D} = 1162.90$$

Step 3: Compute the standard error of the difference.

a. Compute the standard deviation of the difference scores.

$$s_D = \sqrt{\frac{\sum(X - \bar{X})^2}{n-1}}$$

$$s_D = \sqrt{\frac{4{,}995{,}908.90}{10-1}}$$

$$s_D = 745.05$$

b. Plug the result into the standard error of the difference formula.

$$s_{\bar{D}} = \frac{s_D}{\sqrt{n}}$$

$$s_{\bar{D}} = \frac{745.05}{\sqrt{10}}$$

$$s_{\bar{D}} = \frac{745.05}{3.16}$$

$$s_{\bar{D}} = 235.78$$

Step 4: Compute *t* value:

$$t = \frac{\bar{D}}{s_{\bar{D}}}$$

$$t = \frac{1162.90}{235.78}$$

$$t = 4.93$$

Step 5: Compute the degrees of freedom (*df*):

$$df = n - 1$$

$$df = 10 - 1$$

$$df = 9$$

Step 6: Locate the critical *t* value on the *t* distribution table in Appendix A and compare it to the obtained *t*.

The critical *t* value for 9 *df* at alpha (α) = 0.05 is 2.262 (rounded to 2.26) for a two-tailed test. Our obtained *t* is 4.93, exceeding the critical value (see Appendix A), which means our *t*-test is statistically significant and represents a real difference between the two pairs. Therefore we can reject our null hypothesis. This means that if we viewed the *t* distribution for *df* = 9, the middle 95% of the distribution would be marked by −2.26 and 2.26. It should be noted that if the obtained *t* was −4.93, it would also be considered statistically significant because the absolute value of the obtained *t* is compared with the critical *t* value (Gray & Grove, 2021).

SPSS COMPUTATIONS

This is how our dataset looks in SPSS.

File	Edit	View	Data	Transform	Analyze	Graphs	Utilities	Ex

	ID	ImpedBaseline	Imped2Week
1	1	2249	773
2	2	3993	1329
3	3	1422	1113
4	4	3676	1670
5	5	2004	1231
6	6	3271	2660
7	7	2130	1784
8	8	2947	2000
9	9	2000	850
10	10	3021	1674
11			
12			
13			
14			
15			
16			

Data View   Variable View

Step 1: From the "Analyze" menu, choose "Compare Means" and "Paired-Samples T Test."

Step 2: Move both variables over to the right, as in the window shown. Click "OK."

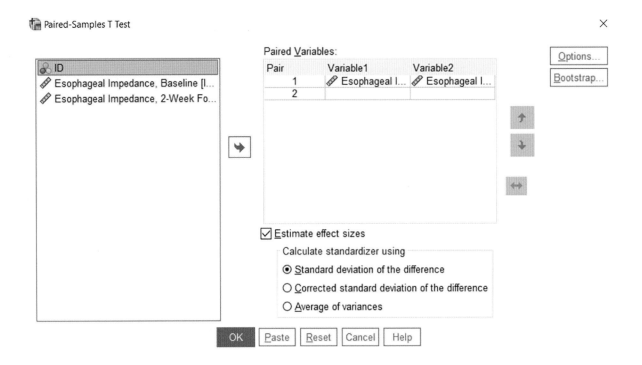

Interpretation of SPSS Output

The following tables are generated from SPSS. The first table contains descriptive statistics for the two variables. The second table contains the Pearson product-moment correlation between the two variables. The last table contains the *t*-test results.

T-Test

Paired Samples Statistics

		Mean	N	Std. Deviation	Std. Error Mean
Pair 1	Esophageal Impedance, Baseline	2671.30	10	832.819	263.360
	Esophageal Impedance, 2-Week Follow-up	1508.40	10	571.268	180.651

Observe the means for the two assessments

Paired Samples Correlations

				Significance	
		N	Correlation	One-Sided p	Two-Sided p
Pair 1	Esophageal Impedance, Baseline & Esophageal Impedance, 2-Week Follow-up	10	.489	.076	.152

Paired Samples Test

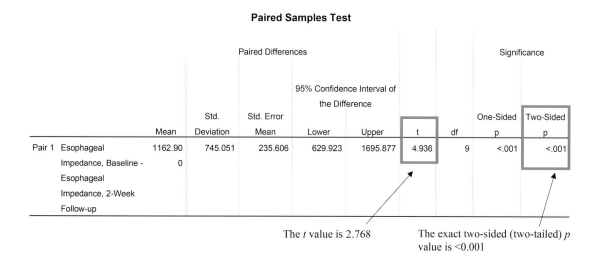

	Mean	Std. Deviation	Std. Error Mean	Lower	Upper	t	df	One-Sided p	Two-Sided p
Pair 1 Esophageal Impedance, Baseline - Esophageal Impedance, 2-Week Follow-up	1162.90 0	745.051	235.606	629.923	1695.877	4.936	9	<.001	<.001

The *t* value is 2.768   The exact two-sided (two-tailed) *p* value is <0.001

The first table displays descriptive statistics that include the means at baseline and follow-up. This table is important because we can observe that the mean impedance at baseline was 2,671.30, and the mean impedance at follow-up was 1,508.40, indicating a decrease in esophageal impedance. Recall that higher numbers are indicative of healthy esophageal functioning, and therefore a decrease over time is undesirable for persons with GERD.

The second table displays the Pearson product-moment correlation coefficient (*r*) that was computed between the two variables. It is common that the two variables are significantly correlated, because the sample is being assessed twice, and therefore it is logical that a person's follow-up value is affected by his or her baseline value in a repeated measures design. Although this table is a standard part of the SPSS output for a paired samples *t*-test, the contents are not reported in the results of published studies.

The last table contains the actual *t*-test value, along with the values that compose the *t*-test formula. Note that the first value in the table, 1,162.90, was the mean difference that we computed in Step 2 of our hand calculations. The next two values in the table, 745.05 and 235.61, were the values we computed in Steps 3a and 3b of our hand calculations. The *t*-test value of 4.936 is slightly higher than what we obtained in our hand calculations. This is because we rounded to the hundredth decimal place in our hand calculations, when the standard error value is actually 235.606, which yields a *t*-test value of $1,162.90 \div 235.606 = 4.936$. Therefore 4.936 (rounded to 4.94) is more accurate and will be reported as 4.94 in the interpretation below.

The last value in the table is the two-sided *p* value, otherwise known as the probability of obtaining a statistical value at least as extreme or as close to the one that was actually observed, assuming that the null hypothesis is true. SPSS has printed a value of "<.001," indicating a less than 0.10% probability of obtaining a *t*-test value at least as extreme or as close to the one that was actually observed, assuming that the null hypothesis is true (Gray & Grove, 2021). In this example, the two-sided *p* value (also known as *two-tailed p value*) will be reported instead of the one-sided *p* value. This is because the one-sided *p* value only allows for a one-sided or directional hypothesis, where the hypothesized difference is only tested in one direction or one tail of the normal curve. For a two-sided test, we allow for the possibility that the baseline dependent variable values could either be higher or lower than the follow-up dependent variable values.

FINAL INTERPRETATION IN AMERICAN PSYCHOLOGICAL ASSOCIATION FORMAT

The following interpretation is written as it might appear in a research article, formatted according to American Psychological Association (APA, 2020) guidelines. It should be noted that all statistical values reported here are rounded to two decimal places, with the exception of the *p* value, which is rounded to three decimal places.

A paired samples *t*-test computed on esophageal impedance revealed that the patients with GERD undergoing the withdrawal of PPIs had significantly lower impedance from baseline to posttreatment, $t(9) = 4.94$, $p < 0.001$; $\bar{X} = 2{,}671.30$ versus $1{,}508.40$, respectively. Thus the removal of PPI medications appeared to play a role in the deterioration of the esophageal mucosal integrity.

STUDY QUESTIONS

1. Use SPSS to create a frequency distribution for the two study variables of esophageal impedance at baseline and follow-up. Describe the appearance of the distributions.

2. Use SPSS to compute the Shapiro-Wilk tests of normality for those two variables (esophageal impedance at baseline and follow-up) as demonstrated in Exercise 27.

3. Do the data meet criteria for paired samples? Provide a rationale for your answer.

4. On average, did esophageal impedance improve or deteriorate over time? Provide a rationale for your answer.

5. What was the exact likelihood of obtaining a *t*-test value at least as extreme or as close to the one that was actually observed, assuming that the null hypothesis is true?

6. Identify the Pearson correlation (r) between the two study variables. Why do you think the baseline and follow-up variables were correlated?

7. What is the numerator for the paired samples *t*-test in this example? What does the numerator of the paired samples *t*-test represent?

8. What is the denominator for the paired samples *t*-test in this example? What does the denominator of the paired samples *t*-test represent?

9. Why would a one-sample crossover design also be suitable for a paired samples *t*-test?

10. The researchers concluded that the removal of PPI medications appeared to deteriorate the mucosal integrity of the esophagus. What are some alternative explanations for these changes? (These alternative scientific explanations would apply to any one-sample repeated measures design.) Document your response.

Answers to Study Questions

1. See the two SPSS frequency distributions below. Because the sample size is very small ($n = 10$), the shapes of the distributions do not follow a normal bell-shaped curve, but contain gaps in the x-axis.

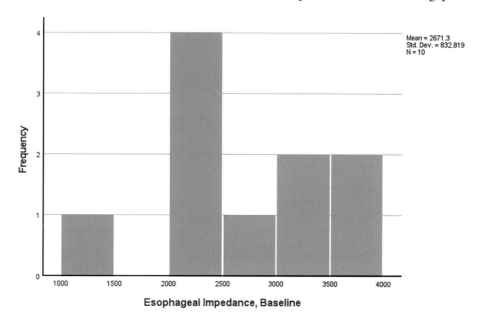

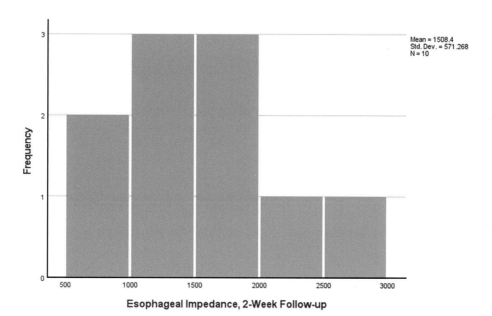

2. The Shapiro-Wilk *p* values for baseline and follow-up esophageal impedance were 0.67 and 0.70, respectively, indicating that the two frequency distributions did not significantly deviate from normality. Moreover, visual inspection of the frequency distributions in the answer to Question 1 indicates that the variables are approximately normally distributed.

Tests of Normality

	Kolmogorov-Smirnov[a]			Shapiro-Wilk		
	Statistic	df	Sig.	Statistic	df	Sig.
Esophageal Impedance, Base-line	.194	10	.200[*]	.950	10	.670
Esophageal Impedance, 2-Week Follow-up	.123	10	.200[*]	.953	10	.701

*. This is a lower bound of the true significance.

a. Lilliefors Significance Correction

3. Yes, the data meet criteria for paired samples because the two esophageal impedance values were collected from the same single group of study participants over time.

4. The mean impedance at baseline was 2,671.30, and the mean impedance at follow-up was 1,508.40, indicating a decrease in esophageal impedance, and therefore an undesirable trend for persons with GERD. As noted earlier, higher numbers are more desirable and indicative of healthy esophageal functioning.

5. The exact likelihood of obtaining a *t*-test value at least as extreme as or as close to the one that was actually observed, assuming that the null hypothesis is true, is less than 0.10%.

6. The baseline and follow-up variables were correlated ($r = 0.489$) because the sample of patients was assessed twice, and therefore it is logical that a person's follow-up value is affected by his or her baseline value in a repeated measures design (Kim et al., 2022).

7. As shown in the SPSS output, the numerator of the paired samples *t*-test in this example is 1,162.90. The numerator represents the mean difference between the two variables (see formula for the paired samples *t*-test in this exercise).

8. As shown in the SPSS output, the denominator of the paired samples *t*-test in this example is 235.606 (rounded to 235.61). The denominator represents the extent to which there is dispersion among the entire dataset's values.

9. A one-sample crossover design also would be suitable for a paired samples *t*-test because one group of participants is exposed to one level of an intervention and then those scores are compared with the same participants' responses to another level of the intervention. This meets criteria for paired samples because the two variables were collected from the same single group of people (Gliner et al., 2017).

10. When changes occur in a one-sample pretest–posttest design, we cannot be certain that the intervention caused the changes. Other explanations may include the passing of time, the inadvertent use of other treatments during the time elapsed from baseline to posttreatment, or statistical regression (a phenomenon that refers to artificially high baseline levels that naturally decrease to the actual population mean at posttreatment, or vice versa) (Gliner et al., 2017; Gray & Grove, 2021; Shadish et al., 2002).

DATA FOR ADDITIONAL COMPUTATIONAL PRACTICE

Using an example from a study examining the gastroesophageal reflux among 12 adults with GERD, changes over time were investigated (Dunbar et al., 2016). These data are presented in Table 33.2. The independent variable in this example is intervention over time, meaning that all of the participants were followed over time while being required to be free of all PPI medications for 2 weeks (the intervention). The dependent variable was esophageal reflux symptoms, measured by the GERD Health-Related Quality of Life (HRQL) questionnaire, a validated instrument for GERD symptom severity, with higher scores representing more GERD symptoms (Velanovich, 2007). The data in Table 33.2 were transformed to approximate normality. The null hypothesis is: *There is no change in esophageal reflux symptoms from baseline to follow-up for patients with GERD.*

Compute the paired samples *t*-test on the data in Table 33.2 below.

TABLE 33.2   ESOPHAGEAL SYMPTOM SCORES AT BASELINE AND 2-WEEK FOLLOW-UP

Participant #	Esophageal Symptom Scores, Baseline	Esophageal Symptom Scores, 2-Week Follow-Up	Difference Scores
1	.00	3.00	3.00
2	5.00	4.69	−.31
3	4.12	5.39	1.26
4	1.00	1.73	.73
5	4.36	4.47	.11
6	3.32	4.00	.68
7	.00	3.74	3.74
8	1.41	2.00	.59
9	.00	2.24	2.24
10	1.41	2.00	.59
11	2.00	4.24	2.24
12	.00	2.00	2.00

Questions for Additional Study

EXERCISE 33

Name: _____ Class: _____

Date: _____

Answer the following questions with hand calculations using the data presented in Table 33.2 or the SPSS dataset called "Exercise 33 Example 2.sav" available on the Evolve website. Follow your instructor's directions to submit your answers to the following questions for additional study. Your instructor may ask you to write your answers below and submit them as a hard copy for evaluation. Alternatively, your instructor may ask you to submit your answers online.

1. Do the example data meet the assumptions for the paired samples *t*-test? Provide a rationale for your answer.

2. If you have access to SPSS, compute the Shapiro-Wilk tests of normality for the two variables, baseline and follow-up GERD Health-Related Quality of Life (HRQL) questionnaire scores (as demonstrated in Exercise 27).

3. What are the means for the baseline and follow-up GERD HRQL questionnaire scores, respectively?

4. What is the paired samples *t*-test value?

5. Is the *t*-test significant at $\alpha = 0.05$? Use the table in Appendix A to specify how you arrived at your answer.

6. If using SPSS, what is the exact likelihood of obtaining a *t*-test value at least as extreme as or as close to the one that was actually observed, assuming that the null hypothesis is true?

7. On average, did the GERD HRQL scores improve or deteriorate over time? Provide a rationale for your answer.

8. Write your interpretation of the results as you would in an APA-formatted journal (American Psychological Association, 2020).

9. What do the results indicate regarding the effect of the removal of PPI s among persons with GERD?

10. What are the weaknesses of the design in this example?

Calculating the Mann-Whitney *U* Test

One of the most common nonparametric statistical tests chosen to investigate significant differences between two independent samples is the **Mann-Whitney *U* test**. When assumptions are not met for an independent samples *t*-test, such as equal group variances and/or non-normality, the Mann-Whitney *U* test is an appropriate alternative (Terrell, 2021). The samples are independent if the study participants in one group are unrelated or different participants than those in the second group. Exercise 12 provides an algorithm that will assist you in determining whether the Mann-Whitney *U* is an appropriate statistical technique. It should be noted that the Mann-Whitney *U* test is also known as the **Wilcoxon rank-sum test**, which is not to be confused with the **Wilcoxon signed-rank test**, which is covered in Exercise 22.

RESEARCH DESIGNS APPROPRIATE FOR THE MANN-WHITNEY *U* TEST

Research designs that may use the Mann-Whitney *U* test include the randomized experimental, quasi-experimental, and comparative designs (Gray & Grove, 2021; Gliner et al., 2017). The independent variable (the *grouping* variable) may be active or attributional. An **active independent variable** refers to an intervention, treatment, or program. An **attributional independent variable** refers to a characteristic of the participant, such as gender, diagnosis, or ethnicity. Regardless of the nature of the independent variable, the Mann-Whitney *U* test only compares two groups at a time.

Example 1: Researchers conduct a randomized experimental study where the participants are randomized to either a novel weight loss intervention or a placebo. The number of pounds lost from baseline to posttreatment for both groups is measured. The research question is: *Is there a difference between the two groups in weight loss?* The active independent variable is the weight loss intervention, and the dependent variable is the number of pounds lost over the treatment span. The frequency distribution of the dependent variable significantly deviates from normality.

Null hypothesis: *There is no difference in weight loss between the intervention group exposed to a novel weight loss program and the comparison (placebo) group receiving a standard diet.*

Example 2: Researchers conduct a retrospective comparative descriptive study where a chart review of patients is done to identify patients who recently underwent a colonoscopy. The patients were divided into two groups: those who used statin drugs continuously in the past year, and those who did not. The dependent variable is the number of polyps found during the colonoscopy, and the independent variable is statin drug use. The frequency distribution of the dependent variable significantly deviates from normality. The research question is: *Is there a difference between the statin drug users and nonusers in number of colon polyps found?*

Null hypothesis: *There is no difference between the group taking statin drugs versus the group not taking statins (control) in number of colon polyps found.*

STATISTICAL FORMULA AND ASSUMPTIONS

Unlike the independent samples *t*-test, the use of the Mann-Whitney *U* test makes no assumptions regarding the variances or the distributions of the data. The only assumption required by the Mann-Whitney *U* test is that all observations within each sample are independent (Daniel, 2000).

To calculate the value of *U*, the data of both samples are combined, and each data value is assigned a rank. The lowest value is ranked 1, the next value is ranked 2, and so forth until all values are ranked, regardless from which sample the score was obtained. The idea is that if two distributions came from the same population, the average of the ranks of values would be equal as well.

When calculating the Mann-Whitney *U* by hand, one must compute *two U* values, and choose the smallest of the two *U* values when determining significance of the result (Daniel, 2000). Therefore when reporting the Mann-Whitney *U* test results, researchers should identify the sample size of each of the independent groups, the value of the *z* statistic (converted from the smallest *U* value) and its associated *p* value, and the medians for the two groups (Terrell, 2021). The *z* statistic for the Mann-Whitney *U* test represents the extent to which the two groups differ on the dependent variable. The higher the *z* statistic, the more likely the groups significantly differ on the values of the dependent variable (Gray & Grove, 2021).

A median can be more informative than a mean in describing a variable when the variable's frequency distribution is positively or negatively skewed. Although the mean is sensitive to or increases or decreases based on the values of the outliers, the median is relatively unaffected (see Exercises 27 and 28).

The formula for the Mann-Whitney *U* test is:

$$U = \sum R - \frac{n(n+1)}{2}$$

where
R = the ranked values

n = sample size for one group

As noted previously, one must apply this *U* formula twice: once for each of the two groups. Therefore when computing the *U* by hand, one must compute *two U* values.

HAND CALCULATIONS

Deng and colleagues (2021) conducted a cross-sectional study (*n* = 260) to describe and compare fear of childbirth, in-labor pain intensity, and pain relief between primipara and multipara women living in Guangzhou, China. A simulated subset (*n* = 10) was created for this example so that the computations would be small and manageable (Table 34.1). In actuality, studies involving Mann-Whitney *U* tests need to be adequately powered, as determined by a power analysis (Aberson, 2019; Cohen, 1988). See Exercises 24 and 25 for more information regarding statistical power.

The independent variable in this example is primipara (i.e., the individual had given birth for the first time) in group 1 or multipara (i.e., the individual had given birth more than once) in group 2. The dependent variable was the duration (hours) of analgesia during labor. The null hypothesis is: *There is no difference between the primipara and multipara groups on the duration of analgesia during labor.*

TABLE 34.1   DURATION OF LABOR ANALGESIA BY GROUP

Primipara Group		Multipara Group	
Participant #	**Duration of Labor Analgesia**	**Participant #**	**Duration of Labor Analgesia**
1	6.20	6	5.20
2	8.10	7	6.30
3	19.00	8	2.50
4	19.40	9	3.30
5	7.20	10	2.30

The computations for the Mann-Whitney *U* test are as follows:

Step 1: Rank-order the dependent variable, regardless of group or condition.

Group	Ordered Value, Lowest to Highest	Assigned Rank
2	2.30	1
2	2.50	2
2	3.30	3
2	5.20	4
1	6.20	5
2	6.30	6
1	7.20	7
1	8.10	8
1	19.00	9
1	19.40	10

Step 2: Add the ranks for each group separately.

Primipara group (group 1): 5 + 7 + 8 + 9 + 10 = 39

Multipara group (group 2): 1 + 2 + 3 + 4 + 6 = 16

Step 3: Compute U_1 where ΣR_1 = the sum of ranks for group 1 and $n_1 = n$ for group 1. It should be noted that it does not matter which of the groups is assigned "group 1" and "group 2." In this example, the primipara group is coded as "1" and the multipara group is coded as "2," but the results would not differ if these designations were to be switched.

$$U_1 = \sum R_1 - \frac{n_1(n_1+1)}{2}$$

$$U_1 = 39 - \frac{5(5+1)}{2}$$

$$U_1 = 39 - 15$$

$$U_1 = 24$$

Step 4: Compute U_2 where ΣR_2 = the sum of ranks for group 2 and $n_2 = n$ for group 2

$$U_2 = \sum R_2 - \frac{n_2(n_2+1)}{2}$$

$$U_2 = 16 - \frac{5(5+1)}{2}$$

$$U_2 = 16 - 15$$

$$U_2 = 1$$

Step 5: Choose the *smaller* of the U values for your observed U.

The two computed U values are 24 and 1, respectively. The smaller U is 1.

Step 6: Compare the observed (calculated) U to the tabled critical U (Plichta & Kelvin, 2013, pp. 523–524). If the observed U is *smaller* than the critical U, then the observed U is statistically significant and indicates a difference between the two groups. The critical U value for $n_1 = 5$ and $n_2 = 5$ at alpha (α) = 0.05 is 2, and the observed (smaller) U value is 1. Therefore the U is statistically significant and represents a real difference between the two groups. Therefore we can reject the null hypothesis: *There is no difference between the primipara and multipara groups on the duration of analgesia during labor.*

SPSS COMPUTATIONS

This is how the dataset looks in SPSS.

	ID	Group	DurationAnalgesia	var
1	1	1	6.20	
2	2	1	8.10	
3	3	1	19.00	
4	4	1	19.40	
5	5	1	7.20	
6	6	2	5.20	
7	7	2	6.30	
8	8	2	2.50	
9	9	2	3.30	
10	10	2	2.30	
11				

Step 1: From the "Analyze" menu, choose "Nonparametric Tests," "Legacy Dialogs," and "2 Independent Samples." Move the dependent variable, "Duration Analgesia" (duration of labor analgesia), over to the right as shown and click "OK."

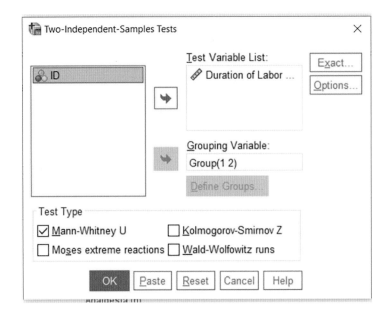

Step 2: Move the independent variable, group, into the space titled "Grouping Variable." Click "Define Groups" and enter "1" and "2" to represent the coding chosen to differentiate between the two groups. Click "Continue" and "OK."

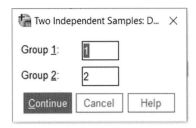

INTERPRETATION OF SPSS OUTPUT

The following tables are generated from SPSS. The first table contains descriptive statistics for duration of labor analgesia, separated by the two groups. The second table contains the Mann-Whitney *U* test results.

NPar Tests

Mann-Whitney Test

Ranks

	Group	N	Mean Rank	Sum of Ranks
Duration of Labor Analgesia (h)	Primiparas	5	7.80	39.00
	Multiparas	5	3.20	16.00
	Total	10		

Observe the mean ranks (not the mean original values) for the two groups

The first table displays descriptive statistics that allow us to observe the mean ranks for both groups. This table does not display the means of the original values, because nonparametric tests assume potentially non-normally distributed data. Recall that the mean is sensitive to increases or decreases based on the values of the outliers (Exercises 27 and 28). This table is important because it indicates that the participants in the primipara group had a mean rank of 7.80, and the participants in the multipara group had a mean rank of 3.20, indicating that the primipara group had the higher ranked values of labor analgesia durations. The *median* labor analgesia duration for the primipara group was 8.10, compared with 3.30 for the multipara group.

Test Statistics[a]

	Duration of La-bor Analgesia (h)
Mann-Whitney U	1.000
Wilcoxon W	16.000
Z	-2.402
Asymp. Sig. (2-tailed)	.016
Exact Sig. [2*(1-tailed Sig.)]	.016[b]

a. Grouping Variable: Group

b. Not corrected for ties.

Note that only the smallest of the two *U* values is reported here

The exact *p* value is the correct *p* to report for small samples

The second table contains the Mann-Whitney *U* test value, the *z* statistic, and two *p* values. Note that only the smallest of the two *U* values is reported here (1.0). The *z* statistic, which was created with a formula involving the smallest of the *U* values and sums of ranks, is often reported in published articles instead of the *U* value. The first *p* value ($p = 0.016$) is the asymptotic *p* value for large samples. The last *p* value ($p = 0.016$) is an exact *p* value and is the more appropriate *p* to report for small samples. Sometimes these values slightly differ, and other times these values are the same, as in this example. The exact two-sided *p* value is 0.016, otherwise known as the probability of obtaining a statistical value at least as extreme or close to the one that was actually observed, assuming that the null hypothesis is true.

In this example, the two-sided *p* value (also known as *two-tailed p value*) is being reported instead of the one-sided *p* value. This is because the one-sided *p* value only allows for a one-sided or directional hypothesis, where the hypothesized difference is only tested in one direction or one tail of the normal curve. For a two-sided test, we allow for the possibility that one group could either be higher or lower than the other group on the dependent variable. Because the exact two-sided *p* value is 0.016, which is less than the alpha of 0.05, we can reject our null hypothesis (Gray & Grove, 2021).

FINAL INTERPRETATION IN AMERICAN PSYCHOLOGICAL ASSOCIATION FORMAT

The following interpretation is written as it might appear in a research article, formatted according to American Psychological Association (APA) guidelines (2020). It should be noted that all statistical values reported here are rounded to two decimal places, with the exception of the *p* value, which is rounded to three decimal places.

A Mann-Whitney *U* test revealed that the primipara group had a significantly longer duration of labor analgesia than the multipara group, $z = -2.40$, $p = 0.016$, *Mdn* = 8.10 versus 3.30 hours, respectively. Thus parity may have an influence on the duration of labor analgesia and associated pain management. Further research is needed in this area.

STUDY QUESTIONS

1. Use SPSS to obtain the frequency distribution and skewness statistic for duration of labor analgesia as demonstrated in Exercise 27. What do the results indicate?

2. Use SPSS to compute the Shapiro-Wilk test of normality for the dependent variable, duration of labor analgesia in hours (h), as demonstrated in Exercise 27. What do the results indicate?

3. Do the data meet criteria for independent samples? Provide a rationale for your response.

4. What is the null hypothesis in this example?

5. Use SPSS to determine the exact likelihood of obtaining a *U* value at least as extreme or close to the one that was actually observed, assuming that the null hypothesis is true. Report the answer as a percentage.

6. What scale of measurement is used for the duration of labor analgesia?

7. Why were medians reported in the interpretation of the results instead of means?

8. If the dependent variable duration of labor analgesia was normally distributed, what would be the appropriate statistic to compare the two groups?

9. What kind of design was implemented in the example? Does this design allow causal statements to be made for the effect of number of births on labor analgesia and pain management?

10. Was the sample size adequate to detect differences between the two groups in this example? Provide a rationale for your answer.

Answers to Study Questions

1. As shown here, the frequency distribution appears to be non-normally distributed. The skewness statistic is 1.359, indicating substantial positive skewness.

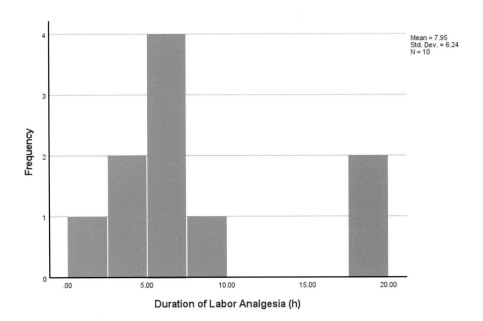

Statistics

Duration of Labor Analgesia (h)

N	Valid	10
	Missing	0
Skewness		1.359
Std. Error of Skewness		.687

2. As shown here, the Shapiro-Wilk *p* value for duration of labor analgesia in hours (h) was 0.008, indicating that the distribution significantly deviated from normality.

Tests of Normality

	Kolmogorov-Smirnov[a]			Shapiro-Wilk		
	Statistic	df	Sig.	Statistic	df	Sig.
Duration of Labor Analgesia (h)	.290	10	.017	.779	10	.008

a. Lilliefors Significance Correction

3. Yes, the data meet criteria for independent samples because the dependent variable data were collected from two mutually exclusive groups of study participants. In addition, the definition of the independent variable (primipara versus multipara) specifies that a participant must belong to either one category or the other, which makes the groups independent (Grove & Gray, 2023).

4. The null hypothesis is: *There is no difference between the primipara and multipara groups on the duration of analgesia during labor (in hours).*

5. The exact likelihood of obtaining a *U* value at least as extreme or close to the one that was actually observed, assuming that the null hypothesis is true, is 1.60%. This value can be found in the "Test Statistics" table in the SPSS output, where the exact *p* value is reported as 0.016. The value is calculated as follows: $0.016 \times 100\% = 1.60\%$.

6. The variable duration of labor analgesia is defined as the number of hours elapsed when analgesia was used. Because number of hours has numerically equal intervals and an absolute zero point, it is considered a ratio (see Exercise 1; Grove & Gray, 2023).

7. Medians are reported instead of means because the data were non-normally distributed. When the dependent variable is non-normally distributed, a nonparametric test is more appropriate. Moreover, a median can be more informative than a mean in describing a variable when the variable's frequency distribution is positively or negatively skewed. Although the mean is sensitive to or increases or decreases based on the values of the outliers, the median is relatively unaffected (see Exercises 27 and 28).

8. If duration of labor analgesia was normally distributed, the appropriate statistic to compare the two groups would be the independent samples *t*-test. The duration of labor analgesia was measured in hours, which is ratio-level data. As described earlier, the two groups are independent. Thus the independent samples *t*-test is the appropriate analysis technique to conduct if the data were normally distributed (Gray & Grove, 2021; Waltz et al., 2017).

9. The study design in the example was a cross-sectional quasi-experimental design. The independent variable (primipara versus multipara) was an attributional independent variable because it was a characteristic of the participant. No, this kind of design does not allow causal statements to be made for the effect of parity on labor analgesia and pain management. However, the findings of this study can serve as a foundation for a larger and more in-depth study of the association between parity and analgesic/pain management needs (Gliner et al., 2017; Kazdin, 2022).

10. The sample size was adequate to detect differences between the two groups because a significant difference was found, $p = 0.016$. However, this sample is considered small, and as emphasized in Exercises 24 and 25, it is strongly recommended that a power analysis be conducted before the study begins in order to avoid the risk of Type II error (Aberson, 2019; Cohn, 1988; Taylor & Spurlock, 2018).

DATA FOR ADDITIONAL COMPUTATIONAL PRACTICE

This example involves additional data collected in the same study by Deng et al. (2021). The independent variable in this example is primipara (i.e., the individual had given birth for the first time) or multipara (i.e., the individual had given birth more than once). The dependent variable was hourly analgesic consumption (milliliters per hour, or mL/h) during labor. The null hypothesis is: *There is no difference between the primipara and multipara groups on hourly analgesic consumption during labor.* A simulated subset of 10 observations was created for this example. The data are presented in Table 34.2.

TABLE 34.2   HOURLY ANALGESIC CONSUMPTION BY GROUP

Primipara Group		Multipara Group	
Participant #	Hourly Analgesic Consumption	Participant #	Hourly Analgesic Consumption
1	12.79	6	15.88
2	14.37	7	16.12
3	10.46	8	27.19
4	11.28	9	27.43
5	10.68	10	15.22

Questions for Additional Study

<table>
<tr><td>Name:</td><td>Class:</td></tr>
<tr><td>Date:</td><td></td></tr>
</table>

Answer the following questions with hand calculations using the data presented in Table 34.2 or the SPSS dataset called "Exercise 34 Example 2.sav" available on the Evolve website. Follow your instructor's directions to submit your answers to the following questions for additional study. Your instructor may ask you to write your answers below and submit them as a hard copy for evaluation. Alternatively, your instructor may ask you to submit your answers online.

1. Use SPSS to obtain the frequency distribution and skewness statistic for the dependent variable of hourly analgesic consumption (mL/h), as demonstrated in Exercise 27. What do the results indicate?

2. Use SPSS to compute the Shapiro-Wilk test of normality for the dependent variable, hourly analgesic consumption (mL/h), as demonstrated in Exercise 27. What do the results indicate?

3. Compute the Mann-Whitney *U* test using the formula provided. List the *U* value for the primipara group.

4. Compute the Mann-Whitney *U* test using the formula provided. List the *U* value for the multipara group.

5. Is the Mann-Whitney *U* test significant at $\alpha = 0.05$? Specify how you arrived at your answer.

6. Use SPSS to determine the exact likelihood of obtaining a *U* value at least as extreme or as close to the one that was actually observed, assuming that the null hypothesis is true. Report as a percentage.

7. Identify the median hourly analgesic consumption (mL/h) for each group (primipara and multipara). Show your work.

8. Write your interpretation of the results as you would in an APA-formatted journal (American Psychological Association, 2020).

9. Collectively, what do the results from the two computational examples (duration of labor analgesia and hourly analgesic consumption) indicate regarding the effect of parity on pain management during labor?

10. Was the sample size adequate to detect significant differences between the two groups in this example? Provide a rationale for your answer.

Calculating Analysis of Variance (ANOVA) and Post Hoc Analyses After ANOVA

Analysis of variance (ANOVA) is a statistical procedure that compares data between two or more groups or conditions to investigate the presence of differences between those groups on some continuous dependent variable (see Exercise 18). In this exercise, we will focus on the **one-way ANOVA**, which involves testing one independent variable and one dependent variable (as opposed to other types of ANOVAs, such as factorial ANOVAs that incorporate multiple independent variables).

Why ANOVA and not a *t*-test? Remember that a *t*-test is formulated to compare two sets of data or two groups at one time (see Exercise 23 for guidance on selecting appropriate statistics). Thus data generated from a clinical trial that involves four groups—treatment 1, treatment 2, treatments 1 and 2 combined, and a control—would require six *t*-tests. Consequently, the chance of making a Type I error (alpha error) increases substantially (or is inflated) because so many computations are being performed. Specifically, the chance of making a Type I error is the number of comparisons multiplied by the alpha level. Thus ANOVA is the recommended statistical technique for examining differences between more than two groups (Tabachnick & Fidell, 2019; Zar, 2010).

ANOVA is a procedure that culminates in a value called the *F* statistic. It is this value that is compared against an *F* distribution (see Appendix C) to determine whether the groups significantly differ from one another on the dependent variable. The formulas for ANOVA actually compute two estimates of variance: one estimate represents differences between the groups/conditions, and the other estimate represents differences among (within) the data.

RESEARCH DESIGNS APPROPRIATE FOR THE ONE-WAY ANOVA

Research designs that may use the one-way ANOVA include the randomized experimental, quasi-experimental, and comparative designs (Gliner et al., 2017). The independent variable (the grouping variable for the ANOVA) may be active or attributional. An active independent variable refers to an intervention, treatment, or program. An attributional independent variable refers to a characteristic of the participant, such as gender, diagnosis, or ethnicity. The ANOVA can compare two groups or more. In the case of a two-group design, the researcher can either select an independent samples *t*-test or a one-way ANOVA to answer the research question. The results will always yield the same conclusion, regardless of which test is computed; however, when examining differences between more than two groups, the one-way ANOVA is the preferred statistical test (Tabachnick & Fidell, 2019).

Example 1: A researcher conducts a randomized experimental study wherein she randomizes participants to receive a high-dosage weight loss pill, a low-dosage weight loss pill, or a placebo. She assesses the number of pounds lost from baseline to posttreatment for the three groups. Her research question is: *Is there a difference between the three groups in weight loss?*

The independent variables are the treatment conditions (high-dose weight loss pill, low-dose weight loss pill, and placebo) and the dependent variable is number of pounds lost over the treatment span.

Null hypothesis: *There is no difference in weight lost among the high-dose weight loss pill, low-dose weight loss pill, and placebo groups in a population of overweight adults.*

Example 2: A nurse researcher working in dermatology conducts a retrospective comparative study wherein she conducts a chart review of patients and divides them into three groups: psoriasis, psoriatic symptoms, or control. The dependent variable is health status, and the independent variable is disease group: psoriasis, psoriatic symptoms, and control. Her research question is: *Is there a difference between the three groups on levels of health status?*

Null hypothesis: *There is no difference in health status among the psoriasis, psoriatic, and control groups of selected patients.*

STATISTICAL FORMULA AND ASSUMPTIONS

Use of the ANOVA involves the following assumptions (Zar, 2010):

1. Sample means from the population are normally distributed.
2. The groups are mutually exclusive.
3. The dependent variable is measured at the interval/ratio level.
4. The groups should have equal variance, termed *homogeneity of variance*.
5. All observations within each sample are independent.

The dependent variable in an ANOVA must be scaled as interval or ratio. If the dependent variable is measured with a Likert scale and the frequency distribution is approximately normally distributed, these data are usually considered interval-level measurements and are appropriate for an ANOVA (see Exercise 1; de Winter & Dodou, 2010; Rasmussen, 1989; Waltz et al., 2017).

The basic formula for the F without numerical symbols is:

$$F = \frac{\text{Mean Square Between Groups}}{\text{Mean Square Within Groups}}$$

The term *mean square* (*MS*) is used interchangeably with the word *variance*. The formulas for ANOVA compute two estimates of variance: the between-groups variance and the within-groups variance. The **between-groups variance** represents differences between the groups/conditions being compared, and the **within-groups variance** represents differences among (within) each group's data. Therefore the formula is $F = MS$ between$/MS$ within.

HAND CALCULATIONS

This example involves a study of patients with inflammatory bowel disease (IBD) who underwent various types of treatment for prostate cancer (Feagins et al., 2020). A retrospective multisite cohort study investigated three different types of treatment received for prostate cancer among persons with IBD: external radiotherapy (XRT), brachytherapy (a type of internal radiation therapy), or treatments that did not involve radiation, such as chemotherapy and hormonal therapy. Persons in the nonradiation group received hormonal therapy, chemotherapy, both hormonal and chemotherapy, or some other type of treatment that did not involve radiation.

The data are presented in Table 35.1. A simulated subset was selected for this example so that the computations would be small and manageable. In actuality, studies involving one-way

TABLE 35.1   GLEASON SCORES BY TREATMENT GROUP FOR PATIENTS WITH INFLAMMATORY BOWEL DISEASE AND PROSTATE CANCER

Participant#	XRT	Participant #	Brachytherapy	Participant #	Nonradiation
1	7	11	7	21	6
2	9	12	8	22	5
3	6	13	5	23	8
4	8	14	5	24	7
5	8	15	6	25	6
6	6	16	7	26	4
7	9	17	6	27	7
8	7	18	5	28	5
9	7	19	5	29	6
10	6	20	7	30	6

XRT, external radiotherapy.

ANOVAs need to be adequately powered (Aberson, 2019; Cohen, 1988). See Exercises 24 and 25 for more information regarding statistical power.

The independent variable in this example is type of treatment (XRT, brachytherapy, or nonradiation treatment), and the dependent variable is a grading score related to prostate cancer cells, the Gleason score. The Gleason score ranges from 2 to 10, with higher numbers reflecting faster cancer growth and aggression (Prostate Cancer Foundation, 2022).

The null hypothesis is: *There is no difference between the treatment groups (XRT, brachytherapy, and nonradiation treatment) on prostate cancer grading scores among persons with IBD.*

The computations for the ANOVA are as follows:

Step 1: Compute correction term, C.

Square the grand sum (G), and divide by total N:

$$C = \frac{194^2}{30} = 1254.53$$

Step 2: Compute the Total sum of squares (SS).

Square every value in dataset, sum, and subtract C:

$$(7^2 + 9^2 + 6^2 + 8^2 + 8^2 + 6^2 + 6^2 + \cdots 6^2) - 1254.53$$

$$= 1300.00 - 1254.53 = 45.47$$

Step 3: Compute Between-groups sum of squares.

Square the sum of each column and divide by N. Add each, and then subtract C:

$$\frac{73^2}{10} + \frac{61^2}{10} + \frac{60^2}{10} - 1020.83$$

$$(532.90 + 372.10 + 360.00) - 1254.53 = 10.47$$

Step 4: Compute Within-groups sum of squares.

Subtract the between-groups sum of squares (Step 3) from Total sum of squares (Step 2):

$$45.47 - 10.47 = 35.00$$

TABLE 35.2 ANOVA SUMMARY TABLE				
Source of Variation	**SS**	**df**	**MS**	**F**
Between groups	10.47	2	5.24	4.03
Within groups	35.00	27	1.30	
Total	45.47	29		

Step 5: Create ANOVA summary table (see Table 35.2).

a. Insert the sum of squares values in the first column.

b. The degrees of freedom (*df*) are in the second column. Because the *F* is a ratio of two separate statistics (mean square between groups and mean square within groups) both have different *df* formulas—one for the *numerator* and one for the *denominator*:

$$\text{Mean square between-groups } df = \text{number of groups} - 1$$

$$\text{Mean square within-groups } df = N - \text{number of groups}$$

For this example, the *df* for the numerator is $3 - 1 = 2$.

The *df* for the denominator is $30 - 3 = 27$.

c. The mean square between groups and mean square within groups are in the third column. These values are computed by dividing the *SS* by the *df*. Therefore the *MS* between $= 10.47 \div 2 = 5.235$ rounded to 5.24. The *MS* within $= 35.00 \div 27 = 1.30$.

d. The *F* is the final column and is computed by dividing the *MS* between by the *MS* within. Therefore $F = 5.24 \div 1.30 = 4.03$.

Step 6: Locate the critical *F* value on the *F* distribution table (see Appendix C) and compare it to our obtained $F = 4.03$ value. The critical *F* value for 2 and 27 *df* at $\alpha = 0.05$ is 3.35, which indicates the *F* value in this example exceeds the critical value in the table. Thus the *F* is statistically significant and the population means are not equal. Therefore we can reject our null hypothesis that *the three groups do not differ on prostate cancer grading scores among persons with IBD*. However, the *F* does not indicate which groups differ from one another, and this *F* value does not identify which groups are significantly different from one another. Further testing, termed *multiple comparison tests* or *post hoc tests*, is required to complete the ANOVA process and determine all the significant differences among the study groups (Field, 2013; Tabachnick & Fidell, 2019).

Post Hoc Tests

Post hoc tests have been developed specifically to determine the location of group differences after ANOVA is performed on data from more than two groups. These tests were developed to reduce the incidence of a Type I error. Frequently used post hoc tests are the Newman-Keuls test, the Tukey Honestly Significant Difference (HSD) test, the Scheffé test, and the Dunnett test (Zar, 2010; see Exercise 18 for examples). When these tests are calculated, the alpha level is reduced in proportion to the number of additional tests required to locate statistically significant differences. For example, for several of the aforementioned post hoc tests, if many groups' mean values are being compared, the magnitude of the difference is set higher than if only two groups are being compared. Thus post hoc tests are tedious to perform by hand and are best handled with statistical computer software programs. Accordingly, the rest of this example will be presented with the assistance of SPSS.

SPSS COMPUTATIONS

This is how our dataset looks in SPSS.

	ParticipantID	TreatmentGroup	Gleasonscore	va
1	1	1	7	
2	2	1	9	
3	3	1	6	
4	4	1	8	
5	5	1	8	
6	6	1	6	
7	7	1	9	
8	8	1	7	
9	9	1	7	
10	10	1	6	
11	11	2	7	
12	12	2	8	
13	13	2	5	
14	14	2	5	
15	15	2	6	
16	16	2	7	

Data View Variable View

Step 1: Because the dependent variable, Gleason score, is measured ordinally, it must be examined for normality prior to submitting the data for a one-way ANOVA. Normality will be examined for all treatment groups, and within each treatment group. As reviewed in Exercise 27, from the "Analyze" menu, choose "Descriptive Statistics" and "Explore." Move Gleason score over to the box labeled "Dependent List." Click "Plots." Check "Normality plots with tests." Click "Continue" and "OK." As shown, the distribution of Gleason scores did not significantly deviate from normality according to the Shapiro-Wilk test ($p = 0.081$).

Tests of Normality

	Kolmogorov-Smirnov[a]			Shapiro-Wilk		
	Statistic	df	Sig.	Statistic	df	Sig.
Gleason Score Post-Treatment	.179	30	.016	.938	30	.081

a. Lilliefors Significance Correction

Step 2: Subsequently, normality of the Gleason scores will be examined within each treatment group. From the "Analyze" menu, choose "Descriptive Statistics" and "Explore." Move Gleason score over to the box labeled "Dependent List" and move "Treatment Group" over to the box labeled "Factor List." Click "Plots." Check "Normality plots with tests." Click "Continue" and "OK."

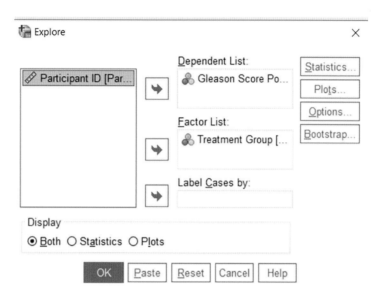

As shown, the distribution of Gleason scores did not significantly deviate from normality for any of the groups according to the Shapiro-Wilk test, with *p* values ranging from 0.067 for the brachytherapy group to 0.703 for the nonradiation group. Therefore we will proceed with the one-way ANOVA analysis.

Tests of Normality

	Treatment Group	Kolmogorov-Smirnov[a]			Shapiro-Wilk		
		Statistic	df	Sig.	Statistic	df	Sig.
Gleason Score Post-Treatment	XRT	.202	10	.200*	.878	10	.124
	Brachytherapy	.241	10	.103	.855	10	.067
	Non-Radiation	.200	10	.200*	.953	10	.703

*. This is a lower bound of the true significance.

a. Lilliefors Significance Correction

Step 3: From the "Analyze" menu, choose "Compare Means" and "One-Way ANOVA." Move the dependent variable, "Gleason Score", over to the right, as shown.

Step 4: Move the independent variable, "Treatment Group", to the right in the space labeled "Factor."

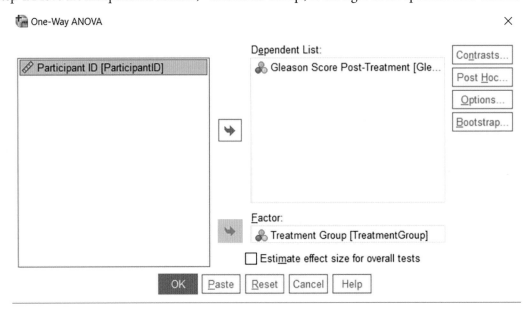

Step 5: Click "Options." Check the boxes next to "Descriptive" and "Homogeneity of variance test." Click "Continue" and "OK."

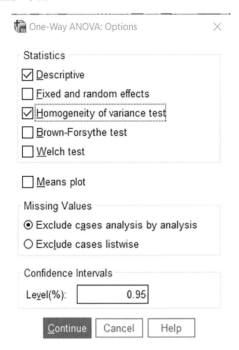

INTERPRETATION OF SPSS OUTPUT

The following tables are generated from SPSS. The first table contains descriptive statistics for Gleason score, separated by the three groups. The second table contains the Levene's test of homogeneity of variances. The third table contains the ANOVA summary table, along with the F and p values.

The first table displays descriptive statistics that allow us to observe the means for the three groups. This table is important because it indicates that the patients who received XRT had a mean Gleason score of 7.30, compared with 6.10 for patients who received brachytherapy, and 6.00 for patients who received nonradiation treatment. Recall that the higher the Gleason score, the more aggressive and rapid growing are the prostate cancer cells.

Oneway

Descriptives

Gleason Score Post-Treatment

	N	Mean	Std. Deviation	Std. Error	95% Confidence Interval for Mean Lower Bound	95% Confidence Interval for Mean Upper Bound	Minimum	Maximum
XRT	10	7.30	1.160	.367	6.47	8.13	6	9
Brachytherapy	10	6.10	1.101	.348	5.31	6.89	5	8
Non-Radiation	10	6.00	1.155	.365	5.17	6.83	4	8
Total	30	6.47	1.252	.229	6.00	6.93	4	9

The second table contains the Levene's test for equality of variances. The Levene's test is a statistical test of the equal variances assumption (Field, 2013; Tabachnick & Fidell, 2019). As is shown on the first row of the table, the p value is 0.843, indicating there was no significant difference among the three groups' variances; thus the data have met the equal variances assumption for ANOVA.

Tests of Homogeneity of Variances

		Levene Statistic	df1	df2	Sig.
Gleason Score Post-Treatment	Based on Mean	.171	2	27	.843
	Based on Median	.067	2	27	.935
	Based on Median and with adjusted df	.067	2	25.338	.935
	Based on trimmed mean	.155	2	27	.857

The last table contains the contents of the ANOVA summary table, which looks much like Table 35.2. It should be noted that the F value of 4.037 in the output table differs slightly from our hand calculations of 4.03 because we used two decimal places in our hand calculations, while SPSS uses many decimals in computations and is therefore more accurate. Thus when reporting results, the values from the SPSS output should be reported because they have higher accuracy. This table also contains an additional value that we did not compute by hand—the exact p value, which is 0.029. Because the SPSS output indicates that we have a significant ANOVA, post hoc testing must be performed.

ANOVA

Gleason Score Post-Treatment

	Sum of Squares	df	Mean Square	F	Sig.
Between Groups	10.467	2	5.233	4.037	.029
Within Groups	35.000	27	1.296		
Total	45.467	29			

Return to the ANOVA window and click "Post Hoc." You will see a window similar to the one shown. Select the "LSD" and "Tukey" options. Click "Continue" and "OK."

The following output is added to the original output. This table contains post hoc test results for two different tests: the Least Significant Difference (LSD) test and the Tukey HSD test. The LSD test, the original post hoc test, explores all possible pairwise comparisons of means using the equivalent of multiple t-tests. However, the LSD test, in performing a set of multiple t-tests, may report inaccurate p values because they have not been adjusted for multiple computations (Zar, 2010). Consequently, researchers should exercise caution when choosing the LSD post hoc test after completing an ANOVA.

The Tukey HSD comparison test, on the other hand, is a more *conservative* test, meaning that it requires a larger difference between two groups to indicate a significant difference than some of the other post hoc tests available. By requiring a larger difference between the groups, the Tukey HSD procedure might yield more accurate p values to reflect the multiple comparisons (Kim et al., 2022; Zar, 2010).

Post Hoc Tests

Multiple Comparisons

Dependent Variable: Gleason Score Post-Treatment

	(I) Treatment Group	(J) Treatment Group	Mean Difference (I-J)	Std. Error	Sig.	95% Confidence Interval Lower Bound	95% Confidence Interval Upper Bound
Tukey HSD	XRT	Brachytherapy	1.200	.509	.065	-.06	2.46
		Non-Radiation	1.300*	.509	.043	.04	2.56
	Brachytherapy	XRT	-1.200	.509	.065	-2.46	.06
		Non-Radiation	.100	.509	.979	-1.16	1.36
	No Radiation	XRT	-1.300*	.509	.043	-2.56	-.04
		Brachytherapy	-.100	.509	.979	-1.36	1.16
LSD	XRT	Brachytherapy	1.200*	.509	.026	.16	2.24
		Non-Radiation	1.300*	.509	.017	.26	2.34
	Brachytherapy	XRT	-1.200*	.509	.026	-2.24	-.16
		Non-Radiation	.100	.509	.846	-.94	1.14
	No Radiation	XRT	-1.300*	.509	.017	-2.34	-.26
		Brachytherapy	-.100	.509	.846	-1.14	.94

*. The mean difference is significant at the 0.05 level.

Observe the "Mean Difference" column. Any difference noted with an asterisk (*) is significant at $p < 0.05$. The p values of each comparison are listed in the "Sig." column, and values below 0.05 indicate a significant difference between the pair of groups. Observe the p values for the comparison of the XRT group versus the brachytherapy group. The Tukey HSD test indicates no significant difference between the groups, with a p of 0.065; however, the LSD test indicates that the groups significantly differed, with a p of 0.026. This example enables you to see the difference in results obtained when calculating a conservative versus a lenient post hoc test. However, it should be noted that this simulated dataset is limited to 30 observations, and therefore it is a possibility that these analyses are underpowered. See Exercises 24 and 25 for more information regarding the consequences of low statistical power.

According to the Tukey HSD test results, the only significant difference that emerged was that of the XRT versus nonradiation comparison ($p = 0.043$). The difference between XRT and brachytherapy was not significant ($p = 0.065$), nor was the difference between brachytherapy and nonradiation ($p = 0.979$). According to the LSD test results, the difference between XRT and nonradiation was significant ($p = 0.017$), as was the difference between XRT and brachytherapy ($p = 0.026$). The difference between brachytherapy and nonradiation was not significant ($p = 0.846$).

FINAL INTERPRETATION IN AMERICAN PSYCHOLOGICAL ASSOCIATION FORMAT

The following interpretation is written as it might appear in a research article, formatted according to American Psychological Association (APA) guidelines (2020). It should be noted that all statistical values reported here are rounded to two decimal places, with the exception of the p value, which is rounded to three decimal places.

A one-way ANOVA performed on Gleason scores revealed significant differences among the three groups, $F(2,27) = 4.04$, $p = 0.029$. Post hoc comparisons using the Tukey HSD comparison test indicated that the patients who received XRT had significantly higher Gleason scores that those who received nonradiation treatment ($\bar{X} = 7.30$ versus 6.00, respectively). There were no significant differences in Gleason scores between the XRT group and the brachytherapy group ($\bar{X} = 7.30$ versus 6.10), nor between the brachytherapy group and the nonradiation group ($\bar{X} = 6.10$ versus 6.00).

It should be noted that the design of this study was a retrospective cohort study, and not a randomized controlled trial (RCT). Therefore our ability to make a causal link between the type of treatment received and the study outcomes is limited (Gliner et al., 2017). With cohort studies, there can be factors that affect the reasons why a person belongs to a particular cohort, and those factors can affect study outcomes (Celentano & Szklo, 2018). In RCTs, participants are randomly assigned to the treatment group, and this eliminates the aforementioned factors responsible for cohort membership (Gliner et al., 2017). For example, our results from this example indicate that persons receiving treatment that did not involve radiation had the lowest mean Gleason scores. Persons in the nonradiation group received hormonal therapy, chemotherapy, both hormonal and chemotherapy, or some other type of treatment that did not involve radiation. A certain type of treatment received by a person in the nonradiation group could have lowered the group's overall Gleason score. However, we would not be able to pinpoint the effect of this treatment unless we performed subsequent subgroup analyses. Ultimately there are a multitude of factors that could explain the differences between the groups in this retrospective cohort study.

STUDY QUESTIONS

1. What are the means for the three groups' Gleason scores, and why are those values important in the interpretation of the ANOVA results?

2. What are the two instances that must occur to warrant post hoc testing after an ANOVA?

3. Do the data in this example meet criteria for homogeneity of variance? Provide a rationale for your answer.

4. What is the null hypothesis in the example?

5. What was the exact likelihood of obtaining an F value at least as extreme as or as close to the one that was actually observed, assuming that the null hypothesis is true?

6. Do the data meet criteria for mutual exclusivity? Provide a rationale for your answer.

7. What does the numerator of the *F* ratio represent?

8. What does the denominator of the *F* ratio represent?

9. How would our final interpretation of the results have changed if we had chosen to report the LSD post hoc test instead of the Tukey HSD test? Rewrite the post hoc interpretation portion of the results.

10. Was the sample size adequate to detect differences among the three groups in this example? Provide a rationale for your answer.

Answers to Study Questions

1. The group means for XRT, brachytherapy, and nonradiation were 7.30, 6.10, and 6.00, respectively. The means are important because in any statistically significant findings, means indicate which group had the highest and lowest mean values. When writing the results of post hoc tests, group comparisons can be described with phrases like "significantly higher/more than" and "significantly lower/less than."

2. The two instances that must occur to warrant post hoc testing after an ANOVA are (1) the ANOVA was performed on data comparing more than two groups, and (2) the F value is statistically significant (Field, 2013; Tabachnick & Fidell, 2019).

3. Yes, the data met criteria for homogeneity of variance because the Levene's test for equality of variances yielded a p of 0.843 (see the "Tests of Homogeneity of Variances" table in this exercise), indicating no significant differences in variance between the groups.

4. The null hypothesis is: *There is no difference between the treatment groups (XRT, brachytherapy, and nonradiation treatment) on prostate cancer grading scores among persons with IBD.*

5. The exact likelihood of obtaining an F value at least as extreme as or as close to the one that was actually observed, assuming that the null hypothesis is true, is 2.90%. This value can be found in the "ANOVA" table in the SPSS output, where the exact p value is reported as 0.029. The value is calculated as follows: $0.029 \times 100\% = 2.90\%$.

6. Yes, the data met criteria for mutual exclusivity because a patient could only belong to one of the three cohorts of treatment (XRT, brachytherapy, or nonradiation). Patients who received more than one type of treatment were excluded from the study.

7. The numerator of the F ratio represents the between-groups variance or the differences between the groups/conditions being compared.

8. The denominator of the F ratio represents within-groups variance or the extent to which there is dispersion among the dependent variable's values.

9. The final interpretation of the results would have changed if we had chosen to report the LSD post hoc test instead of the Tukey HSD test. Review the results of the "Multiple Comparisons" table in this exercise to assist with the answer. The results of the LSD test indicated that the difference between XRT and nonradiation was significant ($p = 0.017$), as was the difference between XRT and brachytherapy ($p = 0.026$).

10. The sample size was most likely adequate to detect differences among the three groups overall because a significant difference was found, $p = 0.029$. However, there was a discrepancy between the results of the LSD post hoc test and the Tukey HSD test. The difference between the XRT and brachytherapy groups was significant according to the results of the LSD test but not the Tukey HSD test. Therefore it is possible that with only 30 participants in this example, the data were underpowered for the multiple comparisons after the ANOVA (Aberson, 2019; Cohen, 1988).

DATA FOR ADDITIONAL COMPUTATIONAL PRACTICE

Using the same simulated example from Feagins and colleagues (2020), a retrospective multisite cohort study investigated three different types of treatment received for prostate cancer among persons with IBD. The independent variable in this example is type of treatment (XRT, brachytherapy, or nonradiation treatment), and the dependent variable is the number (raw count) of IBD flares experienced by the patient during the span of 2 years posttreatment. An IBD flare is defined as a reappearance of IBD symptoms (Feagins et al., 2020).

The null hypothesis is: *There is no difference between the treatment groups (XRT, brachytherapy, and nonradiation treatment) on number of posttreatment IBD flares among persons with IBD.*

Compute the ANOVA on the data in Table 35.3.

TABLE 35.3   NUMBER OF INFLAMMATORY BOWEL DISEASE FLARES BY TREATMENT GROUP

Participant #	XRT	Participant #	Brachytherapy	Participant #	Nonradiation
1	5	11	5	21	1
2	3	12	2	22	2
3	2	13	5	23	2
4	4	14	4	24	0
5	3	15	3	25	2
6	4	16	4	26	3
7	7	17	7	27	3
8	3	18	3	28	2
9	2	19	6	29	1
10	6	20	1	30	3

XRT, external radiotherapy.

Name: _____ Class: _____

Date: _____

Answer the following questions with hand calculations using the data presented in Table 35.3 or the SPSS dataset called "Exercise 35 Example 2.sav" available on the Evolve website. Follow your instructor's directions to submit your answers to the following questions for additional study. Your instructor may ask you to write your answers below and submit them as a hard copy for evaluation. Alternatively, your instructor may ask you to submit your answers online.

1. Do the data meet criteria for homogeneity of variance? Provide a rationale for your answer.

2. Use SPSS to compute the Shapiro-Wilk test of normality for the dependent variable, number of posttreatment inflammatory bowel disease (IBD) flares. What do the results indicate?

3. What are the means for three treatment groups' numbers of IBD flares?

4. What are the *F* value and the group and error degrees of freedom (*df*) for this set of data?

5. Is the *F* significant at $\alpha = 0.05$? Specify how you arrived at your answer.

6. If using SPSS, what is the exact likelihood of obtaining an *F* value at least as extreme or close to the one that was actually observed, assuming that the null hypothesis is true?

7. Write your interpretation of the results as you would in an APA-formatted journal.

8. Is there a difference in your final interpretation when comparing the results of the Least Significant Difference (LSD) post hoc test versus the Tukey HSD test? Provide a rationale for your answer.

9. What was the design of the Feagins et al. (2020) study? How does the design of the study affect our ability to make causal statements about the type of treatment received by the patients?

10. If the researcher decided to combine the two groups that involved radiation to represent an overall radiation treatment group, then there would be two groups to compare: radiation treatment versus nonradiation treatment. What would be the appropriate statistic to address the difference in number of posttreatment IBD flares between the two groups? Provide a rationale for your answer.

Calculating Sensitivity and Specificity

An important part of building evidence-based practice is the ability to differentiate between people who have a disease and those who do not. This is accomplished by using the most accurate and precise measure or test to promote quality outcomes. Regardless of whether the test is used by clinicians or researchers, the same issue is raised—how good is the screening test in separating patients with and without a disease? This question is best answered by current, quality research to determine the sensitivity and specificity of the test (Celentano & Szklo, 2018).

The accuracy of a screening test or a test used to confirm a diagnosis is evaluated in terms of its ability to correctly assess the presence or absence of a disease or condition compared with a gold standard. The **gold standard** is the most accurate means of currently diagnosing a particular disease and serves as a basis for comparison with newly developed diagnostic or screening tests (Campo et al., 2010; Celentano & Szklo, 2018). As shown in Table 36.1, there are four possible outcomes of a screening test for a disease: (1) **sensitivity**, or true positive, which accurately identifies the presence of a disease; (2) **false positive**, which indicates a disease is present when it is not; (3) **specificity**, or true negative, which indicates accurately that a disease is not present; or (4) **false negative**, which indicates that a disease is not present when it is (Celentano & Szklo, 2018; Straus et al., 2019).

STATISTICAL FORMULA AND ASSUMPTIONS

Sensitivity and Specificity

Sensitivity and specificity can be calculated based on research findings and clinical practice outcomes to determine the most accurate diagnostic or screening tool to use in identifying the presence or absence of a disease for a population of patients. The calculations for sensitivity and specificity are provided as follows. Table 36.2 displays the following notation to assist the researcher in calculating the sensitivity and specificity of a screening test, where:

TABLE 36.1 RESULTS OF SENSITIVITY AND SPECIFICITY OF SCREENING TESTS

	Disease Present	Disease Not Present
Positive test	True positive = sensitivity	False positive
Negative test	False negative	True negative = specificity

TABLE 36.2 STRUCTURE OF DATA FOR SENSITIVITY AND SPECIFICITY CALCULATIONS

	Disease Present	Disease Not Present
Positive test	a	b
Negative test	c	d

a = The number of people who have the disease and the test is positive (true positive)

b = The number of people who do not have the disease and the test is positive (false positive)

c = The number of people who have the disease and the test is negative (false negative)

d = The number of people who do not have the disease and the test is negative (true negative)

The disease variable (present/absent) is often called the *state* variable. It is always dichotomous. The screening test variable can be either dichotomous or continuous (such as a lab value). If the screening test is continuous, sensitivity and specificity are repeatedly calculated for each individual test value (Melnyk & Fineout-Overholt, 2023; Straus et al., 2019).

Sensitivity calculation = probability of having the disease

$$= a/(a + c)$$

= true positive rate

Specificity calculation = probability of the absence of disease

$$= d/(b + d)$$

= true negative rate

False positive calculation = probability of no disease but having a positive test

$$= b/(b + d)$$

= false positive rate

False negative calculation = probability of having the disease but having a negative test

$$= c/(c + a)$$

= false negative rate

Sensitivity is the proportion of patients with the disease who have a positive test result, or true positive. The ways the researcher or clinician might refer to the test sensitivity include the following:

- A highly sensitive test is very good at identifying the patient with a disease.
- If a test is highly sensitive, it has a low percentage of false negatives.
- A low-sensitivity test is limited in identifying the patient with a disease.
- If a test has low sensitivity, it has a high percentage of false negatives.
- If a sensitive test has negative results, the patient is less likely to have the disease.

Specificity of a screening or diagnostic test is the proportion of patients without the disease who have a negative test result, or true negative. The ways the researcher or clinician might refer to the test specificity include the following:

- A highly specific test is very good at identifying patients without a disease.
- If a test is very specific, it has a low percentage of false positives.
- A low-specificity test is limited in identifying patients without a disease.
- If a test has low specificity, it has a high percentage of false positives.
- If a specific test has positive results, the patient is more likely to have the disease.

Likelihood Ratios

Likelihood ratios (LRs) are additional calculations that can help researchers to determine the accuracy of diagnostic or screening tests, which are based on the sensitivity and specificity results. LRs are calculated to determine the likelihood that a positive test result is a true positive and a negative test result is a true negative.

The ratio of the true positive results to false positive results is known as the **positive LR** (Melnyk & Fineout-Overholt, 2023). The positive LR is calculated as follows:

Positive LR = Sensitivity ÷ (1 – Specificity)

The ratio of true negative results to false negative results is known as the **negative LR**, and it is calculated as follows:

Negative LR = (1 – Sensitivity) ÷ Specificity

A LR greater than 1.0 represents an increase in the likelihood of the disease, while a LR of less than 1.0 represents a decrease in the likelihood of the disease. The very high LRs (or LRs that are >10) rule in the disease or indicate that the patient has the disease. The very low LRs (or LRs that are <0.1) virtually rule out the chance that the patient has the disease (Campo et al., 2010; Celentano & Szklo, 2018). Understanding sensitivity, specificity, and LR increases the researcher's ability to read clinical studies and to determine the most accurate diagnostic test to use in research and clinical practice (Celentano & Szklo, 2018; Elmore et al., 2020).

Receiver Operating Characteristic Curves

In studies that compute sensitivity and specificity, a receiver operating characteristic (ROC), or ROC curve, is often created. An **ROC curve** is a descriptive graph that plots the true positive rate against the false positive rate. The x-axis represents the false positive rate ($1 -$ specificity), and the y-axis represents the true positive rate (sensitivity). The actual rates are plotted and a line is drawn between the numbers. The larger the area under that line, the more accurate the test. The actual area under the line can be calculated by a value called the C statistic. The **C statistic**, or area under the curve, is the probability that the test result from a randomly selected person with the disease will be positive (Austin & Steyerberg, 2012; Elmore et al., 2020).

Hand Calculations

This example uses simulated data involving the alpha fetoprotein (AFP) test and its ability to identify a prenatal diagnosis of neural tube defects (NTDs). AFP testing involves the detection of AFP levels in amniotic fluid, and the results yield either a normal or abnormal result (Mayo Foundation for Medical Education and Research, 2022). As shown in Table 36.3, to analyze the sensitivity and specificity of these data, a pregnancy outcome of NTD will be considered the disease, also known as the *state* variable. The screening test variable is the presence of an abnormal AFP test result or a normal AFP test result.

TABLE 36.3 ALPHA FETOPROTEIN TEST RESULTS AND NEURAL TUBE DEFECTS AS A PREGNANCY OUTCOME		
	NTDs	**Normal**
Abnormal AFP test	127	180
Normal AFP test	20	99,673

AFP, alpha fetoprotein; NTDs, neural tube defects.

The computations for sensitivity, specificity, positive LR, and negative LR are as follows: Sensitivity calculation

$$\textbf{Sensitivity = a/(a + c)}$$

$$\frac{127}{127+20} = 0.8639 \times 100\% = 86.39\%$$

Specificity calculation

$$\textbf{Specificity = d/(b + d)}$$

$$\frac{99,673}{180+99,673} = 0.9982 \times 100\% = 99.82\%$$

Positive LR calculation

$$\textbf{Positive LR = Sensitivity} \div \textbf{(1 − Specificity)}$$

$$0.8639 \div (1 - 0.9982) = 479.94$$

Negative LR calculation

$$\textbf{Negative LR = (1−Sensitivity)} \div \textbf{Specificity}$$

$$(1-0.8639) \div 0.9982 = 0.1363$$

The sensitivity of the test was 86.39%, indicating that the proportion of pregnancy outcomes identified as NTD who were correctly identified as positive by their AFP tests was 86.39%. The specificity of the test was 99.82%, indicating that the proportion of patients with normal pregnancy outcomes who were correctly identified as normal by their AFP test was 99.82%. The positive LR was 479.94, indicating a large likelihood of NTDs among those with abnormal AFP test results. The negative LR was 0.1363, indicating a very low likelihood of NTDs among those who with normal AFP test results (Celentano & Szklo, 2018).

SPSS COMPUTATIONS

This is how our dataset looks in SPSS. The data for observations 17 through 100,000 are viewable by scrolling down in the SPSS screen. The values in the dataset must be coded as "1" or "0" for the state variable and the test variable, where a "1" indicates the presence of NTD for the pregnancy outcome and the presence of an abnormal AFP test, respectively.

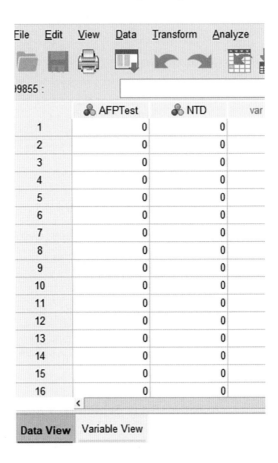

Step 1: From the "Analyze" menu, choose "Descriptive Statistics" and "Crosstabs." Move the two variables to the right, where either variable can be in the "Row" or "Column" space. Click "OK."

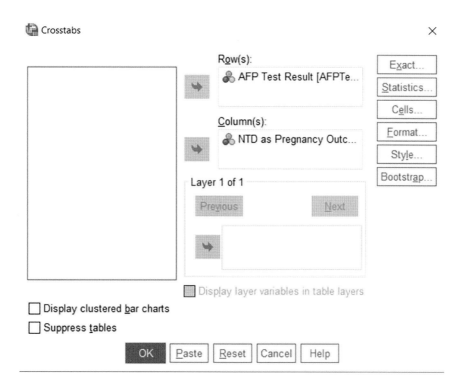

Step 2: From the "Analyze" menu, choose "Classify," and "ROC Curve." Move AFP test to the box labeled test variable, and move NTD to the box labeled "State Variable." Enter the number "1" next to the box labeled "Value of State Variable." Check all of the boxes underneath ("ROC Curve," "With diagonal reference line," "Standard error and confidence interval," and "Coordinate points of the ROC Curve"). Click "OK."

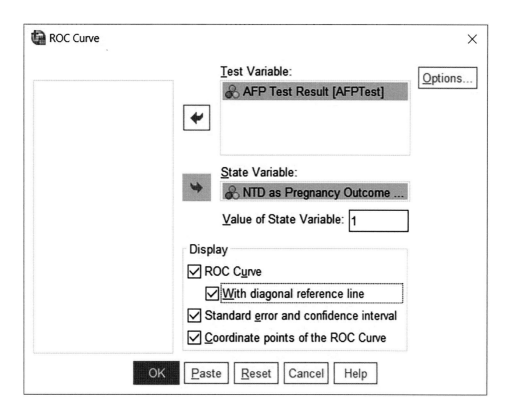

INTERPRETATION OF SPSS OUTPUT

The following tables are generated from SPSS. The first table contains the contingency table, similar to Table 36.3, presented previously. The following tables and figure are generated from the "ROC Curve" menu.

Crosstabs

AFP Test Result * NTD as Pregnancy Outcome Crosstabulation

Count

		NTD as Pregnancy Outcome		Total
		Normal	NTD	
AFP Test Result	Normal	99673	20	99693
	Abnormal	180	127	307
Total		99853	147	100000

The first table is the cross-tabulation table of the two variables. The values are the same as in Table 36.3. The next set of output is generated from the ROC menu selections. The first table contains the number of women whose pregnancy outcomes were positive and negative for NTDs.

ROC Curve

Case Processing Summary

NTD as Pregnancy Outcome[a]	Valid N (listwise)
Positive[b]	147
Negative	99853

Larger values of the test result variable(s) indicate stronger evidence for a positive actual state.

The second table contains the ROC curve, where the x-axis represents the false positive rate $(1 - \text{specificity})$, and the y-axis represents the true positive rate (sensitivity). The blue line represents our actual data, and the black line is the reference line that represents a 50/50 chance of accurately predicting NTDs. The greater the distance the blue line is from the black line, the more accurate the test.

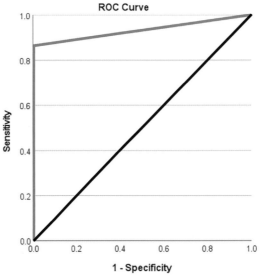

ROC Curve

Diagonal segments are produced by ties.

In the table titled "Area Under the Curve," the first value labeled "Area" is also considered the *C* statistic. The area under the curve is the probability that the AFP test from a randomly selected pregnancy outcome of NPDs will be abnormal. For the example data, the probability that an AFP test from a randomly selected pregnancy outcome of NTD will be abnormal is 0.931 or 93.1%. The *p* value is listed as ".000," which is interpreted as $p < 0.001$, indicating that knowing the AFP test value (abnormal AFP test) is significantly better than guessing. The 95% confidence interval for the *C* statistic was 0.898 to 0.964, which can be interpreted as the interval of 89.8% to 96.4% estimates the population *C* statistic with 95% confidence (Kline, 2004; United States Census, 2021).

Area Under the Curve

Test Result Variable(s): AFP Test Result

Area	Std. Error[a]	Asymptotic Sig.[b]	Asymptotic 95% Confidence Interval Lower Bound	Upper Bound
.931	.017	.000	.898	.964

The *C* statistic is 0.931, or 93.10%

The last table contains the sensitivity and $1 -$ specificity of AFP tests, which is listed as 0.864 and 0.002, respectively. Because $1 -$ specificity is 0.002, the specificity equals 0.998, or 99.8%.

Coordinates of the Curve

Test Result Variable(s): AFP Test Result

Positive if Greater Than or Equal To	Sensitivity	1 - Specificity
-1.00	1.000	1.000
.50	.864	.002
2.00	.000	.000

Sensitivity is 86.4%, and 1 – Specificity (false positive rate) is 0.2%, indicating that specificity is 99.8%

STUDY QUESTIONS

1. Discuss the sensitivity of a screening test and its importance in diagnosing a disease.

2. Discuss the specificity of a screening test and its importance in diagnosing a disease.

3. Define false positive rate.

4. What is the difference between a *test* variable and a *state* variable when calculating sensitivity and specificity?

5. Define the C statistic and how it relates to sensitivity and specificity.

6. The specificity of the screening test for the AFP test was 99.82%. What are the implications for the ability of the test to identify patients with a normal AFP test result?

7. What was the false positive rate of the AFP test?

8. What was the false negative rate of the AFP test?

9. In the ROC curve for the AFP test example, what were the coordinates used to represent the blue line?

10. List the 95% confidence interval of the C statistic and state your interpretation of that interval.

Answers to Study Questions

1. Sensitivity indicates the portion of patients with the disease and who have positive test results. The higher the sensitivity of a screening test, the more likely the test is to be positive when a person has a disease: true positive (Celentano & Szklo, 2018; Elmore et al., 2020).

2. Specificity of a test indicates the proportion of the patients who do not have a disease and have negative test results. The higher the specificity of a screening test, the more likely the test is to be negative when a person does not have a disease: true negative. A test that is both sensitive and specific identifies the patients with disease and rules out those who do not have disease (Celentano & Szklo, 2018; Elmore et al., 2020).

3. The false positive rate is defined as the number of people who do not have the disease and the test is positive for the disease.

4. The *test* variable is the screening variable, and the *state* variable is the disease state or the gold standard. It is important to define these two variables so that the calculations for sensitivity and specificity are correct.

5. The *C* statistic is the actual area under a ROC curve. The *C* statistic is created when a line is drawn with coordinates from the false positive rate (1 − specificity, represented on the *x*-axis) and the true positive rate (sensitivity, represented on the *y*-axis). The larger the area under that line, the larger the *C* statistic and the more accurate the test.

6. The specificity of the AFP test, or true negative rate, was 99.82%. Thus the AFP test was excellent and highly accurate in identifying pregnancy outcomes without NTD.

7. The calculation for the false positive rate (probability of no disease but having a positive test) is: b/(b + d). The false positive rate of the AFP test is calculated as: 180/(180 + 99,673) = 0.002 or 0.20%. This rate can also be computed by subtracting the specificity of the AFP test from 1.00: 1.00 − 0.9982 = 0.002 or 0.20%.

8. The calculation for the false negative rate (probability of disease but having a negative test) is: c/(c + a). The false negative rate of the AFP test is calculated as: 20/(20 + 127) = 0.1361 or 13.61%. This rate can also be computed by subtracting the sensitivity of the AFP test from 1.00: 1.00 − 0.8639 = 0.1361 or 13.61%.

9. The coordinates of the ROC curve that were used to represent the blue line are 0,0 and 0.864,0.002. The line was subsequently drawn to connect these two coordinates.

10. The 95% confidence interval of the *C* statistic was 0.898–0.964, or 89.8% to 96.4%. Thus the interval of 89.8% to 96.4%. estimates the population *C* statistic with 95% confidence. These values are identified in the SPSS table "Area Under the Curve."

DATA FOR ADDITIONAL COMPUTATIONAL PRACTICE

This additional example uses simulated data presented by Flowers et al. (2022) in a retrospective study to examine predictors of nursing student performance on the National Council Licensure Examination for Registered Nurses (NCLEX-RN). One of the predictors tested was performance on the Health Education Systems Incorporated (HESI) exam. Most nursing programs use comprehensive examinations such as the HESI exit exam to assess students' preparedness for the NCLEX-RN. The two variables in this example are HESI exam pass or fail and NCLEX-RN pass or fail at first attempt. The state variable, or gold standard, in this example is NCLEX-RN pass or fail. The screening test variable is HESI pass or fail. These data are presented in Table 36.4 as a contingency table.

TABLE 36.4   HESI AND NCLEX-RN EXAM PERFORMANCE

	NCLEX-RN Pass	NCLEX-RN Fail
HESI exam pass	66	7
HESI exam fail	11	6

HESI, Health Education Systems Incorporated; NCLEX-RN, National Council Licensure Examination for Registered Nurses.

Questions for Additional Study

Name: _____ Class: _____

Date: _____

Answer the following questions with hand calculations using the data presented in Table 36.4 or the SPSS dataset called "Exercise 36 Example 2.sav" available on the Evolve website. Follow your instructor's directions to submit your answers to the following questions for additional study. Your instructor may ask you to write your answers below and submit them as a hard copy for evaluation. Alternatively, your instructor may ask you to submit your answers online.

1. Compute the sensitivity value using the data from Table 36.4. Show your calculations and explain the meaning of the results.

2. Compute the specificity value. Show your calculations and explain the meaning of the results.

3. Compute the false positive rate. Show your calculations and explain the meaning of the results.

4. Compute the false negative rate. Show your calculations and explain the meaning of the results.

5. Using SPSS, create a receiver operating characteristic (ROC) curve and list the C statistic. How would you interpret the value?

6. What does the p value for the C statistic indicate?

7. What is the 95% confidence interval of the C statistic? State your interpretation of that interval.

8. In the ROC curve for the NCLEX-RN example, what were the coordinates used to represent the blue line?

9. What was the positive likelihood ratio (LR), and how would you interpret that value?

10. What was the negative LR, and how would you interpret that value?

Calculating the Pearson Chi-Square

The **Pearson chi-square test** (χ^2) compares differences between groups on variables measured at the nominal level. The chi-square compares the frequencies that are observed with the frequencies that are expected. When a study requires that researchers compare proportions (percentages) in one category versus another category, the chi-square is a statistic that will reveal if the difference in proportion is statistically improbable.

A **one-way chi-square** is a statistic that compares different levels of one variable only. For example, a researcher may collect information on gender and compare the proportions of males to females. If the one-way chi-square is statistically significant, it would indicate that proportions of one gender are significantly higher than proportions of the other gender than what would be expected by chance (Daniel, 2000; Pett, 2016). If more than two groups are being examined, the chi-square does not determine where the differences lie; it only determines that a significant difference exists. Further testing on subgroups of the data with the Pearson chi-square test would then be warranted to identify the significant differences.

A **two-way chi-square** is a statistic that tests whether proportions in levels of one nominal variable are significantly different from proportions of the second nominal variable. For example, Conlon and colleagues (2021) conducted a large retrospective cohort study to examine demographic and clinical differences between those who tested negative versus positive for novel coronavirus of 2019 (COVID-19) (see Exercise 19). One of the null hypotheses tested was: *There is no difference between persons who tested negative versus positive for COVID-19 on the presence of diabetes.* The results of the chi-square test indicated that the rates of diabetes were significantly higher among those who tested positive for COVID-19 (Conlon et al., 2021), suggesting that diabetes may be a risk factor for developing COVID-19. Further examples of two-way chi-square tests are reviewed in Exercise 19.

RESEARCH DESIGNS APPROPRIATE FOR THE PEARSON CHI-SQUARE

Research designs that may use the Pearson chi-square include the randomized experimental, quasi-experimental, and comparative designs (Gliner et al., 2017). The variables may be active, attributional, or a combination of both. An active variable refers to an intervention, treatment, or program. An attributional variable refers to a characteristic of the participant, such as gender, diagnosis, or race/ethnicity. Regardless of the whether the variables are active or attributional, all variables submitted to chi-square calculations must be measured at the nominal level.

STATISTICAL FORMULA AND ASSUMPTIONS

Use of the Pearson chi-square involves the following assumptions (Daniel, 2000):

1. Only one datum entry is made for each participant in the sample. Therefore if repeated measures from the same participant are being used for analysis, such as pretests and posttests, chi-square is not an appropriate test.
2. The variables must be categorical (nominal), either inherently or transformed to categorical from quantitative values.
3. For each variable, the categories are mutually exclusive and exhaustive. No cells may have an *expected* frequency of zero. In the actual data, the *observed* cell frequency may be zero. However, the Pearson chi-square test is not sensitive to small sample sizes, and other tests, such as the Fisher exact test, are more appropriate when testing very small samples (Daniel, 2000; Yates, 1934).

The test is distribution free, or nonparametric, which means that no assumption has been made for a normal distribution of values in the population from which the sample was taken (Daniel, 2000).

The formula for a two-way chi-square is:

$$\chi^2 = \frac{n[(A)(D) - (B)(C)]^2}{(A+B)(C+D)(A+C)(B+D)}$$

A **contingency table** displays the relationship between two or more categorical variables (Daniel, 2000). The contingency table is labeled as follows.

Rows	Columns	
	A	B
	C	D

With any chi-square analysis, the degrees of freedom (*df*) must be calculated to determine the significance of the value of the statistic. The following formula is used for this calculation:

$$df = (R-1)(C-1)$$

where

$$R = \text{Number of rows}$$

$$C = \text{Number of columns}$$

HAND CALCULATIONS

Conlon and colleagues (2021) conducted a retrospective cohort study to assess the role of the influenza vaccine on COVID-19 susceptibility and severity. The primary study aim was the comparison of positive and negative COVID-19 testing in those who received the influenza vaccine versus those who did not. Other study variables included baseline patient characteristics and the presence of comorbidities. Over 4.5 million unique patient charts within the Michigan Medicine healthcare system were extracted, and of those, 27,201 patients received laboratory testing for COVID-19.

The data are presented in Table 37.1. The null hypothesis is: *There is no difference between persons who tested negative versus those who tested positive for COVID-19 on history of a recent influenza vaccine.*

TABLE 37.1   COVID-19 TEST RESULTS BY INFLUENZA VACCINE

	COVID–19 Positive (n = 1218)	COVID–19 Negative (n = 25,983)	Totals	
Influenza vaccine	525	12,472	12,997	
No influenza vaccine	693	13,511	14,204	
Totals	1,218	25,983	27,201	←Total N

COVID-19, novel coronavirus of 2019.

The computations for the Pearson chi-square test are as follows:

Step 1: Create a contingency table of the two nominal variables (see Table 37.1).

Step 2: Fit the cells into the formula:

$$\chi^2 = \frac{n[(A)(D)-(B)(C)]^2}{(A+B)(C+D)(A+C)(B+D)}$$

$$\chi^2 = \frac{27,201[(525)(13,511)-(12,472)(693)]^2}{(525+12,472)(693+13,511)(525+693)(12,472+13,511)}$$

$$\chi^2 = \frac{27,201(-1,549,821)^2}{(12,997)(14,204)(1,218)(25,983)}$$

$$\chi^2 = \frac{65,335,309,536,647,200}{5,842,387,577,196,070}$$

$$\chi^2 = 11.18$$

Step 3: Compute the *df*:

$$df = (2-1)(2-1) = 1$$

Step 4: Locate the critical chi-square value in the chi-square distribution table (Appendix D) and compare it to the obtained chi-square value.

The table in Appendix D includes the critical values of chi-square for specific *df* at selected levels of significance. If the value of the statistic is equal to or greater than the value identified in the chi-square table, the difference between the two variables is statistically significant. The critical chi-square for *df*=1 is 3.8415, which was rounded to 3.84, and our obtained chi-square is 11.18. Thus the obtained chi-square value exceeds the critical value, which indicates a significant difference between persons who tested negative versus positive for COVID-19 on history of a recent influenza vaccine.

Furthermore we can compute the rates of influenza vaccines among those with positive and negative COVID-19 tests by using the numbers in the contingency table from Step 1. The influenza vaccine rate among those who tested positive can be calculated as 525 ÷ 1218 = 0.4310 × 100% = 43.1%. The influenza vaccine rate among those who tested negative can be calculated as 12,472 ÷ 25,983 = 0.4800 × 100% = 48.0%.

SPSS COMPUTATIONS

The following screenshot is a replica of what the SPSS dataset will look like. The data for participants 17 through 27,201 are viewable by scrolling down in the SPSS screen.

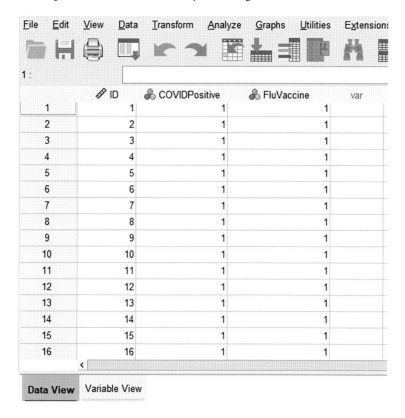

Step 1: From the "Analyze" menu, choose "Descriptive Statistics" and "Crosstabs." Move the two variables to the right, where either variable can be in the "Row" or "Column" space.

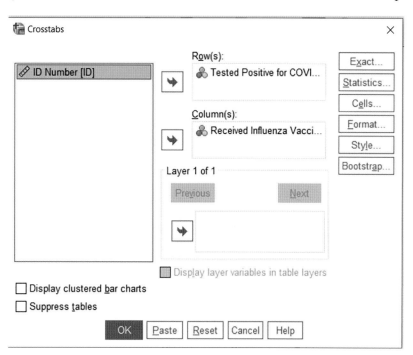

Step 2: Click "Statistics" and check the box next to "Chi-square." Click "Continue" and "OK."

INTERPRETATION OF SPSS OUTPUT

The following tables are generated from SPSS. The first table contains the contingency table, similar to Table 37.1, presented previously. The second table contains the chi-square results.

Crosstabs

Received Influenza Vaccine * Tested Positive for COVID-19 Crosstabulation

Count

		Tested Positive for COVID-19		Total
		Negative	Positive	
Received Influenza Vaccine	Did Not Receive Influenza Vaccine	13511	693	14204
	Received Influenza Vaccine	12472	525	12997
Total		25983	1218	27201

Chi-Square Tests

	Value	df	Asymptotic Significance (2-sided)	Exact Sig. (2-sided)	Exact Sig. (1-sided)
Pearson Chi-Square	11.183[a]	1	<.001		
Continuity Correction[b]	10.988	1	<.001		
Likelihood Ratio	11.228	1	<.001		
Fisher's Exact Test				<.001	<.001
Linear-by-Linear Association	11.183	1	<.001		
N of Valid Cases	27201				

a. 0 cells (0.0%) have expected count less than 5. The minimum expected count is 581.98.

b. Computed only for a 2x2 table

The last table contains the chi-square value in addition to other statistics that test associations between nominal variables. The Pearson chi-square test is located in the first row of the table, which contains the chi-square value, *df*, and *p* value.

FINAL INTERPRETATION IN AMERICAN PSYCHOLOGICAL ASSOCIATION FORMAT

The following interpretation is written as it might appear in a research article, formatted according to American Psychological Association (APA) guidelines (2020). It should be noted that all statistical values reported here are rounded to two decimal places, with the exception of the *p* value, which is rounded to three decimal places.

A Pearson chi-square analysis indicated that those who tested negative for COVID-19 had significantly higher rates of influenza vaccines than those who tested positive for COVID-19, chi-square(1, $N = 27{,}201$) = 11.18, $p < 0.001$ (48.00% versus 43.10%, respectively). This finding suggests that receiving a recent influenza vaccine may be a protective factor for acquiring COVID-19, and further research is needed to investigate the effect of influenza vaccines on testing positive for COVID-19.

STUDY QUESTIONS

1. Do the example data meet the assumptions for the Pearson chi-square test? Provide a rationale for your answer.

2. State the null hypothesis. Was the null hypothesis accepted or rejected? Provide a rationale for your answer.

3. What is the exact likelihood of obtaining a chi-square value at least as extreme or close to the one that was actually observed, assuming that the null hypothesis is true?

4. Using the numbers in the contingency table, calculate the percentage of people who tested positive for COVID-19 among those who received a recent influenza vaccine. In other words, calculate the COVID-19 positivity rate among those who received an influenza vaccine. Show your calculations.

5. Using the numbers in the contingency table, calculate the percentage of people who tested negative for COVID-19 among those who received a recent influenza vaccine. In other words, calculate the COVID-19 negativity rate among those who received an influenza vaccine. Show your calculations.

6. Using the numbers in the contingency table, calculate the percentage of people who tested positive for COVID-19 among those who did *not* receive a recent influenza vaccine. In other words, calculate the COVID-19 positivity rate for those who did not receive an influenza vaccine. Show your calculations.

7. Using the numbers in the contingency table, calculate the percentage of people who tested negative for COVID-19 among those who did *not* receive a recent influenza vaccine. In other words, calculate the COVID-19 negativity rate among those who did not receive an influenza vaccine. Show your calculations.

8. Was this an appropriate research design for a Pearson chi-square analysis? Provide a rationale for your answer.

9. What result would have been obtained if the variables in the SPSS "Crosstabs" window had been switched, with the COVID-19 test variable placed in the "Row" and the influenza vaccine variable placed in the "Column"?

10. Was the sample size adequate to detect differences between the two groups in this example? Provide a rationale for your answer.

Answers to Study Questions

1. Yes, the data meet the assumptions of the Pearson chi-square:

   a. Only one datum per participant was entered into the contingency table, and no participant was counted twice.

   b. Both COVID-19 test result (positive/negative) and influenza vaccine (yes/no) are categorical (nominal-level data).

   c. For each variable, the categories are mutually exclusive and exhaustive. It was not possible for a participant to belong to both groups, and the two categories (COVID-19 positive and negative tests) included all study participants.

2. The null hypothesis is: *There is no difference between persons who tested negative versus those who tested positive for COVID-19 on history of a recent influenza vaccine.* The null hypothesis is rejected. The critical chi-square value for 1 *df* at alpha (α) = 0.05 is 3.84 (see Appendix D, which includes the critical values for the chi-square distribution). Our obtained chi-square is 11.18, exceeding the critical value in the table. Moreover, the SPSS reported the exact p value as <0.001. This value can be found in the "Chi-Square Tests" table in the SPSS output. This p value is less than α = 0.05, indicating a significant result.

3. The exact likelihood of obtaining a chi-square value at least as extreme as or close to the one that was actually observed, assuming that the null hypothesis is true, is less than 0.10%. This value can be found in the "Chi-Square Tests" table in the SPSS output, where the exact p value is reported as "<.001." The value is calculated as follows: 0.001 × 100% = <0.10%.

4. The percentage of people who tested positive for COVID-19 among those who received a recent influenza vaccine is calculated as 525 ÷ 12,997 = 0.0404 × 100% = 4.04%.

5. The percentage of people who tested negative for COVID-19 among those who received a recent influenza vaccine is calculated as 12,472 ÷ 12,997 = 0.9596 × 100% = 95.96%.

6. The percentage of people who tested positive for COVID-19 among those who did *not* receive a recent influenza vaccine is calculated as 693 ÷ 14,204 = 0.0488 × 100% = 4.88%.

7. The percentage of people who tested negative for COVID-19 among those who did *not* receive a recent influenza vaccine is calculated as 13,511 ÷ 14,204 = 0.9512 × 100% = 95.12%.

8. The study design in the example was a retrospective cohort design (Gliner et al., 2017; Gray & Grove, 2021). Both of the variables (COVID-19 test result and influenza vaccination) were nominal (yes/no). Therefore the design was appropriate for a Pearson chi-square analysis.

9. Switching the variables in the SPSS "Crosstabs" window would have resulted in the exact same chi-square result. It does not matter which variable is placed in the column section and which is placed in the row section.

10. The sample size is $N = 27{,}201$, which is extremely large, and the vast majority of the statistical results were significant, indicating adequate statistical power (see Exercises 24 and 25; Aberson, 2019; Cohen, 1988).

DATA FOR ADDITIONAL COMPUTATIONAL PRACTICE

This example uses additional data from Conlon and colleagues (2021), who conducted a retrospective cohort study to compare patients who tested positive with patients who tested negative for COVID-19 on key clinical and demographic variables. In this example, persons who tested positive versus negative for COVID-19 were compared on the presence (rate) of diabetes. The null hypothesis is: *There is no difference between persons who tested negative versus positive for COVID-19 on the presence of diabetes.* These data are presented in Table 37.2 as a contingency table.

TABLE 37.2   COVID-19 TEST RESULTS BY PRESENCE OF DIABETES

	COVID–19 Positive (*n* = 1,218)	COVID–19 Negative (*n* = 25,983)	Totals	
Diabetes	262	2,556	2,818	
No diabetes	956	23,427	24,383	
Totals	1,218	25,983	27,201	← Total *N*

COVID-19, novel coronavirus of 2019.

Questions for Additional Study

Name: _____ Class:_____

Date: _____

Answer the following questions with hand calculations using the data presented in Table 37.2 or the SPSS dataset called "Exercise 37 Example 2.sav" available on the Evolve website. Follow your instructor's directions to submit your answers to the following questions for additional study. Your instructor may ask you to write your answers below and submit them as a hard copy for evaluation. Alternatively, your instructor may ask you to submit your answers online.

1. Calculate the degrees of freedom (*df*) for the Pearson chi-square test comparing novel coronavirus 2019 (COVID-19) test result (positive/negative) by diabetes (present/absent). Show your calculations.

2. Compute the chi-square test using the chi-square formula. Show your calculations.

3. Is the chi-square significant at $\alpha = 0.05$? Specify how you arrived at your answer.

4. Use SPSS to determine the exact likelihood of obtaining a chi-square value at least as extreme or as close to the one that was actually observed, assuming that the null hypothesis is true. Report the answer as a percentage.

5. Using the numbers in the contingency table, calculate the percentage of persons with diabetes among those who tested positive for COVID-19. In other words, calculate the rate of diabetes among those who were positive for COVID-19. Show your calculations.

6. Using the numbers in the contingency table, calculate the percentage of persons with diabetes among those who tested negative for COVID-19. In other words, calculate the rate of diabetes among those who were negative for COVID-19. Show your calculations.

7. Using the numbers in the contingency table, calculate the percentage of people who tested positive for COVID-19 among only the persons with diabetes. In other words, calculate the COVID-19 positivity rate among diabetics. Show your calculations.

8. Using the numbers in the contingency table, calculate the percentage of people who tested positive for COVID-19 among only the persons *without* diabetes. In other words, calculate the COVID-19 positivity rate among those without diabetes. Show your calculations.

9. Write your interpretation of the results as you would in an APA-formatted journal (American Psychological Association, 2020).

10. Does a statistically significant chi-square result provide evidence of causation between the variables? Provide a rationale for your answer.

EXERCISE 38

Calculating Odds Ratio and 95% Confidence Intervals

When both the predictor and the dependent variable are dichotomous (having only two values), the **odds ratio (OR)** is a commonly used statistic to obtain an indication of association. The OR is defined as the ratio of the odds of an event occurring in one group to the odds of it occurring in another group (Celentano & Szklo, 2018). Put simply, the OR is a way of comparing whether the odds of a certain event is the same for two groups. For example, dropped courses and persistence were examined in a large sample of registered nurse–to–bachelor of science in nursing (RN-to-BSN) and prelicensure BSN nursing students (Cipher & Urban, 2022). The OR was 5.58, indicating that students in an RN-to-BSN program were significantly more likely to have dropped a course than students in a prelicensure BSN program (specifically, 5.58 times as likely).

The OR can also be computed when the dependent variable is dichotomous and the predictor is continuous and would be computed by performing logistic regression analysis. **Logistic regression** analysis tests a predictor (or set of predictors) with a dichotomous dependent variable. The output yields an adjusted OR, meaning that each predictor's OR represents the relationship between that predictor and y after adjusting for the presence of the other predictors in the model (Tabachnick & Fidell, 2019). As is the case with multiple linear regression, each predictor serves as a covariate to every other predictor in the model. Logistic regression is best conducted using a statistical software package. Full explanations and examples of the mathematical computations of logistic regression are presented in Tabachnick and Fidell (2019). This exercise only focuses on the odds ratio that involves two dichotomous variables.

RESEARCH DESIGNS APPROPRIATE FOR THE ODDS RATIO

Research designs that may use the OR include the randomized experimental, quasi-experimental, comparative, and associational designs (Gliner et al., 2017). The variables may be active, attributional, or a combination of both. An **active variable** refers to an intervention, treatment, or program. An **attributional variable** refers to a characteristic of the participant, such as gender, diagnosis, or race/ethnicity. Regardless of whether the variables are active or attributional, the dependent variable submitted to OR calculations must be dichotomous.

STATISTICAL FORMULA AND ASSUMPTIONS

Use of the OR involves the following assumptions (Celentano & Szklo, 2018):

1. Only one datum entry is made for each subject in the sample. Therefore if repeated measures from the same subject are being used for analysis, such as pretests and posttests, the OR is not an appropriate test.
2. The variables must be dichotomous, either inherently or transformed to categorical from quantitative values.

The formula for the *OR* is:

$$OR = \frac{ad}{bc}$$

The formula for the *OR* designates the predictor's ratios of 1s to 0s within the positive outcome in the numerator, and the predictor's ratios of 1s to 0s within the negative outcome in the denominator. Note that the values must be coded accordingly. Table 38.1 displays the following notation to assist you in calculating the *OR*. Note that the *a* cell represents the presence of both variables. Both variables should be coded as 1 for presence and 0 for absence.

HAND CALCULATIONS

A retrospective multisite cohort study was conducted on 100 patients with inflammatory bowel disease (IBD) who underwent various types of treatment for prostate cancer (Feagins et al., 2020). The treatments were categorized into two categories: treatments involving radiation (including either external or internal radiation) and treatments that did not involve radiation, such as chemotherapy and hormonal therapy. Persons in the nonradiation group received hormonal therapy, chemotherapy, both hormonal and chemotherapy, or some other type of treatment that did not involve radiation.

The two variables in this example are dichotomous: radiation treatment (yes/no) and the presence of an IBD flare posttreatment (yes/no). The data are presented in Table 38.2. The null hypothesis is: *There is no association between radiation treatment and IBD flares among persons with IBD and prostate cancer.*

TABLE 38.1   STRUCTURE OF DATA FOR ODDS RATIO CALCULATION

	Yes (Presence)	No (Absence)
Yes (Presence)	*a*	*b*
No (Absence)	*c*	*d*

TABLE 38.2   PROSTATE CANCER TREATMENT AND INFLAMMATORY BOWEL DISEASE FLARES

	IBD Flare	No IBD Flare
Radiation treatment	14	36
Nonradiation treatment	5	45

IBD, inflammatory bowel disease.

The computations for the *OR* are as follows:

Step 1: Fit the cell values into the *OR* formula:

$$OR = \frac{ad}{bc} = \frac{(14)(45)}{(36)(5)} = \frac{630}{180} = 3.50$$

$$OR = 3.50$$

Step 2: Compute the 95% confidence interval (CI) for the *OR*. As demonstrated in Exercise 28, the CI for any statistic is composed of three components: the statistic $+/- SE(t)$, where *SE* is the standard error of the statistic. To compute a 95% CI for the *OR*, the *OR* must first be converted into the natural logarithm of the *OR*. The natural logarithm of a number X is the power to which e would have to be raised to equal X (where e is approximately 2.718288). For example, the natural logarithm of e itself would be 1, because $e^1 = 2.718288$.

Convert the *OR* to the *ln(OR)*

$$ln(3.50) = 1.25$$

Step 3: Compute the standard error of *ln(OR)*. Note that four decimal places in the following calculations are being retained so that the resulting values for the remaining steps will be more accurate.

$$SE_{ln(OR)} = \sqrt{\frac{1}{a} + \frac{1}{b} + \frac{1}{c} + \frac{1}{d}}$$

$$SE_{ln(OR)} = \sqrt{\frac{1}{14} + \frac{1}{36} + \frac{1}{5} + \frac{1}{45}}$$

$$SE_{ln(OR)} = \sqrt{0.0714 + 0.0278 + 0.2000 + 0.0222}$$

$$SE_{ln(OR)} = \sqrt{0.3214}$$

$$SE_{ln(OR)} = 0.5669$$

Step 4: Create the CI still using the *ln(OR)*, with a t of 1.96:

$$95\% \ CI = ln(OR) +/-SE(t)$$

$$95\% \ CI = 1.25 +/- 0.5669(1.96)$$

$$95\% \ CI = 0.1389 \ to \ 2.3611$$

rounded to:

$$95\% \ CI = 0.14 \ to \ 2.36 \ or \ (0.14, 2.36)$$

Step 5: Convert the lower and upper limits of the CI back to the original *OR* unit:

$$e^{0.14} = 1.15$$

$$e^{2.36} = 10.59$$

This means that the interval of (1.15, 10.59) estimates the population *OR* with 95% confidence (Kline, 2004; Pett, 2016). Moreover, because the CI does not include the number 1.0, the *OR* indicates a significant association between radiation treatment and the presence of IBD flares among persons with prostate cancer.

Step 6: Interpret the directionality of the *OR*:

An *OR* of $\cong 1.0$ indicates that exposure (to radiation treatment) does not affect the odds of the outcome (presence of an IBD flare).

An *OR* of >1.0 indicates that exposure (to radiation treatment) is associated with a higher odds of the outcome (presence of an IBD flare).

An *OR* of <1.0 indicates that exposure (to radiation treatment) is associated with a lower odds of the outcome (presence of an IBD flare).

The *OR* for the study was 3.50, indicating the odds of having experienced an IBD flare among persons receiving radiation treatment for prostate cancer was higher than those who did not receive radiation treatment. We can further note that persons receiving radiation treatment were over three times as likely, or 250% more likely, to have experienced an IBD flare posttreatment (Feagins et al., 2020). This value was computed by subtracting 1.0 from the *OR* (3.50 − 1.00 = 2.50 × 100% = 250%). The difference between the obtained *OR* and 1.00 represents the extent of the lesser or greater likelihood of the event occurring.

SPSS COMPUTATIONS

This is how our dataset looks in SPSS. The remaining data (rows 17 through 100) are viewable by scrolling down in the SPSS screen. The values in the dataset must be coded as "1" or "0."

File Edit View Data Transform Analyze Graphs Utilities			
	ID	TreatmentGroup	IBDFlare
1	1	1	1
2	2	0	1
3	3	1	1
4	4	0	0
5	5	0	0
6	6	1	0
7	7	1	1
8	8	1	0
9	9	1	0
10	10	0	0
11	11	0	0
12	12	0	0
13	13	1	0
14	14	1	0
15	15	1	1
16	16	1	0

Data View   Variable View

Step 1: From the "Analyze" menu, choose "Descriptive Statistics" and "Crosstabs." Move the two variables to the right, where either variable can be in the "Row" or "Column" space.

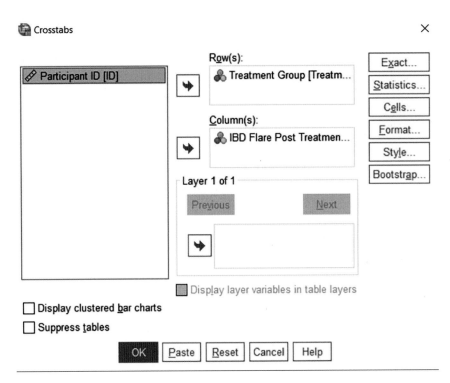

Step 2: Click "Statistics" and check the box next to "Risk." Click "Continue" and "OK."

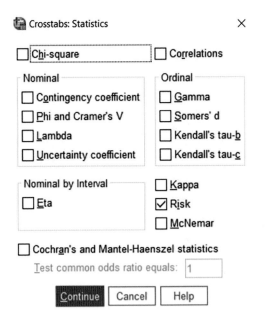

INTERPRETATION OF SPSS OUTPUT

The following tables are generated from SPSS. The first table contains the contingency table, similar to Table 38.2, presented previously. The order of the values in the contingency table is different than that of Table 38.2, but the actual values are the same. The second table contains the *OR* results.

Crosstabs

Treatment Group * IBD Flare Post Treatment Crosstabulation

Count

		IBD Flare Post Treatment		Total
		No IBD Flare	IBD Flare	
Treatment Group	Non-radiation Treatment	45	5	50
	Radiation Treatment	36	14	50
Total		81	19	100

Risk Estimate

	Value	95% Confidence Interval	
		Lower	Upper
Odds Ratio for Treatment Group (Non-radiation Treatment / Radiation Treatment)	3.500	1.152	10.633
For cohort IBD Flare Post Treatment = No IBD Flare	1.250	1.028	1.521
For cohort IBD Flare Post Treatment = IBD Flare	.357	.139	.917
N of Valid Cases	100		

The last table contains the *OR* value in addition to the lower and upper limits of the 95% CI, respectively. The *OR* is located in the first row of the table. Note that there is no *p* value, because *OR*s are not traditionally reported accompanied by a *p* value; rather, the 95% CI is reported. The CI values calculated by SPSS are slightly different than the hand-calculated values of 1.15 and 10.59 because of rounding error.

FINAL INTERPRETATION IN AMERICAN PSYCHOLOGICAL ASSOCIATION FORMAT

The following interpretation is written as it might appear in a research article, formatted according to American Psychological Association (APA, 2020) guidelines.

An *OR* was computed to assess the association between radiation treatment and the presence of posttreatment IBD flares among persons with prostate cancer. Persons receiving radiation treatment were over three times as likely to have experienced an IBD flare posttreatment (28.0% versus 10.0%, respectively; *OR* = 3.50, 95% CI [1.15, 10.53]).

It should be noted that the design of this study was a retrospective cohort study, and not a randomized controlled trial (RCT). Therefore the ability to make a causal link between the type of treatment received and the study outcomes is limited (Gliner et al., 2017). With cohort studies, there can be factors that affect the reasons why a person belongs to a particular cohort, and those factors can affect study outcomes (Celentano & Szklo, 2018). In RCTs, participants are randomly assigned to the treatment group, and this eliminates the aforementioned factors responsible for cohort membership (Gliner et al., 2017). For example, our results from this example indicate that persons receiving radiation treatment were significantly more likely to experience an IBD flare. This finding could be attributed to the radiation, or it could be attributed to the possibility that persons who received radiation had a more severe level of disease at baseline, or a multitude of other characteristics that may have affected the outcomes.

STUDY QUESTIONS

1. What does an *OR* of 1.0 indicate?

2. Using the numbers in the contingency table, calculate the percentage of the radiation treatment cohort that experienced an IBD flare. Show your calculations.

3. Using the numbers in the contingency table, calculate the percentage of the nonradiation treatment cohort that experienced an IBD flare. Show your calculations.

4. Using the numbers in the contingency table, calculate the percentage of the radiation treatment cohort that did *not* experience an IBD flare. Show your calculations.

5. A 95% CI was computed for an *OR* of 0.70. The lower and upper limits were 0.55 to 0.85, respectively. What do the results indicate?

6. A 95% CI was computed for an *OR* of 0.70. The lower and upper limits were 0.35 to 1.05, respectively. What do the results indicate?

7. A 95% CI was computed for an *OR* of 1.23. The lower and upper limits were 1.15 to 1.31, respectively. What do the results indicate?

8. What kind of design was used in the example? Was this design appropriate for conducting an *OR* analysis? Provide a rationale for your answers.

9. A researcher recodes the variable of IBD flare from binary to a four-category nominal variable: 1 = 0 flares, 2 = 1 to 2 flares, 3 = 3 to 4 flares, 4 = more than 4 flares. The researcher wants to compare the radiation treatment cohort to the nonradiation treatment cohort on the newly recoded variable. What would be an appropriate statistical approach?

10. What result would have been obtained if the variables in the SPSS "Crosstabs" window had been switched, with IBD flare being placed in the "Row" and treatment group being placed in the "Column"?

Answers to Study Questions

1. An *OR* of 1.0 indicates no significant association between the two variables (Celentano & Szklo, 2018).

2. There were 50 patients who received radiation treatment, 14 of which experienced an IBD flare. Therefore the percentage of the radiation treatment cohort who experienced an IBD flare is calculated as $14 \div 50 = 0.280 \times 100\% = 28.0\%$.

3. There were 50 patients who received nonradiation treatment, 5 of which experienced an IBD flare. Therefore the percentage of the nonradiation treatment cohort who experienced an IBD flare is calculated as $5 \div 50 = 0.100 \times 100\% = 10.0\%$.

4. There were 50 patients who received radiation treatment, 36 of which did *not* experience an IBD flare. Therefore the percentage of the radiation treatment cohort that did *not* experience an IBD flare is calculated as $36 \div 50 = 0.720 \times 100\% = 72.0\%$.

5. An *OR* of 0.70 with 95% CI of 0.55 to 0.85 indicates a significant association between the two variables, because the CI does not contain 1.0. The probability of the event is 30% lower among the exposure/test group (Celentano & Szklo, 2018).

6. An *OR* of 0.70 with 95% CI of 0.35 to 1.05 indicates that there is no significant association between the two variables, because the CI contains 1.0 (Celentano & Szklo, 2018).

7. An *OR* of 1.23 with 95% CI of 1.15 to 1.31 indicates a significant association between the two variables, because the CI does not contain 1.0. The probability of the event is 23% higher among the exposure/test group.

8. The study design in the example was a retrospective cohort design, because the data were a retrospective examination of groups of patients receiving types of treatment that did not involve randomization. Moreover, both variables (radiation treatment/nonradiation treatment and flare/no flare) were nominal and binary. Therefore the research design was appropriate for an *OR* calculation (Celentano & Szklo, 2018).

9. The appropriate statistical approach would no longer be an *OR* because one of the variables is not binary. Rather, the newly recoded variable is ordinal. To compare two groups on an ordinal variable, a Mann-Whitney *U* test would be appropriate (see Exercises 21 and 23; Kim et al., 2022).

10. Switching the variables in the SPSS "Crosstabs" window would have resulted in the exact same *OR* value and 95% CI values.

DATA FOR ADDITIONAL COMPUTATIONAL PRACTICE

This example uses additional data from the retrospective cohort study by Feagins and colleagues (2020), who investigated different types of treatment received for prostate cancer among persons with IBD. In this example, the type of treatment consists of external radiotherapy (XRT) and brachytherapy (a type of internal radiation therapy). The two variables in this example are dichotomous: type of treatment received (XRT/brachytherapy) and the presence of an IBD flare posttreatment (yes/no). The null hypothesis is: *There is no association between type of radiation treatment and posttreatment IBD flares among persons with IBD and prostate cancer.* These simulated data are presented in Table 38.3 as a contingency table.

TABLE 38.3   PROSTATE CANCER TREATMENT AND INFLAMMATORY BOWEL DISEASE

	IBD Flare	No IBD Flare
XRT treatment	14	54
Brachytherapy treatment	8	24

XRT, external radiotherapy; IBD, inflammatory bowel disease.

Name: _____ Class: _____

Date: _____

Answer the following questions with hand calculations using the data presented in Table 38.3 or the SPSS dataset called "Exercise 38 Example 2.sav" available on the Evolve website. Follow your instructor's directions to submit your answers to the following questions for additional study. Your instructor may ask you to write your answers below and submit them as a hard copy for evaluation. Alternatively, your instructor may ask you to submit your answers online.

1. Are the data in Table 38.3 appropriate to compute an odds ratio (*OR*)? Provide a rationale for your answer.

2. Compute the *OR*. Show your calculations.

3. Compute the 95% confidence interval (CI) for the *OR* calculated in Question 2. Show your calculations.

4. Does the *OR* represent a significant association between type of treatment received and IBD flares? Specify how you arrived at your answer.

5. Using the numbers in the contingency table, calculate the percentage of the external radiation (XRT) cohort that experienced an IBD flare. Show your calculations.

6. Using the numbers in the contingency table, calculate the percentage of the brachytherapy cohort that experienced an IBD flare. Show your calculations.

7. Using the numbers in the contingency table, calculate the percentage of the XRT cohort that did *not* experience an IBD flare. Show your calculations.

8. Using the numbers in the contingency table, calculate the percentage of the brachytherapy cohort that did *not* experience an IBD flare. Show your calculations.

9. Write your interpretation of the results as you would in an APA-formatted journal (American Psychological Association, 2020).

10. Was the sample size adequate to detect an association between the two variables in this example? Provide a rationale for your answer.

References

Aberson, C. L. (2019). *Applied power analysis for the behavioral sciences* (2nd ed.). Routledge Taylor & Francis Group.

Aday, L., & Cornelius, L. J. (2006). *Designing and conducting health surveys* (3rd ed.). John Wiley & Sons.

Aiken, L. S., & West, S. G. (1991). *Multiple regression: Testing and interpreting interactions*. Sage.

Allison, P. D. (1999). *Multiple regression: A primer*. Pine Forge Press.

Al-Rawajfah, O. M., Al Hadid, L., Madhavanprabhakaran, G. K., Francis, F. & Khalaf, A. (2022). Predictors of effective clinical teaching—nursing educators' perspective. *BMC Nursing, 21*(1), 1–9. https://doi.org/10.1186/s12912-022-00836-y

American Psychological Association (APA). (2020). *Publication manual of the American Psychological Association* (7th ed.). American Psychological Association.

Aponte, J. (2010). Key elements of large survey data sets. *Nursing Economics, 28*(1), 27–36.

Armenta, B. E., Hartshorn, K. J., Whitbeck, L. B., Crawford, D. M., & Hoyt, D. R. (2014). A longitudinal examination of the measurement properties and predictive utility of the Center for Epidemiologic Studies Depression Scale among North American indigenous adolescents. *Psychological Assessment, 26*(4), 1347–1355. https://doi.org/10.1037/a0037608

Austin, P. C., & Steyerberg, E. W. (2012). Interpreting the concordance statistic of a logistic regression model: Relation to the variance and odds ratio of a continuous explanatory variable. *BMC Medical Research Methodology, 12*(82), 1–8. https://doi.org/10.1186/1471-2288-12-82

Ayar, D., & Sabancioğullari, S. (2022). The effect of a solution-oriented therapy on the depression levels and the perceived social support of depressive patients. *Archives of Psychiatric Nursing, 36,* 62–69. https://doi.org/10.1016/j.apnu.2021.11.004

Bandalos, D. L. (2018). *Measurement theory and applications for the social sciences*. Guilford Press.

Bannigan, K., & Watson, R. (2009). Reliability and validity in a nutshell. *Journal of Clinical Nursing, 18*(23), 3237–3243. https://doi.org/10.1111/j.1365-2702.2009.02939.x

Bartlett, J. W., & Frost, C. (2008). Reliability, repeatability and reproducibility: Analysis of measurement errors in continuous variables. *Ultrasound Obstetric Gynecology, 31*(4), 466–475. https//doi.org/10.1002/uog.5256

Batra, K., Singh, T. P., Sharma, M., Batra, R., & Schvaneveldt, N. (2020). Investigating the psychological impact of COVID-19 among healthcare workers: A meta-analysis. *International Journal of Environmental Research and Public Health, 17*(23), 9096. https://doi.org/10.3390/ijerph17239096

Bender, R., & Lange, S. (1999). Multiple test procedures other than Bonferroni's deserve wider use. *British Medical Journal, 318*(7183), 600–601. https://doi.org/10.1136/bmj.318.7183.600a

Bialocerkowski, A., Klupp, N., & Bragge, P. (2010). Research methodology series: How to read and critically appraise a reliability article. *International Journal of Therapy & Rehabilitation, 17*(3), 114–120. https://doi.org/10.12968/ijtr.2010.17.3.46743

Bradley, K. L., Bagnell, A. L., & Brannen, C. L. (2010). Factorial validity of the Center for Epidemiological Studies Depression-10 in adolescents. *Issues in Mental Health Nursing, 31*(6), 408–412. https://doi.org/10.3109/01612840903484105

Breusch, T. S., & Pagan, A. R. (1979). A simple test for heteroscedasticity and random coefficient variation. *Econometrica, 47*(5), 1287–1294. https://doi.org/10.2307/1911963

Brino, K. A. S., Derouin, A. L., & Silva, S. G. (2022). Problematic Internet use in adolescents and implementation of a social media hygiene protocol. *Journal of Pediatric Nursing, 63,* 84–89. https://doi.org/10.1016/j.pedn.2021.10.011

Bronas, L. G., Hanna, M., Lash, J. P., Ajilore, O., Zhou, X. J., & Lamar, M. (2022). Exercise training and cognitive function in kidney disease: Protocol for a pilot randomized controlled trial. *Nursing Research, 71*(1), 75–82. https://doi.org/10.1097/NNR.0000000000000554

Caceres, B. A., Doan, D., Barcelona, V., & Suero-Tejeda, N. (2022). Lifetime trauma and cardiovascular health in Latinas. *Nursing Research, 71*(1), 66–74. https://doi.org/10.1097/NNR.0000000000000560

Campo, M., Shiyko, M., & Lichtman, S. W. (2010). Sensitivity and specificity: A review of related statistics and current controversies in physical therapist education. *Journal of Physical Therapy Education, 24*(3), 69–78. https://doi.org/10.1097/00001416-201007000-00009

Celentano, D. D. & Szklo, M. (2018). *Gordis epidemiology* (6th ed.). Elsevier.

Centers for Disease Control and Prevention (CDC). U.S. Department of Health and Human Services (2015). *Body mass index.* Retrieved from https://www.cdc.gov/healthyweight/assessing/bmi/index.html

Charmaz, K. (2014). *Constructing grounded theory: A practical guide through qualitative analysis* (2nd ed.). Sage.

Chatreewatanakul, B., Othaganont, P., & Hickman, R. (2022). Early symptom recognition and symptom management among exacerbation COPD patients: A qualitative study. *Applied Nursing Research, 63,* 151522. https://doi.org/10.1016/j.apnr.2021.151522

Cheema, J. R. (2014). A review of missing data handling methods in education research. *Review of Educational Research, 84*(4), 487–508. https://doi.org/10.3102/0034654314532697

Cipher, D. J. (2023). Statistical decision tree for selecting an appropriate analysis technique. In S. K. Grove & J. R. Gray (Eds.), *Understanding nursing research: Building an evidence-based practice* (8th ed., p. 338). Elsevier.

Cipher, D. J., & Urban, R. W. (2022). Course drops and persistence in online undergraduate nursing programs. *Journal of Nursing Education, 61*(11), 609–615. https://doi.org/10.3928/01484834-20220803-07

Cipher, D. J., & Urban, R. W. (2022). Discontinuation and the intention to reenroll in undergraduate nursing education. *Journal of Nursing Education, 61*(2), 97–100. https://doi.org/10.3928/01484834-20211213-06

Coddington, R. D. (1972). The significance of life events as etiologic factors in the diseases of children—II a study of a normal population. *Journal of Psychosomatic Research, 16*(3), 205–213. http://dx.doi.org/10.1016/0022-3999(72)90045-1

Cohen, J. (1962). The statistical power of abnormal–social psychological research: A review. *Journal of Abnormal Psychology, 65,* 145–153. https://doi.org/10.1037/h0045186

Cohen, J. (1988). *Statistical power analysis for the behavioral sciences* (2nd ed.). Academic Press.

Cohen, J., & Cohen, P. (1983). *Applied multiple regression/correlation analysis for the behavioral sciences* (2nd ed.). Erlbaum.

Conlon, A., Ashur, C., Washer, L., Eagle, K. A., & Bowman, M. A. H. (2021). Impact of the influenza vaccine on COVID-19 infection rates and severity. *American Journal of Infection Control, 49*(6), 694–700. https://doi.org/10.1016/j.ajic.2021.02.012

Cosco, T. D., Prina, M., Stubbs, B., & Wu, Y. T. (2017). Reliability and validity of the Center for Epidemiologic Studies Depression Scale in a population-based cohort of middle-aged U.S. adults. *Journal of Nursing Measurement, 25*(3), 476–485. https://doi.org/10.1891/1061-3749.25.3.476

Creswell, J. W., & Báez, J. C. (2021). *30 essential skills for the qualitative research* (2nd ed.). Sage.

Creswell, J. W., & Clark, V. L. (2018). *Designing and conducting mixed methods research* (3rd ed.). Sage.

Creswell, J. W., & Creswell, J. D. (2023). *Research design: Qualitative, quantitative, and mixed methods approaches* (6th ed.). Sage.

Creswell, J. W., & Poth, C. N. (2018). *Qualitative inquiry & research design: Choosing among five approaches* (4th ed.). Sage.

Currin-McCulloch, J., Kaushik, S., & Jones, B. (2022). When will I feel normal? *Cancer Nursing, 45*(2), E355–E363. https://doi.org/10.1097/NCC.0000000000000977

Daniel, W. W. (2000). *Applied nonparametric statistics* (2nd ed.). Duxbury Press.

Deng, Y., Lin, Y., Yang, L., Liang, Q., Fu, B., Li, H., Zhang, H., & Liu, Y. (2021). A comparison of maternal fear of childbirth, labor pain intensity and intrapartum analgesic consumption between primiparas and multiparas: A cross-sectional study. *International Journal of Nursing Science, 8*(4), 380–387. https://doi.org/10.1016/j.ijnss.2021.09.003

DeVon, H. A., Block, M. E., Moyle-Wright, P., Ernst, D. M., Hayden, S. J., Lazzara, D. J., Savoy, S. M., & Kostas-Polston, E. (2007). A psychometric toolbox for testing validity and reliability. *Journal of Nursing Scholarship*, *39*(2), 155–164. https//doi.org/10.1111/j.1547-5069.2007.00161.x

de Winter, J. C. F., & Dodou, D. (2010). Five-point Likert items: *t*-test versus Mann-Whitney-Wilcoxon. *Practical Assessment, Research, and Evaluation*, *15*(11), 1–16. https://doi.org/10.7275/bj1p-ts64

Dickson, V. V., Jun, J., & Melkus, G. D. (2021). A mixed methods study describing the self-care practices in an older working population with cardiovascular disease (CVD): Balancing work, life, and health. *Heart & Lung, 50*(3), 447–454. https://doi.org/10.1016/j.hrtlng.2021.02.001 0147-9563

Ding, S., Lei, Q., Wu, W., Xiao, Z., Wu, Z., Chen, M., & Chen, L. (2022). Changes in lifestyle, mood, and disease management among community-dwelling older adults during the COVID-19 pandemic in China. *Aging and Health Research*, *2*(1), 100059. https://doi.org/10.1016/j.ahr.2022.100059

Donnelly, M. R., Grigorian, A., Swentek, L., Arora, J., Kuza, C. M., Inaba, K., Kim, D., Lekawa, M., & Nahmias, J.(2022). Firearm violence against children in the United States: Trends in the wake of the COVID-19 pandemic. *Journal of Trauma & Acute Care Surgery, 92*(1), 65–68. https://doi.org/10.1097/TA.0000000000003347

Dunbar, K. B., Agoston, A. T., Odze, R. D., Huo, X., Pham, T. H., Cipher, D. J., Castell, D. O., Genta, R. M., Souza, R. F., & Spechler, S.J. (2016). Association of acute gastroesophageal reflux disease with esophageal histologic changes. *Journal of the American Medical Association*, *315*(19), 2104–2112. https://doi.org/10.1001/jama.2016.5657

Elixhauser, A., Steiner, C., Harris, D. R., & Coffey, R. M. (1998). Comorbidity measures for use with administrative data. *Medical Care, 36*(1), 8–27. https://doi.org/10.1097/00005650-199801000-00004

Elmore, J., Wild, D., Nelson, H. D., & Katz, D. L. (2020). *Jekel's epidemiology, biostatistics, preventive medicine, and public health* (5th ed.). Elsevier.

Fadlilah, S., Setiawan, D. I., Murdhiono, W. R., Wiyani, C., Mindarsih, E., Lustiyati, E. D., & Susanto, R. (2022). The anxiety facing the 1st dose of COVID-19 vaccination and related factors. *International Medical Journal, 29*(1), 38–42.

Faith, M. A., Boone, D. M., Kalin, J. A., Healy, A. S., Rawlins, J. & Mayes, S. (2021). Improvements of psychosocial outcomes following a summer camp for youth with bleeding disorders and their siblings. *Journal of Pediatric Nursing, 61,* 144–150. https://doi.org/10.1016/j.pedn.2021.05.001

Faria, G., Santos, P. B., Marinho, R. S., Firmino, S. M., Rizzatti, F. P., Mendes, R. G., Borghi-Silva, A., & Roscani, M. G. (2022). Association of right ventricle diastolic diameter with pulmonary function, exercise tolerance and exacerbation period in patients with chronic obstructive pulmonary disease: A prospective study. *Heart & Lung, 55,* 11–15. https://doi.org/10.1016/j.hrtlng.2022.04.003

Faul, F., Erdfelder, E., Buchner, A., & Lang, A. G. (2009). Statistical power analyses using G*Power 3.1: Tests for correlation and regression analyses. *Behavior Research Methods*, *41*(4), 1149–1160. https://doi.org/10.3758/BRM.41.4.1149

Feagins, L. A., Kim, J., Chandrakumaran, A., Gandle, C., Naik, K., Cipher D. J., Hou, J. K., Yao, M. D., & Gaidos, J. K. (2020). Rates of adverse IBD-related outcomes for patients with IBD and concomitant prostate cancer treated with radiation therapy. *Inflammatory Bowel Diseases, 26*(5), 728-733. https://doi.org/10.1093/ibd/izz175

Field, A. (2013). *Discovering statistics using IBM SPSS Statistics* (4th ed.). Sage.

Flowers, M., Olenick, M., Maltseva, T., Simon, S., Diez-Sampedro, A., & Allen, L. R. (2022). Academic factors predicting NCLEX-RN success. *Nursing Education Perspectives*, *43*(2), 112–114. https://doi.org/10.1097/01.NEP.0000000000000788

Gaskin, C. J., & Happell, B. (2014). Power, effects, confidence, and significance: An investigation of statistical practices in nursing research. *International Journal of Nursing Studies*, *51*(5), 795–806. https://doi.org/10.1016/j.ijnurstu.2013.09.014

Gliner, J. A., Morgan, G. A., & Leech, N. L. (2017). *Research methods in applied settings* (3rd ed.). Routledge.

Gray, J. R., & Grove, S. K. (2021). *The practice of nursing research: Appraisal, synthesis, and generation of evidence* (9th ed.). Elsevier.

Grove, S. K., & Gray, J. R. (2023). *Understanding nursing research: Building an evidence-based practice* (8th ed.). Elsevier.

Ha, F. J., Toukhsati, S. R., Cameron, J. D., Yates, R., & Hare, D. L. (2018). Association between the 6-minute walk test and exercise confidence in patients with heart failure: A prospective observational study. *Heart & Lung, 47*(1), 54–60. https://doi.org/10.1016/j.hrtlng.2017.09.006

Han, C. J., Korde, L. A., Reding, S., Allott, K., Doren, M. V. Schwarz, Y., Vaughan, C., & Reding, K. W. (2018). Investigation of a lifestyle intervention in women at high risk of breast cancer. *Western Journal of Nursing Research, 40*(7), 976–996. https://doi.org/10.1177/0193945917697227

Hartson, K. R., Gance-Cleveland, B., Amura, C. R., & Schmiege, S. (2018). Correlates of physical activity and sedentary behaviors among overweight Hispanic school-aged children. *Journal of Pediatric Nursing, 40*(1), 1–6. https://doi.org/10.1016/j.pedn.2018.01.019

Hayat, M. J. (2013). Understanding sample size determination in nursing research. *Western Journal of Nursing Research, 35*(7), 943–956. https://doi.org/10.1177/0193945913482052

Heavey, E. (2019). *Statistics for nursing: A practical approach* (3rd ed.). Jones & Bartlett Learning.

Hendricks, E., Ajmeri, A. N., Singh, M. M., Mongalo, M.., Goebel, L. J. (2021). A Randomized open-label study of two methods of proton pump inhibitors discontinuation. *Cureus, 13*(5):e15022. https://doi.org/10.7759/cureus.15022.

Hersch, R. K., Cook, R. F., Deitz, D. K., Kaplan, S., Hughes, D., Friesen, M. A., & Vezina, M. (2016). Reducing nurses' stress: A randomized controlled trial of a web-based stress management program for nurses. *Applied Nursing Research, 32*(1), 18–25. https://doi.org/10.1016/j.apnr.2016.04.003

Holmes Jr., L. (2018). *Applied biostatistical principles and concepts: Clinicians' guide to data analysis and interpretation*. Routledge.

Hulley, S. B., Cummings, S. R., Browner, W. S., Grady, D. G., & Newman, T. B. (2013). *Designing clinical research* (4th ed.). Lippincott Williams & Wilkins.

Hurley, S., Edwards, J., Cupp, J., & Phillips, M. (2018). Nurses' perceptions of self as a role model of health. *Western Journal of Nursing Research, 40*(8), 1131–1147. https://doi.org/10.1177/0193945917701396

Hunt, C., Peters, L., & Rapee, R. M. (2012). Development of a measure of of being bullied in youth. *Psychological Assessment, 24*(1), 156–165. http://dx.doi.org/10.1037/a0025178

IBM Corp. (2022). *IBM SPSS Statistics for Windows, Version 29.0*. Armonk: IBM Corp.

Inayati, A., Lee, B., Wang, R., Chen, S., Hsu, H., Lu, C., & Head, Y. L. (2022). Determinants of fear of falling in older adults with diabetes. *Geriatric Nursing, 46,* 7–12. https://doi.org/10.1016/j.gerinurse.2022.04.017

Jafri, S. H., Imran, T. F., Medbury, E., Ursillo, J., Ahmad, K., Imran, H., Drwal, K., & Wu, W. (2022). Cardiovascular outcomes of patients referred to home based cardiac rehabilitation. *Heart & Lung, 52,* 1–7. https://doi.org/10.1016/j.hrtlng.2021.11.005

Jiang, L., Wang, Y., Zhang, Y, Li, R., Wu, H., Le, C., & Wu, Y. (2019). The reliability and validity of the Center for Epidemiological Studies Depression Scale (CES-D) for Chinese university students. *Frontiers in Psychiatry, 10,* Article 315. https://doi.org/10.3389/fpsyt.2019.00315

Jones, M., deValpine, M., McDonal, M., & Schubert, C. (2021). Use of statistical tests in Doctor of Nursing Practice projects. *Journal for Nurse Practitioners, 17,* 118–1121. https://doi.org/10.1016/j.nurpra.2021.06.006

Kagee, A., Bantijes, J., Saal, W., & Sterley, A. (2020). Predicting caseness of major depressive disorder using the Center for Epidemiological Studies Depression Scale (CESD-R) among patients receiving HIV care. *General Hospital Psychiatry, 67,* 70–76. https://doi.org/10.1016/j.genhosppsych.2020.09.005

Kazdin, A. E. (2022). *Research design in clinical psychology* (5th ed.). Pearson.

Kim, H. J., & Hwang, S. Y. (2022). Effect of website-based learning on improved monitoring and adverse drug reactions by clinical nurses. *Asian Nursing Research, 16,* 45–51. https://doi.org/10.1016/j.anr.2021.12.004

Kim, M., Mallory, C., & Valerio, T. (2022). *Statistics for evidence-based practice in nursing*. Jones & Bartlett Learning.

King, A. P., & Eckersley, R. J. (2019). *Statistics for biomedical engineers and scientist*. Elsevier Academic Press.

Kline, R. B. (2004). *Beyond significance testing*. American Psychological Association.

Knapp, H. (2017). *Practical statistics for nursing using SPSS*. Sage.

Koo, T. K., & Li, M. Y. (2016). A guideline of selecting and reporting intraclass correlation coefficients for reliability research. *Journal of Chiropractic Medicine, 15*(2), 155–163. https://doi.org/10.1016/j.jcm.2016.02.012

Kozel, E., Barnoy, S., & Itzhaki, M. (2022). Emotion management of women at risk for premature birth: The association with optimism and social support. *Applied Nursing Research, 64,* 151568. https://doi.org/10.1016/j.apnr.2022.151568

Kuroki, M. (2022). Healthcare coverage and out-of-pocket medical expenses: Evidence from the 2017 Tax Cuts and Jobs Act and the medical expense deduction. *Public Health, 205,* 58–62. https://doi.org/10.1016/j.puhe.2022.01.022

Lee, H., Nguyen, H. Q., Jarrett, M. E., Mitchell, P. H., Pike, K. C., & Fan, V. S. (2018). Effect of symptoms on physical performance in COPD. *Heart & Lung, 47*(2), 149–156. https://doi.org/10.1016/j.hrtlng.2017.12.007

Lee, J., Nguyen, H. Q., Jarrett, M. E., Mitchell, P. H., Pike, K. C., & Fan, V. S. (2018). Effect of symptoms on physical performance in COPD. *Heart & Lung, 47*(2), 149–156. https://doi.org/10.1016/j.hrtlng.2017.12.007

Lee, S. J., Kang, K. J., & Lee, J. H. (2021). Safe patient handling legislation and changes in programs, practices, perceptions, and experience of musculoskeletal disorders by hospital characteristics: A repeated cross-sectional survey study. *International Journal of Nursing Studies, 113,* 103791. https://doi.org/10.1016/j.ijnurstu.2020.103791

Lehmann, R. (2013). 3σ-rule for outlier detection from the viewpoint of geodetic adjustment. *Journal of Surveying Engineering, 139*(4), 157–165. https://doi.org/10.1061/(ASCE)SU.1943-5428.0000112

Levine, M., & Ensom, M. H. (2001). Post hoc power analysis: an idea whose time has passed? *Pharmacotherapy, 21*(4), 405–409. https://doi.org/10.1592/phco.21.5.405.34503

Li, Y. Scherer, N., Felix, L., & Kuper, H. (2021). Prevalence of depression, anxiety, and post-traumatic stress disorder in healthcare workers during the COVID-19 pandemic: A systematic review and meta-analysis. *PLoS One, 16*(3), Article e0246454. https://doi.org/10.1371/journal.pone.0246454

Little R. J. A. (1988). A test of missing completely at random for multivariate data with missing values. *Journal of the American Statistical Association, 83*(404), 1198–1202. https://doi.org/10.1080/01621459.1988.10478722

Little, R. J. A., & Rubin, D. B. (1987). *Statistical analysis with missing data.* John Wiley & Sons.

Loew, N., Mackin, M. L., & Ayres, L. (2018). Collegiate women's definitions of responsible sexual behavior. *Western Journal of Nursing Research, 40*(8), 1148–1162. https://doi.org/10.1177/0193945917706508

Lohr, S. L. (2022). *Sampling: Design and analysis* (3rd ed.). CRC Press.

Macartney, G., Simoncic, V., Goulet, K., & Aglipay, M. (2018). Concussion symptoms prevalence, severity, and trajectory: Implications for nursing practice. *Journal of Pediatric Nursing, 40*(1), 58–62. https://doi.org/10.1016/j.pedn.2018.03.006

Mansfield, L. N., Onsomu, E. O., Merwin, E., Hall, N. M., & Harper-Harrison, A. (2018). Association between parental HPV knowledge and intentions to have their daughters vaccinated. *Western Journal of Nursing Research, 40*(4), 481–501. https://doi.org/10.1177/0193945916682953

Marsaglia, G., Tang, W. W., & Wang, J. (2003). Evaluating Kolmogorov's distribution. *Journal of Statistical Software, 8*(18),1–4. https://doi.org/10.18637/jss.v008.i18

Mayo Foundation for Medical Education and Research. (2022). *Alpha-fetoprotein (AFP), single marker screen, maternal, serum*. Retrieved from https://www.mayocliniclabs.com/test-catalog/Overview/113382

McCarthy, V. J., Wills, T., & Crowley, S. (2018). Nurses, age, job demands and physical activity at work and at leisure: A cross-sectional study. *Applied Nursing Research, 40,* 116–121. https://doi.org/10.1016/j.apnr.2018.01.010

Meehan, C. D., & Barker, N. (2021). Remediation for NCLEX-RN success in high-risk nursing students. *Teaching and Learning in Nursing, 16,* 254–257. https://doi.org/10.1016/j.teln.2021.02.003

Melnyk, B. M., & Fineout-Overholt, E. (2023). *Evidence-based practice in nursing & healthcare: A guide to best practice* (5th ed.). Wolters Kluwer.

Mensinger, J. L., Brom, H., Havens, D. S., Costello, A., D'Annunzio, C., Durning, J. D., Bradley, P. K., Copel, L., Maldonado, L., Smeltzer, S., Yost, J., & Kaufmann, P. (2022). Psychological responses of hospital-based nurses working during the COVID-19 pandemic in the United States: A crosssectional study. *Applied Nursing Research, 63,* 151517. https://doi.org/10.1016/j.apnr.2021.151517

Oshvandi, K., Movaheditabar, E., Naghshtabrizi, B., Mohammadi, Y., & Shamsizadeh, M. (2021). The effect of video-based educational program on satisfaction and comfort in patients undergoing transradial coronary angiography: A single-blinded, randomized controlled trial. *Journal of Vascular Nursing, 39*(2), 27–32. https://doi.org/10.1016/j.jvn.2021.01.001

Page, M. J., McKenzie, J. E., Bossuyt, P. M., Boutron, I., Hoffmann, T. C., Mulrow, C. D., Shamseer, L., Tetzlaff, J. M., Akl, E. A., Brennan, S. E., Chou, R., Glanville, J., Grimshaw, J. M., Hobjartsson, A., Lalu, M. M., Li, T., Loder, E. W., Mayo-Wilson, E., McDonald, S., … Moher, D. (2021). The PRISMA 2020 statement: An updated guideline for reporting systematic reviews. *Systematic Reviews, 10*:89. https://doi.org/10.1186/s13643-021-01626-4

Pett, M. A. (2016). *Nonparametric statistics for health care research: Statistics for small sample and unusual distributions* (2nd ed.). Sage.

Plichta, S. B., & Kelvin, E. (2013). *Munro's statistical methods for health care research* (6th ed.). Lippincott Williams & Wilkins.

Prion, S. K., & Haerling, K. A. (2020). Making sense of methods and measurements: Simple linear regression. *Clinical Simulation in Nursing, 48*, 94–95. https://doi.org/10.1016/j.ecns.2020.07.004

Prostate Cancer Foundation. (2022). *Gleason Score and Grade Group*. Retrieved from https://www.pcf.org/about-prostate-cancer/diagnosis-staging-prostate-cancer/gleason-score-isup-grade

Radloff, L. S. (1977). The CES-D scale: A self-report depression scale for research in the general population. *Applied Psychological Measures, 1*, 385–394.

Rasmussen, J. L. (1989). Analysis of Likert-scale data: A reinterpretation of Gregoire and Driver. *Psychological Bulletin, 105*, 167–170. https://doi.org/10.1037/0033-2909.105.1.167

Rekisso, A. D., Mengistu, Z., & Wurjine, T. H. (2022). Nurses' attitudes towards the nursing profession and associated factors in selected public hospitals, Addis Ababa, Ethiopia, 2021: A cross-sectional study. *BMC Nursing, 21*(1), 1–9. https://doi.org/10.1186/s12912-022-00808-2

Riegel, B., Dickson, V. V., Lee, C. S., Daus, M., Hill, J., Irani, E., Lee, S., Wald, J. W., Moelter, S. T., Rathman, L., Streur, M., Baah, F. O., Ruppert, L., Schwartz, D. R., & Bove, A. (2018). A mixed methods study of symptom perception in patients with chronic heart failure. *Heart & Lung, 47*(2), 107–114. https://doi.org/10.1016/j.hrtlng.2017.11.002

Robinson, E. M., Baker, R., & Hossain, M. (2018). Randomized trial valuating the effectiveness of coloring on decreasing anxiety among parents in a pediatric surgical waiting area. *Journal of Pediatric Nursing, 41*(1), 80–83. https://doi.org/10.1016/j.pedn.2018.02.001

Rubin, D. B. (1976). Inference and missing data. *Biometrika, 63*(3), 581–592. https://doi.org/10.1093/biomet/63.3.581

Ryan-Wenger, N. A. (2017). Precision, accuracy, and uncertainty of biophysical measurements for research and practice. In C. F. Waltz, O. L. Strickland, & E. R. Lenz (Eds.), *Measurement in nursing and health research* (5th ed., pp. 427–445). Springer Publishing Company.

Salimetrics LLc (2013). *Salivary cortisol*. Retrieved from https://www.salimetrics.com

Shadish, W. R., Cook, T. D., & Campbell, D. T. (2002). *Experimental and quasi-experimental designs for generalized causal inference*. Rand McNally.

Sharp, L. K., & Lipsky, M. S. (2002). Screening for depression across the lifespan: A review of measures for use in primary care settings. *American Family Physician, 66*(6), 1001–1008.

Siddaway, A. P., Wood, A. M., & Taylor, P. J. (2017). The Center for Epidemiologic Studies-Depression (CES-D) scale measures a continuum from well-being to depression: Testing two key predictions of positive clinical psychology. *Journal of Affective Disorders, 213*, 180–186. https://doi.org/10.1016/j.jad.2017.02.015

Stevens, J. P. (2009). *Applied multivariate statistics for the social sciences* (5th ed.). Psychology Press.

Stevens, S. S. (1946). On the theory of scales of measurement. *Science, 103*(2684), 677–680.

Stone, K. S., & Frazier, S. K. (2017). Measurement of physiological variables using biomedical instrumentation. In C. F. Waltz, O. L. Strickland, & E. R. Lenz (Eds.), *Measurement in nursing and health research* (5th ed., pp. 379–425). Springer Publishing Company.

Straus, S. E., Glasziou, P., Richardson, W. S., & Haynes, R. B. (2019). *Evidence-based medicine: How to practice and teach it* (5th ed.). Elsevier.

Tabachnick, B. G., & Fidell, L. S. (2019). *Using multivariate statistics* (7th ed.). Allyn and Bacon.

Taylor, J., & Spurlock, D. (2018). Statistical power in nursing education research. *Journal of Nursing Education, 57*(5), 262–264. https://doi.org/10.3928/01484834-20180420-02

Terrell, S. R. (2021). *Statistics translated: A step-by-step guide to analyzing and interpreting data* (2nd ed.). Guilford Press.

Todkar, S., Padwal, R., Michaud, A., & Cloutier, L. (2021). Knowledge, perception, and practice of health professionals regarding blood pressure measurement methods: A scoping review. *Journal of Hypertension, 39*(3), 391–399. https://doi.org/10.1097/HJH.0000000000002663

Urban, R. W., Rogers, M. R., Eades, T. L., Allard, P. M., Porter, M. T., & Cipher, D. J. (2023). Resilience, stress, anxiety, and depression: exploring mental health in new graduate nurses transitioning to practice during COVID-19. *Journal of Continuing Education in Nursing, 53*(12), 533–543. https://doi.org/10.3928/00220124-20221107-05

Urban, R. W., Smith, J., Wilson, S., & Cipher, D. J. (2021). Relationships among stress, resilience, and incivility in undergraduate nursing students and faculty during the COVID-19 pandemic: Policy implications for nurse leaders. *Journal of Professional Nursing, 37*(6), 1063–1070. https://doi.org/10.1016/j.profnurs.2021.08.011

U.S. Department of Health and Human Services & U.S. Department of Agriculture (2015). *2015–2020 dietary guidelines for Americans* (8th ed.) Retrieved from http://health.gov/dietaryguidelines/2015/guidelines/

Velanovich, V. (2007) The development of the GERD-HRQL symptom severity instrument. *Diseases of the Esophagus, 20,* 130–134. https://doi.org/10.1111/j.1442-2050.2007.00658.x

Viera, A. J., & Garrett, J. M. (2005). Understanding interobserver agreement: The kappa statistics. *Family Medicine, 37*(5), 36–363. https://doi.org/10.1370/afm.557

Waltz, C. F., Strickland, O. L., & Lenz, E. R. (2017). *Measurement in nursing and health research* (5th ed.). Springer Publishing Company.

Wang, R., Hsu, C., Chen, S., Lee, C., Lee, Y., Ma, S., & Chen. W. (2021). Risk factors of falls and the gender differences in older adults with diabetes at outpatient clinics. *Journal of Advanced Nursing, 77*(6), 2718–2727. https://doi.org/10.1111/jan.14795

Whelton, P. K., Carey, R. M., Aronow, W. S., Casey, D. E., Collins, K. J., Himmelfarb, C. D. DePalma, S. M., Gidding, S., Jamerson, K. A., Jones, D. W., MacLaughlin, E. J., Muntner, P., Ovbiagele, B., Smith, S. C., Spencer, C. C., Stafford, R. S., Taler, S. J., Thomas, R. J., Williams, K. A., ... Wright, J. T. (2018). 2017 Guideline for the Prevention, Detection, Evaluation, and Management of High Blood Pressure in Adults: Executive summary: A report of the American College of Cardiology/American Heart Association task force on clinical practice guidelines. *Hypertension, 71*(6), 1269–1324. https://doi.org/10.1161/HYP.0000000000000066

White, H. (1980). A heteroskedasticity-consistent covariance matrix estimator and a direct test for heteroskedasticity. *Econometrica, 48*(4), 817–838. https://doi.org/10.2307/1912934

Williams, S. G., Turner-Henson, A., Langhinrichsen-Rohling, J., & Azuero, A. (2017). Depressive symptoms in 9th graders: Stress and physiological contributors. *Applied Nursing Research, 34*(1), 24–28. https://doi.org/10.1016/j.apnr.2017.01.001

Williams, T., Kennedy-Malone, L., Thompson, J., & Monge, E. C. (2022). The effect of an exergame on physical activity among older adults residing in a long-term care facility: A pilot study. *Geriatric Nursing, 44,* 48–53. https://doi.org/10.1016/j.gerinurse.2022.01.001

Xiao, Y., Ran, H., Fang, D., Che, Y., Donald, A. R., Wang, S., Peng, J., Chen, L., & Lu, J. (2022). School bullying associated suicidal risk in children and adolescents from Yunnan, China: The mediation of social support. *Journal of Affective Disorders, 300,* 392–399. https://doi.org/10.1016/j.jad.2022.01.032

Yates, F. (1934). Contingency tables involving small numbers and the χ^2 test. *Journal of Royal Statistical Society, 1*(2), 217–235. https://doi.org/10.2307/2983604

Zar, J. H. (2010). *Biostatistical analysis* (5th ed.). Pearson Prentice-Hall.

Critical Values for Student's *t* Distribution

	0.001	0.005	0.01	0.025	0.05	0.10

LEVEL OF SIGNIFICANCE (α), TWO-TAILED TEST

df	0.002	0.01	0.02	0.05	0.10	0.20
2	22.327	9.925	6.965	4.303	2.920	1.886
3	10.215	5.841	4.541	3.182	2.353	1.638
4	7.173	4.604	3.747	2.776	2.132	1.533
5	5.893	4.032	3.365	2.571	2.015	1.476
6	5.208	3.707	3.143	2.447	1.943	1.440
7	4.785	3.499	2.998	2.365	1.895	1.415
8	4.501	3.355	2.896	2.306	1.860	1.397
9	4.297	3.250	2.821	2.262	1.833	1.383
10	4.144	3.169	2.764	2.228	1.812	1.372
11	4.025	3.106	2.718	2.201	1.796	1.363
12	3.930	3.055	2.681	2.179	1.782	1.356
13	3.852	3.012	2.650	2.160	1.771	1.350
14	3.787	2.977	2.624	2.145	1.761	1.345
15	3.733	2.947	2.602	2.131	1.753	1.341
16	3.686	2.921	2.583	2.120	1.746	1.337
17	3.646	2.898	2.567	2.110	1.740	1.333
18	3.610	2.878	2.552	2.101	1.734	1.330
19	3.579	2.861	2.539	2.093	1.729	1.328
20	3.552	2.845	2.528	2.086	1.725	1.325
21	3.527	2.831	2.518	2.080	1.721	1.323
22	3.505	2.819	2.508	2.074	1.717	1.321
23	3.485	2.807	2.500	2.069	1.714	1.319

LEVEL OF SIGNIFICANCE (α), ONE-TAILED TEST—cont'd

	0.001	**0.005**	**0.01**	**0.025**	**0.05**	**0.10**

LEVEL OF SIGNIFICANCE (α), TWO-TAILED TEST

df	0.002	0.01	0.02	0.05	0.10	0.20
24	3.467	2.797	2.492	2.064	1.711	1.318
25	3.450	2.787	2.485	2.060	1.708	1.316
26	3.435	2.779	2.479	2.056	1.706	1.315
27	3.421	2.771	2.473	2.052	1.703	1.314
28	3.408	2.763	2.467	2.048	1.701	1.313
29	3.396	2.756	2.462	2.045	1.699	1.311
30	3.385	2.750	2.457	2.042	1.697	1.310
31	3.375	2.744	2.453	2.040	1.696	1.309
32	3.365	2.738	2.449	2.037	1.694	1.309
33	3.356	2.733	2.445	2.035	1.692	1.308
34	3.348	2.728	2.441	2.032	1.691	1.307
35	3.340	2.724	2.438	2.030	1.690	1.306
36	3.333	2.719	2.434	2.028	1.688	1.306
37	3.326	2.715	2.431	2.026	1.687	1.305
38	3.319	2.712	2.429	2.024	1.686	1.304
39	3.313	2.708	2.426	2.023	1.685	1.304
40	3.307	2.704	2.423	2.021	1.684	1.303
45	3.281	2.690	2.412	2.014	1.679	1.301
50	3.261	2.678	2.403	2.009	1.676	1.299
55	3.245	2.668	2.396	2.004	1.673	1.297
60	3.232	2.660	2.390	2.000	1.671	1.296
65	3.220	2.654	2.385	1.997	1.669	1.295
70	3.211	2.648	2.381	1.994	1.667	1.294
75	3.202	2.643	2.377	1.992	1.665	1.293
80	3.195	2.639	2.374	1.990	1.664	1.292
85	3.189	2.635	2.371	1.988	1.663	1.292
90	3.183	2.632	2.368	1.987	1.662	1.291
95	3.178	2.629	2.366	1.985	1.661	1.291
100	3.174	2.626	2.364	1.984	1.660	1.290
200	3.131	2.601	2.345	1.972	1.653	1.286
300	3.118	2.592	2.339	1.968	1.650	1.284
∞	3.1	2.58	2.33	1.96	1.65	1.28

df = Degrees of freedom.

Critical Values of *r* for Pearson Product-Moment Correlation Coefficient

LEVEL OF SIGNIFICANCE (α), ONE-TAILED TEST

	0.05	0.025	0.01	0.005			0.05	0.025	0.01	0.005

LEVEL OF SIGNIFICANCE (α), TWO-TAILED TEST

df = n − 2	0.10	0.05	0.02	0.01		df = n − 2	0.10	0.05	0.02	0.01
1	0.9877	0.9969	0.9995	0.9999		39	0.2605	0.3081	0.3621	0.3978
2	0.9000	0.9500	0.9800	0.9900		40	0.2573	0.3044	0.3578	0.3932
3	0.8054	0.8783	0.9343	0.9587		41	0.2542	0.3008	0.3536	0.3887
4	0.7293	0.8114	0.8822	0.9172		42	0.2512	0.2973	0.3496	0.3843
5	0.6694	0.7545	0.8329	0.8745		43	0.2483	0.2940	0.3458	0.3801
6	0.6215	0.7067	0.7887	0.8343		44	0.2455	0.2907	0.3420	0.3761
7	0.5822	0.6664	0.7498	0.7977		45	0.2429	0.2876	0.3384	0.3721
8	0.5493	0.6319	0.7155	0.7646		46	0.2403	0.2845	0.3348	0.3683
9	0.5214	0.6021	0.6851	0.7348		47	0.2377	0.2816	0.3314	0.3646
10	0.4973	0.5760	0.6581	0.7079		48	0.2353	0.2787	0.3281	0.3610
11	0.4762	0.5529	0.6339	0.6835		49	0.2329	0.2759	0.3249	0.3575
12	0.4575	0.5324	0.6120	0.6614		50	0.2306	0.2732	0.3218	0.3542
13	0.4409	0.5140	0.5923	0.6411		55	0.2201	0.2609	0.3074	0.3385
14	0.4259	0.4973	0.5742	0.6226		60	0.2108	0.2500	0.2948	0.3248
15	0.4124	0.4821	0.5577	0.6055		65	0.2027	0.2404	0.2837	0.3126
16	0.4000	0.4683	0.5426	0.5897		70	0.1954	0.2319	0.2737	0.3017
17	0.3887	0.4555	0.5285	0.5751		75	0.1888	0.2242	0.2647	0.2919
18	0.3783	0.4438	0.5155	0.5614		80	0.1829	0.2172	0.2565	0.2830
19	0.3687	0.4329	0.5034	0.5487		85	0.1775	0.2108	0.2491	0.2748
20	0.3598	0.4227	0.4921	0.5368		90	0.1726	0.2050	0.2422	0.2673
21	0.3515	0.4132	0.4815	0.5256		95	0.1680	0.1996	0.2359	0.2604
22	0.3438	0.4044	0.4716	0.5151		100	0.1638	0.1946	0.2301	0.2540
23	0.3365	0.3961	0.4622	0.5052		120	0.1496	0.1779	0.2104	0.2324
24	0.3297	0.3882	0.4534	0.4958		140	0.1386	0.1648	0.1951	0.2155
25	0.3233	0.3809	0.4451	0.4869		160	0.1297	0.1543	0.1827	0.2019
26	0.3172	0.3739	0.4372	0.4785		180	0.1223	0.1455	0.1723	0.1905
27	0.3115	0.3673	0.4297	0.4705		200	0.1161	0.1381	0.1636	0.1809
28	0.3061	0.3610	0.4226	0.4629		250	0.1039	0.1236	0.1465	0.1620
29	0.3009	0.3550	0.4158	0.4556		300	0.0948	0.1129	0.1338	0.1480
30	0.2960	0.3494	0.4093	0.4487		350	0.0878	0.1046	0.1240	0.1371
31	0.2913	0.3440	0.4031	0.4421		400	0.0822	0.0978	0.1160	0.1283
32	0.2869	0.3388	0.3973	0.4357		450	0.0775	0.0922	0.1094	0.1210
33	0.2826	0.3338	0.3916	0.4297		500	0.0735	0.0875	0.1038	0.1149
34	0.2785	0.3291	0.3862	0.4238		600	0.0671	0.0799	0.0948	0.1049
35	0.2746	0.3246	0.3810	0.4182		700	0.0621	0.0740	0.0878	0.0972
36	0.2709	0.3202	0.3760	0.4128		800	0.0581	0.0692	0.0821	0.0909
37	0.2673	0.3160	0.3712	0.4076		900	0.0548	0.0653	0.0774	0.0857
38	0.2638	0.3120	0.3665	0.4026		1000	0.0520	0.0619	0.0735	0.0813

df = Degrees of freedom.

APPENDIX C

Critical Values of F for $\alpha = 0.05$ and $\alpha = 0.01$

CRITICAL VALUES OF F FOR $\alpha = 0.05$

df Denominator	\multicolumn{19}{c}{df Numerator}
	1	2	3	4	5	6	7	8	9	10	12	15	20	24	30	40	60	120	∞
1	161.4	199.5	215.7	224.6	230.2	234.0	236.8	238.9	240.5	241.9	243.9	245.9	248.0	249.1	250.1	251.1	252.2	253.3	254.3
2	18.51	19.00	19.16	19.25	19.30	19.33	19.35	19.37	19.38	19.40	19.41	19.43	19.45	19.45	19.46	19.47	19.48	19.49	19.50
3	10.13	9.55	9.28	9.12	9.01	8.94	8.89	8.85	8.81	8.79	8.74	8.70	8.66	8.64	8.62	8.59	8.57	8.55	8.53
4	7.71	6.94	6.59	6.39	6.26	6.16	6.09	6.04	6.00	5.96	5.91	5.86	5.80	5.77	5.75	5.72	5.69	5.66	5.63
5	6.61	5.79	5.41	5.19	5.05	4.95	4.88	4.82	4.77	4.74	4.68	4.62	4.56	4.53	4.50	4.46	4.43	4.40	4.36
6	5.99	5.14	4.76	4.53	4.39	4.28	4.21	4.15	4.10	4.06	4.00	3.94	3.87	3.84	3.81	3.77	3.74	3.70	3.67
7	5.59	4.74	4.35	4.12	3.97	3.87	3.79	3.73	3.68	3.64	3.57	3.51	3.44	3.41	3.38	3.34	3.30	3.27	3.23
8	5.32	4.46	4.07	3.84	3.69	3.58	3.50	3.44	3.39	3.35	3.28	3.22	3.15	3.12	3.08	3.04	3.01	2.97	2.93
9	5.12	4.26	3.86	3.63	3.48	3.37	3.29	3.23	3.18	3.14	3.07	3.01	2.94	2.90	2.86	2.83	2.79	2.75	2.71
10	4.96	4.10	3.71	3.48	3.33	3.22	3.14	3.07	3.02	2.98	2.91	2.85	2.77	2.74	2.70	2.66	2.62	2.58	2.54
11	4.84	3.98	3.59	3.36	3.20	3.09	3.01	2.95	2.90	2.85	2.79	2.72	2.65	2.61	2.57	2.53	2.49	2.45	2.40
12	4.75	3.89	3.49	3.26	3.11	3.00	2.91	2.85	2.80	2.75	2.69	2.62	2.54	2.51	2.47	2.43	2.38	2.34	2.30
13	4.67	3.81	3.41	3.18	3.03	2.92	2.83	2.77	2.71	2.67	2.60	2.53	2.46	2.42	2.38	2.34	2.30	2.25	2.21
14	4.60	3.74	3.34	3.11	2.96	2.85	2.76	2.70	2.65	2.60	2.53	2.46	2.39	2.35	2.31	2.27	2.22	2.18	2.13
15	4.54	3.68	3.29	3.06	2.90	2.79	2.71	2.64	2.59	2.54	2.48	2.40	2.33	2.29	2.25	2.20	2.16	2.11	2.07
16	4.49	3.63	3.24	3.01	2.85	2.74	2.66	2.59	2.54	2.49	2.42	2.35	2.28	2.24	2.19	2.15	2.11	2.06	2.01
17	4.45	3.59	3.20	2.96	2.81	2.70	2.61	2.55	2.49	2.45	2.38	2.31	2.23	2.19	2.15	2.10	2.06	2.01	1.96
18	4.41	3.55	3.16	2.93	2.77	2.66	2.58	2.51	2.46	2.41	2.34	2.27	2.19	2.15	2.11	2.06	2.02	1.97	1.92
19	4.38	3.52	3.13	2.90	2.74	2.63	2.54	2.48	2.42	2.38	2.31	2.23	2.16	2.11	2.07	2.03	1.98	1.93	1.88
20	4.35	3.49	3.10	2.87	2.71	2.60	2.51	2.45	2.39	2.35	2.28	2.20	2.12	2.08	2.04	1.99	1.95	1.90	1.84
21	4.32	3.47	3.07	2.84	2.68	2.57	2.49	2.42	2.37	2.32	2.25	2.18	2.10	2.05	2.01	1.96	1.92	1.87	1.81
22	4.30	3.44	3.05	2.82	2.66	2.55	2.46	2.40	2.34	2.30	2.23	2.15	2.07	2.03	1.98	1.94	1.89	1.84	1.78
23	4.28	3.42	3.03	2.80	2.64	2.53	2.44	2.37	2.32	2.27	2.20	2.13	2.05	2.01	1.96	1.91	1.86	1.81	1.76
24	4.26	3.40	3.01	2.78	2.62	2.51	2.42	2.36	2.30	2.25	2.18	2.11	2.03	1.98	1.94	1.89	1.84	1.79	1.73
25	4.24	3.39	2.99	2.76	2.60	2.49	2.40	2.34	2.28	2.24	2.16	2.09	2.01	1.96	1.92	1.87	1.82	1.77	1.71
26	4.23	3.37	2.98	2.74	2.59	2.47	2.39	2.32	2.27	2.22	2.15	2.07	1.99	1.95	1.90	1.85	1.80	1.75	1.69
27	4.21	3.35	2.96	2.73	2.57	2.46	2.37	2.31	2.25	2.20	2.13	2.06	1.97	1.93	1.88	1.84	1.79	1.73	1.67
28	4.20	3.34	2.95	2.71	2.56	2.45	2.36	2.29	2.24	2.19	2.12	2.04	1.96	1.91	1.87	1.82	1.77	1.71	1.65
29	4.18	3.33	2.93	2.70	2.55	2.43	2.35	2.28	2.22	2.18	2.10	2.03	1.94	1.90	1.85	1.81	1.75	1.70	1.64
30	4.17	3.32	2.92	2.69	2.53	2.42	2.33	2.27	2.21	2.16	2.09	2.01	1.93	1.89	1.84	1.79	1.74	1.68	1.62
40	4.08	3.23	2.84	2.61	2.45	2.34	2.25	2.18	2.12	2.08	2.00	1.92	1.84	1.79	1.74	1.69	1.64	1.58	1.51
60	4.00	3.15	2.76	2.53	2.37	2.25	2.17	2.10	2.04	1.99	1.92	1.84	1.75	1.70	1.65	1.59	1.53	1.47	1.39
120	3.92	3.07	2.68	2.45	2.29	2.17	2.09	2.02	1.96	1.91	1.83	1.75	1.66	1.61	1.55	1.50	1.43	1.35	1.25
∞	3.84	3.00	2.60	2.37	2.21	2.10	2.01	1.94	1.88	1.83	1.75	1.67	1.57	1.52	1.46	1.39	1.32	1.22	1.00

df = Degrees of freedom.

CRITICAL VALUES OF F FOR α = 0.01

df Denominator	df Numerator																		
	1	2	3	4	5	6	7	8	9	10	12	15	20	24	30	40	60	120	∞
1	4052	4999.5	5403	5625	5764	5859	5928	5982	6022	6056	6106	6157	6209	6235	6261	6287	6313	6339	6366
2	98.50	99.00	99.17	99.25	99.30	99.33	99.36	99.37	99.39	99.40	99.42	99.43	99.45	99.46	99.47	99.47	99.48	99.49	99.50
3	34.12	30.82	29.46	28.71	28.24	27.91	27.67	27.49	27.35	27.23	27.05	26.87	26.69	26.60	26.50	26.41	26.32	26.22	26.13
4	21.20	18.00	16.69	15.98	15.52	15.21	14.98	14.80	14.66	14.55	14.37	14.20	14.02	13.93	13.84	13.75	13.65	13.56	13.46
5	16.26	13.27	12.06	11.39	10.97	10.67	10.46	10.29	10.16	10.05	9.89	9.72	9.55	9.47	9.38	9.29	9.20	9.11	9.02
6	13.75	10.92	9.78	9.15	8.75	8.47	8.26	8.10	7.98	7.87	7.72	7.56	7.40	7.31	7.23	7.14	7.06	6.97	6.88
7	12.25	9.55	8.45	7.85	7.46	7.19	6.99	6.84	6.72	6.62	6.47	6.31	6.16	6.07	5.99	5.91	5.82	5.74	5.65
8	11.26	8.65	7.59	7.01	6.63	6.37	6.18	6.03	5.91	5.81	5.67	5.52	5.36	5.28	5.20	5.12	5.03	4.95	4.86
9	10.56	8.02	6.99	6.42	6.06	5.80	5.61	5.47	5.35	5.26	5.11	4.96	4.81	4.73	4.65	4.57	4.48	4.40	4.31
10	10.04	7.56	6.55	5.99	5.64	5.39	5.20	5.06	4.94	4.85	4.71	4.56	4.41	4.33	4.25	4.17	4.08	4.00	3.91
11	9.65	7.21	6.22	5.67	5.32	5.07	4.89	4.74	4.63	4.54	4.40	4.25	4.10	4.02	3.94	3.86	3.78	3.69	3.60
12	9.33	6.93	5.95	5.41	5.06	4.82	4.64	4.50	4.39	4.30	4.16	4.01	3.86	3.78	3.70	3.62	3.54	3.45	3.36
13	9.07	6.70	5.74	5.21	4.86	4.62	4.44	4.30	4.19	4.10	3.96	3.82	3.66	3.59	3.51	3.43	3.34	3.25	3.17
14	8.86	6.51	5.56	5.04	4.69	4.46	4.28	4.14	4.03	3.94	3.80	3.66	3.51	3.43	3.35	3.27	3.18	3.09	3.00
15	8.68	6.36	5.42	4.89	4.56	4.32	4.14	4.00	3.89	3.80	3.67	3.52	3.37	3.29	3.21	3.13	3.05	2.96	2.87
16	8.53	6.23	5.29	4.77	4.44	4.20	4.03	3.89	3.78	3.69	3.55	3.41	3.26	3.18	3.10	3.02	2.93	2.84	2.75
17	8.40	6.11	5.18	4.67	4.34	4.10	3.93	3.79	3.68	3.59	3.46	3.31	3.16	3.08	3.00	2.92	2.83	2.75	2.65
18	8.29	6.01	5.09	4.58	4.25	4.01	3.84	3.71	3.60	3.51	3.37	3.23	3.08	3.00	2.92	2.84	2.75	2.66	2.5
19	8.18	5.93	5.01	4.50	4.17	3.94	3.77	3.63	3.52	3.43	3.30	3.15	3.00	2.92	2.84	2.76	2.67	2.58	2.4
20	8.10	5.85	4.94	4.43	4.10	3.87	3.70	3.56	3.46	3.37	3.23	3.09	2.94	2.86	2.78	2.69	2.61	2.52	2.42
21	8.02	5.78	4.87	4.37	4.04	3.81	3.64	3.51	3.40	3.31	3.17	3.03	2.88	2.80	2.72	2.64	2.55	2.46	2.36
22	7.95	5.72	4.82	4.31	3.99	3.76	3.59	3.45	3.35	3.26	3.12	2.98	2.83	2.75	2.67	2.58	2.50	2.40	2.31
23	7.88	5.66	4.76	4.26	3.94	3.71	3.54	3.41	3.30	3.21	3.07	2.93	2.78	2.70	2.62	2.54	2.45	2.35	2.26
24	7.82	5.61	4.72	4.22	3.90	3.67	3.50	3.36	3.26	3.17	3.03	2.89	2.74	2.66	2.58	2.49	2.40	2.31	2.21
25	7.77	5.57	4.68	4.18	3.85	3.63	3.46	3.32	3.22	3.13	2.99	2.85	2.70	2.62	2.54	2.45	2.36	2.27	2.17
26	7.72	5.53	4.64	4.14	3.82	3.59	3.42	3.29	3.19	3.09	2.96	2.81	2.66	2.58	2.50	2.42	2.33	2.23	2.13
27	7.68	5.49	4.60	4.11	3.78	3.56	3.39	3.26	3.15	3.06	2.93	2.78	2.63	2.55	2.47	2.38	2.29	2.20	2.10
28	7.64	5.45	4.57	4.07	3.75	3.53	3.36	3.23	3.12	3.03	2.90	2.75	2.60	2.52	2.44	2.35	2.26	2.17	2.06
29	7.60	5.42	4.54	4.04	3.73	3.50	3.33	3.20	3.09	3.00	2.87	2.73	2.57	2.49	2.41	2.33	2.23	2.14	2.03
30	7.56	5.39	4.51	4.02	3.70	3.47	3.30	3.17	3.07	2.98	2.84	2.70	2.55	2.47	2.39	2.30	2.21	2.11	2.01
40	7.31	5.18	4.31	3.83	3.51	3.29	3.12	2.99	2.89	2.80	2.66	2.52	2.37	2.29	2.20	2.11	2.02	1.92	1.80
60	7.08	4.98	4.13	3.65	3.34	3.12	2.95	2.82	2.72	2.63	2.50	2.35	2.20	2.12	2.03	1.94	1.84	1.73	1.60
120	6.85	4.79	3.95	3.48	3.17	2.96	2.79	2.66	2.56	2.47	2.34	2.19	2.03	1.95	1.86	1.76	1.66	1.53	1.38
∞	6.63	4.61	3.78	3.32	3.02	2.80	2.64	2.51	2.41	2.32	2.18	2.04	1.88	1.79	1.70	1.59	1.47	1.32	1.00

df = Degrees of freedom.
From: Merrington, M., & Thompson, C. M. (1943). Tables of percentage points of the inverted beta (F) distribution. *Biometrika, 33*(1), 73–78.

Critical Values of the Chi-Square Distribution

df	Alpha (α) Level				
	0.10	0.05	0.025	0.01	0.001
1	2.7055	3.8415	5.0239	6.6349	10.8276
2	4.6052	5.9915	7.3778	9.2103	13.8155
3	6.2514	7.8147	9.3484	11.3449	16.2662
4	7.7794	9.4877	11.1433	13.2767	18.4668
5	9.2364	11.0705	12.8325	15.0863	20.5150
6	10.6446	12.5916	14.4494	16.8119	22.4577
7	12.0170	14.0671	16.0128	18.4753	24.3219
8	13.3616	15.5073	17.5345	20.0902	26.1245
9	14.6837	16.9190	19.0228	21.6660	27.8772
10	15.9872	18.3070	20.4832	23.2093	29.5883
11	17.2750	19.6751	21.9200	24.7250	31.2641
12	18.5493	21.0261	23.3367	26.2170	32.9095
13	19.8119	22.3620	24.7356	27.6882	34.5282
14	21.0641	23.6848	26.1189	29.1412	36.1233
15	22.3071	24.9958	27.4884	30.5779	37.6973
16	23.5418	26.2962	28.8454	31.9999	39.2524
17	24.7690	27.5871	30.1910	33.4087	40.7902
18	25.9894	28.8693	31.5264	34.8053	42.3124
19	27.2036	30.1435	32.8523	36.1909	43.8202
20	28.4120	31.4104	34.1696	37.5662	45.3147
21	29.6151	32.6706	35.4789	38.9322	46.7970
22	30.8133	33.9244	36.7807	40.2894	48.2679
23	32.0069	35.1725	38.0756	41.6384	49.7282
24	33.1962	36.4150	39.3641	42.9798	51.1786
25	34.3816	37.6525	40.6465	44.3141	52.6197
26	35.5632	38.8851	41.9232	45.6417	54.0520
27	36.7412	40.1133	43.1945	46.9629	55.4760
28	37.9159	41.3371	44.4608	48.2782	56.8923
29	39.0875	42.5570	45.7223	49.5879	58.3012
30	40.2560	43.7730	46.9792	50.8922	59.7031
31	41.4217	44.9853	48.2319	52.1914	61.0983
32	42.5847	46.1943	49.4804	53.4858	62.4872
33	43.7452	47.3999	50.7251	54.7755	63.8701
34	44.9032	48.6024	51.9660	56.0609	65.2472
35	46.0588	49.8018	53.2033	57.3421	66.6188
36	47.2122	50.9985	54.4373	58.6192	67.9852
37	48.3634	52.1923	55.6680	59.8925	69.3465
38	49.5126	53.3835	56.8955	61.1621	70.7029
39	50.6598	54.5722	58.1201	62.4281	72.0547
40	51.8051	55.7585	59.3417	63.6907	73.4020
41	52.9485	56.9424	60.5606	64.9501	74.7449
42	54.0902	58.1240	61.7768	66.2062	76.0838
43	55.2302	59.3035	62.9904	67.4593	77.4186
44	56.3685	60.4809	64.2015	68.7095	78.7495
45	57.5053	61.6562	65.4102	69.9568	80.0767

df = Degrees of freedom.
From: Corty, E. (2007). *Using and interpreting statistics: A practical text for the health, behavioral, and social sciences.* St Louis, MO: Mosby.

Index

Page numbers followed by "*f*" indicate figures, and "*t*" indicate tables.